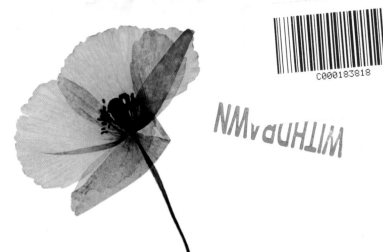

FAST LIVING
SLOW
AGEING

HOW TO AGE LESS · LOOK GREAT · LIVE LONGER · GET MORE

TESTIMONIALS

"The human body is not built for an unlimited lifespan. Yet there are many ways in which we can improve and prolong our health. 'Fast Living, Slow Ageing' is all about embracing those opportunities."
Robin Holliday, author of 'Understanding Ageing' and 'Ageing: The Paradox of Life'

"Today in Australia, we eat too much and move too little. But it is our future that will carry the cost. Our current 'fast' lifestyles will have their greatest impact on our prospects for healthy ageing. This book highlights many of the opportunities we all have to make a difference to our outlook, at a personal and social level."
Professor Stephen Leeder, AO, Director of the Menzies Centre for Health Policy, which leads policy analysis of healthcare

"Healthy ageing can't be found in a single supplement, diet or lifestyle change. It takes an integrated approach across a number of key areas that complement to slowly build and maintain our health. 'Fast Living, Slow Ageing' shows how it is possible to practically develop these kind of holistic techniques and take control of our future."
Professor Marc Cohen, MBBS (Hons), PhD (TCM), PhD (Elec Eng), BMed Sci (Hons), FAMAC, FICAE, Professor, founder of www.thebigwell.com

"SLOW is about discovering that everything we do has a knock-on effect, that even our smallest choices can reshape the big picture. Understanding this can help us live more healthily, more fully and maybe even longer too."
Carl Honoré, author of 'In Praise of Slow'

"We all know about the dangers of fast food. But food is not the only fast thing that is ruining our lives. Slow ageing is about finding important connections in the diet and lifestyle choices we make every day and embracing the possibilities for making real changes - to our own lives - in our own way."
Sally Errey, best-selling author of the cookbook 'Staying Alive!'

"Ageing is a complex process with many different factors combining to determine health and longevity. To slow ageing optimally, we also need to combine a range of lifestyle changes, supplements and other activities. This practical book steers us through the many opportunities we have to change our futures for the better."
Prof Brian J Morris, PhD, DSc, Professor of Molecular Medical Sciences, Basic & Clinical Genomics Laboratory, University of Sydney

'Fast Living, Slow Ageing' delivers a combination of well researched strategies from both Western medicine and complementary therapies to enhance your wellness."
Dr Danika Fietz, MBBS, BN (Hons), GP Registrar

"Forget the plastic surgeons, Botox and makeovers! 'Slow ageing' is really about the practical choices we make every day to stay healthy, fit and vital, to look great and to feel great today and in the years ahead."
Dr David Tye, GP, Kingston Family Clinic, South Brighton, SA

"We all hope that growing old will be part of our lives, although we don't really want to think about it. In fact, 'old' is almost a dirty word in lots of people's minds! 'Fast Living, Slow Ageing' takes you down the path of doing something about how you age, while at the same time providing you with choices and igniting an awareness to start now and take control of how you can age with grace."
Ms Robyn Ewart, businesswoman, mum and household manager

"Ageing is a natural and beautiful process which, all too often, we accelerate through unhealthy attitudes and lifestyle choices. 'Fast Living, Slow Ageing' is all about redressing that balance by making a commitment to mind, body and spirit; to live the fullness of life, while ageing with grace and beauty."
Stephen Penman, President of the Yoga Teachers Association of Australia

"We all want to live longer and healthier lives. 'Fast living, Slow Ageing' shows how this is really possible with minimal fuss and easy ways to incorporate real and long-lasting changes."
Jennifer Aikman, Senior HR Business Partner (MCIPD) and mother of a 7-year-old

"Ageing is determined by the opportunities we take and those we neglect. 'Fast Living, Slow Ageing' is about making the most of these opportunities."
Dr Joe Kosterich, author of 'Dr Joe's DIY Health: Putting You in Charge of Your Health

"I don't know about you, but finding any way to be the best I can be as I age is of great value. I enjoyed applying the practical suggestions and gained immediate benefits from making small, convenient changes in my life."
Margo Field, 53-year-old mother and businesswoman, founder of www.goandseemargo.net

"Ageing starts at the cellular level, so we need to look at the cause of ageing and modify this as much as possible. 'Fast Living, Slow Ageing' does this and explains the principles in everyday language."
Richard Stenlake, B.Pharm, MPS, MRPS

"We spend all our life working for the day when we can slow down, only to find that we haven't taken sufficient care of our body/mind along the way! If we want to live the dreams we have worked so hard for, it is best to do whatever we can NOW to Slow Ageing."
Carolinda Witt, author of 'The 10-Minute Rejuvenation Plan', founder and developer of T5T®, just 10 minutes per day for health, vitality and wellbeing (www.T5T.com)

"This book is well researched and offers practical suggestions that are easy to put into practice by anyone who is determined to make the right choices to stay healthy and age with dignity."
Rosemary Boon, psychologist, nutritionist and teacher

"When first approached to review this book, I worried it was going to be about all the negatives that many people associate with ageing – how to stop it, prevent it or hide it – but it turned out to be a celebration of what we can do to make our ageing a rich and rewarding experience."
Dr Rod Wellard, GP education consultant

"We all have to get older, but this doesn't need to be a rapid, valueless decline. We can all choose a path that maintains vigour and vitality. 'Fast Living, Slow Ageing' gives the directions to follow and succeed!"
Dr Chris Moschou, Adelaide-based GP

"I strongly believe it is our duty to maximise the potential of our brains every day of our lives. For people in their 40s, 50s and 60s, now is the time to really take charge. We are a much larger population compared to the younger people coming through and there is no way they will be able to support us all when we will need it. The longer we can maintain our faculties, the better for us all. If you want to take charge of your brain and enhance your life, this book is a wonderful place to start."
Nerida Saunders, Senior Psychologist and President of the Applied Neuroscience Society of Australasia, and proud grandmother of 4

FAST LIVING SLOW AGEING

www.slowageingbook.com

Text Copyright © 2013 Health Inform Pty Ltd
Published by Health Inform Pty Ltd
PO BOX 2508
Strawberry Hills 2012 Australia
Email: admin@healthinform.com.au

Cover designed by Emma Ross Design
Images by Dreamstime
Printed in China by 1010 Printing International

First published 2009; second edition 2010;
third edition 2011; fourth edition 2013

National Library of Australia
Cataloguing-in-Publication data:
Marie, Kate, 1962-

Fast Living, Slow Ageing : How to age less, look great, live longer, get more
Kate Marie, Merlin Christopher Thomas.
Includes index.
ISBN 978-0-9806339-2-4
1. Ageing. 2. Longevity. 3. Life expectancy. 4. Quality of life.
613

A SPECIAL THANKS TO
JERRY SCHWARTZ;
A DEAR FRIEND.
WITHOUT HIS PERSISTENCE AND ONGOING
SUPPORT, THIS BOOK WOULD
NEVER HAVE BEEN COMPLETED.

AUTHORS & CONTRIBUTORS

What started as a small number of advisors and helpers has developed into what could be the largest collaboration of its kind. By the end of this project we had more than fifty people contributing information and providing expert guidance and support. Because the field of health and ageing is so vast, without this collaboration of scientists, doctors, health professionals and consumers we would never have been able to do it justice. There are many books on the market claiming to help you to slow ageing or even reverse it. Some are good and a handful excellent. The main difference with this book is that through a collaborative effort we've been able to provide the evidence when recommending interventions that work to slow ageing and optimise wellness. We believe we've created a foundation for consumers and doctors alike to methodically review how well they and their patients are, given there are no official guidelines.

Authors

Kate Marie

Professor Merlin Christopher Thomas MD, PhD

Editors

Ian Gillam

Ann-Mary Hromek

Ananda Mahony

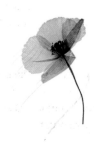

SPECIAL MENTION

Dr Jerry Schwartz

After graduating as a medical doctor from the University of Sydney and spending many years in the public hospital system, Jerry became an early Surgical Fellow of the Australasian College of Cosmetic Surgery. He owns and practices in his thriving ISO2001 accredited surgery in Matraville, Sydney. In addition to his Ophthalmic and Cosmetic Surgery diplomas, Jerry also has a Masters in Public health from Monash University in Melbourne.

Carolen Barripp

Carolen is an innovative Australian-based publisher who creates books of distinction that are acknowledged for their quality and originality.

Dr Ian Gillam
BSc (Hons), MSc, PhD, Dip Phys Ed, AEP, ASP, ESSAF, FSMA

Ian has had more than 25 years an accredited exercise physiologist (AEP), university lecturer and researcher and is a sports physiologist (ASP) and nutritionist. Ian currently works with Exercise and Sports Science Australia (ESSA) in an industry development role and previously at the National Institute of Integrative Medicine. He has also been a consultant sports physiologist and nutritionist to Victorian and Australian Institute of Sport athletes and to a number of professional sports teams including the AFL Demons, Tennis Australia and the Drapac Professional cycling team.

Eva Migdal

Eva is lecturer and course coordinator at RMIT University's School of Health Sciences in the Master of Wellness program. She is also developing the Well School, a social enterprise to support teacher personal wellness literacy, skills and capacity to implement transformative curricula. She has degrees in Physiotherapy, Fine Arts, Masters in Environmental Science and a Dip. Ed. in Health & Media.

Ann-Mary Hromek RN ND

Ann-Mary Hromek is a Registered Nurse, Female Sexual Health Practitioner and Naturopath with 30 years of experience in nutritional and environmental medicine. Ann-Mary has done significant work with ACNEM as the education coordinator for the training programs for GPs and allied health workers.

Dr Ray Welling

Ray is a writer, commentator, consultant and lecturer on online marketing and content strategy. He holds a BS from the Medill School of Journalism at Northwestern University in Chicago, a MA in communications from Macquarie University and a PhD in e-business and marketing from The University of Sydney.

Dr Bill Andrews

Bill is the CEO of Sierra Sciences and is a principal discoverer of human telomerase, the enzyme that lengthens telomeres in human cells. He has spent the last 20 years capitalising on this discovery by developing pharmaceuticals that promise to delay age-related disease.

Dr Michael Lowy

Michael is a men's health physician with a special interest in male sexual dysfunction, relationship counselling and the general health issues of men.

Terry Robson

Terry is a journalist, author, screenwriter, public speaker and qualified naturopath. He has worked as a health journalist for many of the major Australian media outlets focusing on lifestyle and holistic health issues.

Carl Honoré

Carl is a leading champion of the Slow Movement. For information on Carl's work, go to www.carlhonore.com.

Helen Bolger-Harris

Helen is a wellness coach and consultant and has enjoyed a long successful career in the health industry. She has numerous nursing and other health-related qualifications, including a Master of Public Health.

CONTRIBUTORS AND SUPPORTERS

Scientific panel
Prof Robin Holliday, author
'Understanding Ageing' www.robinholliday.com
Prof Brian J. Morris, PhD DSc,
Professor of Molecular Medical Sciences,
http://www.physiol.usyd.edu.au/~brianm/

Academic panel
Prof Marc Cohen,
Professor of Complementary Medicine at RMIT
Prof Stephen Leeder,
Director, Menzies Centre for Health Policy
Dr Rod Wellard, Education Consultant

Nutritional panel
Ann-Mary Hromek RN ND
Sally Errey, Nutritionist, Speaker, Best-selling Author,
www.stayingalivecookbook.com
Rebecca McPhee, BNutr.Diet (Hons), APD, an Accredited
Practicing Dietitian
Andrew Munro B HSc,
Manager - leading Health Sciences company
Brendan Penwarden, Naturopath, www.nutrenews.com

Mind-body and ageing
Donald Moss, PhD, Chair, Mind-Body Medicine Program,
Saybrook Graduate School & Research Center,
http://www.saybrook.edu/contact/con_fac.asp
Margo Field www.goandseemargo.net
Rosemary Boon www.learningdiscoveries.com.au
Wayne Jencke www.i-i.com.au
Stephen Penman
Nerida Saunders www.solstice-mindmatters.com.au
Carolinda Witt www.T5T.com

Skin and ageing
Dr John Arbuckle www.anti-ageingdoctors.com.au
Dr John Flynn Foundation Fellow, Australasian College of
Cosmetic Surgery www.cosmedic.com.au

General sections
Australian Hearing
Matthew Wells, Optometrist & Medical Student

Hormone modulation
Dr Russell Cooper, Board Certified Anti-Aging Medicine,
Fellowships in Nutritional & Environmental Medicine
Dr Ray Kearney (retired),
Infectious Diseases and Immunology
A/Prof Richard Reid www.wips-intl.com
Richard Stenlake www.stenlake.com.au

Genetics panel
Iwona Rudkowska, Ph.D. (McGill University),
Nutritionist-dietitian
and Researcher in Nutrigenomics
Moshe Szyf Ph.D., GlaxoSmithKline
Professor of Pharmacology, McGill University
Jon Cornell, Sierra Sciences www.sierrasci.com

Cosmetic panel
Dr Peter Muzikants, MB BS, specialising in laser and
cosmetic dermatologic procedures,
www.adacosmetic.com.au
Dr Bruce Williamson, Balgowlah Skin Cancer Clinic

Medical practitioner panel
Dr Danika Fietz, MBBS, BN (Hons)
Dr Joe Kosterich, MBBS,
www.drjoesdiyhealth.blogspot.com
Dr Chris Moschou, GP with an interest in hormone
modulation
Dr Ron Tomlins, GP with an interest in health promotion
and disease prevention
Dr David Tye, GP with an interest in allergy

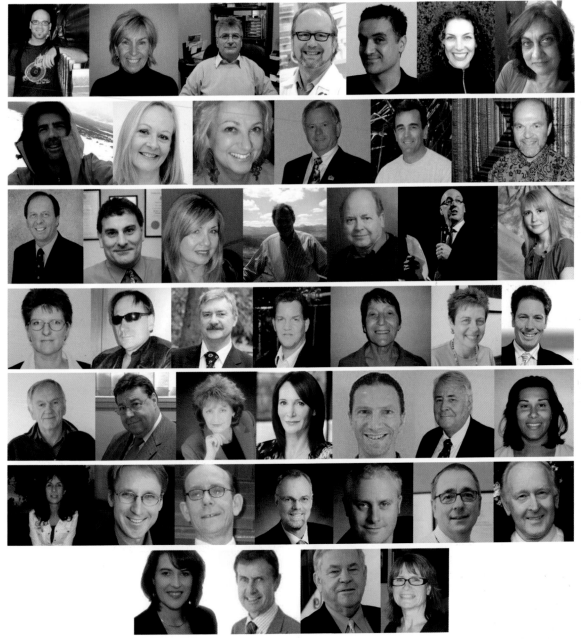

L-R: Line 1 Andrew Munro, Ann-Mary Hromek, Chris Moschou, Merlin Thomas, Carl Honoré, Danika Fietz, Rosemary Boon
L-R: Line 2 Brendan Penwarden, Carolinda Witt, Debbie Verrell, Donald Moss, Stephen Penman, Russell Cooper
L-R: Line 3 Richard Stenlake, Ian Gillam, Robyn Ewart, Ron Tomlins, Robin Holliday, Ray Welling, Iwona Rudkowska
L-R: Line 4 Jennifer Aikman, Wayne Jencke, John Flynn, Marc Cohen, Mary Gurr, Margo Field, Joe Kosterich
L-R: Line 5 Rod Wellard, John Arbuckle, Nerida Saunders, Kate Marie, Jerry Schwartz, Richard Reid, Tania Tissera
L-R: Line 6 Eva Migdal, Peter Muzikants, Moshe Szyf, Bill Andrews, Terry Robson, Michael Lowy, Ray Kearney
L-R: Line 7 Sally Errey, Brian Morris, Stephen Leeder, Helen Bolger-Harris

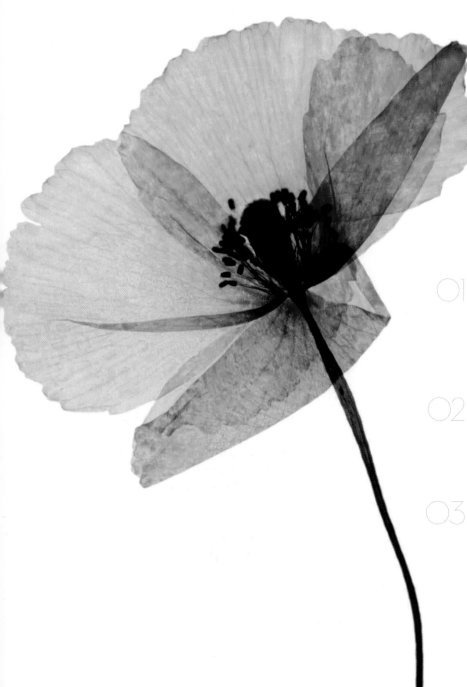

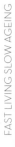

CONTENTS

INTRODUCTION

SOME THINGS SHOULD BE TAKEN SLOWLY.
AGEING IS ONE OF THEM.

There is much to be said for taking it slow. Whether you dream about slow cooking or a 'Slow Boat to China', the same principles that make 'slow' work, apply equally to our lives. It is not just longevity. Vital and fulfilling lives will not automatically come from longer ones. Nor do we expect time to miraculously stand still, but we know it can get away on us. Slow is about taking your time (back).

Ageing is often inexorably linked with disease and decline, rather than being seen as an opportunity for growth and value. Ageing is and should be positive. Old age can be productive, built on the back of wisdom and skills accrued over many years. Our life's journey is a wonderful thing and something to be enjoyed. There a number of opportunities to get here, as there are prospects to lose your way. This book gives you the foundation to look where you are going and find your own way to stay on track.

This book looks at some of the practical ways to apply slow to the ageing process. It is not rocket science. But at the same time it is not about shunning research and technology, rather acknowledging the role many different resources can play in reaching our goals, as well as their limitations. The challenge with getting to grips with ageing is complex. This book is a collaborative effort. More than thirty general and specialist doctors, scientists and other health professionals have contributed to put together its contents. We aim to tell you what you need to know, based on an up-to-date overview of the scientific evidence. Some of the information is technical. This is sometimes the only way in to finding what choices you have and why you would consider making them. Where possible, we have tried to bring the material down to earth, showing real-life examples of how things really work.

Healthy ageing won't happen by mistake. It requires significant planning and investment. This book seeks to put some options before you and a decision-support framework that is directed by you. We don't recommend any particular strategy. There is no miracle 'cure-all solution' in these pages. Instead we aim to assist you in rationally selecting the most appropriate options for your needs and provide the tools and support to stay on track. We have developed this book as a way to navigate the many and varied options you'll come across in your quest to slow ageing and optimise your health and wellness.

We provide a framework so you can make informed decisions in an environment where there is much conflicting and confusing information. In essence, this book's goal is to empower you on your slow ageing journey. It seeks to put you in control and remain proactive in managing your life.

A slow journey means having your eyes wide open to what can happen if you do certain things or if you don't. Many aspects of health and ageing are influenced by the choices you make today. You can actually choose the kind of life you want to live as you age. You don't have to be neurotic, but simply pay attention and make your choices as though they matter. Often very small increments can make a great deal of difference when amplified by many years of practice. We don't advocate anything drastic in this book. These fads are never sustainable and seldom enjoyable. Slow is about taking stock of where you are now and what you are or aren't doing, recognising our personal strengths and weaknesses, as well as our capacity to make real and lasting change. It is also about being realistic in your health planning process; being clear about what you are prepared to do, when, and how, and understanding their consequences. It is never too late to make a difference. The most important thing about this book is that it is all do-able. This book will give you tools you can use today that will make a difference tomorrow.

Unlike many trends, slow ageing is not an alternative approach. In this book, we also look at the practical ways to prevent disease and early death. In this context, strategies to slow ageing are even more important, as longevity without preventing the changes of ageing is a curse not a cure. While successful ageing, like health, is not merely the absence of disease, an effective anti-ageing strategy must always include participation in disease prevention programs and compliance with effective disease management. Equally, the more we strive to prevent disease, the more important it is to examine ways in which slow ageing can also be incorporated into our lives.

This book has been a dream that has been my waking companion for more than a decade. It developed out of my frustration with the 'anti-ageing' industry that sought to dictate my actions with the promise of a miracle cure. I tried many things but came out none the wiser. In the end I wasn't even sure why I bothered. The onus has to be on us, as individuals, to take control. My wish is that this book is a guide and companion as you go about getting to the nub of your desires. I'm assuming that if you have reached for this book that you have an idea of what you want and are ready to do some work. So let's get going.

Kate Marie

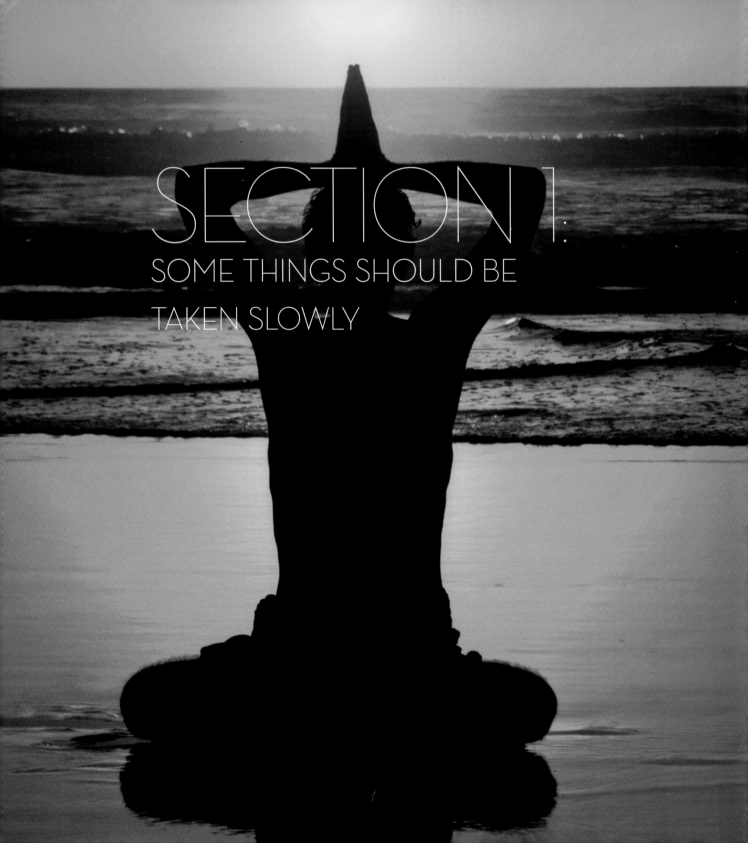

SECTION 1:
SOME THINGS SHOULD BE TAKEN SLOWLY

Some things should be taken slowly. Ageing is one of them. In this first section, we will look at what it means to get older and how this occurs. We will look at the gains and the losses, as well as how our body's attempts to hold things together shapes the signs and symptoms of ageing. We will show that ageing is not something we simply enter into and are taken along for the ride. Our future is something we create, the manifestation of our choices or our inattention. We don't expect time to stand still, but we know it can get away on us. Slow is about taking your time (back).

KATE'S EXPERIENCE
Quite a few things were on my mind at the start of my slow(ing) ageing journey. I had to ask hard questions such as "how am I going to handle this ageing process?", "what does ageing mean to me?", "do I actually want to slow ageing?" and "how am I going to like it, given it is inevitable?" Once I had my head around these questions, next came working out what to do to slow ageing and to know that I was doing it effectively. I found the subsequent intervention selection and change process very much a challenge as there was so much to learn and apply. I initially tried to be completely rules-based, but found this impossible as everyone had a different set of rules for slowing ageing. I also realised that, as with everyone else, I had a unique set of experiences and expectations that would affect my capacity to change and that in the next 50 years the rules would change dramatically. So I constructed my own 'navigation model' to make informed decisions that were right for me. Over time and with help from various people, we ended up with a set of principles and the SLOW ageing philosophy. The SLOW ageing philosophy also pushes back against the fear-driven anti- ageing movement, which treats ageing as the 'anti-Christ'! I wanted to find the joyous side of ageing and develop an approach that paced my journey toward older age more to my liking.

CHAPTER 01

WHAT IS AGEING & WHY SLOW IT DOWN?

Ageing is the sum of the processes that lead us to become old, taking on the characteristics of our elders. We often overlook the positive aspects of ageing, but believe it or not, they do exist! In this book, we explain how to age in a way that will have you living in even better shape than now, in a way that puts you in control of any negative aspects coming your way and in a position to optimise the positive.

A journey to slow the ageing process means taking control and having our eyes wide open to what will definitely happen if we DO certain things or if we DON'T do those things. As with any major decisions in our lives, we need to be aware of our options and recognise our personal strengths and weaknesses, as well as our capacity to make change. Let's face it, if we make conscious decisions now to optimise our state of health, it will be far easier to have a fantastic future as we age. We need to understand ourselves, plan, set goals and objectives, assess, be consistent and become proactive.

AGEING AS LOSS AND DECLINE

Loss is the most recognisable feature of ageing, whether it be memory, hearing or hair. As we age, maintenance and management of these losses becomes increasingly important and this is the most practical way to slow ageing.

When we look in the mirror, many of the features we identify as 'old' are a threshold. The time that it takes to reach this arbitrary threshold is 'ageing' and many factors affect the speed at which this happens. Take the greying of our ageing hair as the cells that pigment our hair become damaged and lost with time. Ageing is not the only factor involved. Smoking, sunlight exposure, inflammation, stress and other factors all act on our hair to shorten the time it takes for the grey to take over. This is how we can appear to get older faster. By preventing this damage, we can appear to age more slowly, even if we never actually change our ageing speed.

AGEING IS GAIN

While ageing is often considered synonymous with decline or loss, some functions are actually enhanced as we get older. We gain and accumulate knowledge, skills and understanding. Many of us muster emotional, intellectual and social reserves unavailable to us when younger. Strengths such as reflection, spirituality, wisdom and caring for others come to the fore. This is the basis for the many success stories of older mentors who are uniquely able to express warmth, understanding and guidance. As we get older, we get much better at opening ourselves to new opportunities, activities and relationships. The goal is to age with these gains outnumbering the losses.

AGEING AS COMPENSATION, REMODELLING AND OVERLOADING

As we get older, there are a number of ways to compensate to keep things ticking over as they should. The human body has a broad range of strategies for its preservation. Ageing increasingly tests our body's limits for adaptation. Many of the changes that we see as ageing are really just remodelling to cope with different demands that ageing places on our body. At its most basic level, all cells do their best to hang on and cling to life, even when severely damaged. This can be achieved by shutting down all but the essential functions, so we can preserve energy and live to fight another day. This kind of compensation is observed in the brain where the nerve fibres shorten and branches and connections disappear, as ageing brain cells conserve the basic functions necessary for survival at the expense of brain power.

RECOGNISING WHAT AGEING IS, AND HOW WE WANT TO AGE, IS THE BEST BASIS TO MOVE FORWARD. BUT WITH MORE CONTROL OVER THE PACE!

AGEING AS LOSS OF RESERVE

While the ageing body can seem healthy, often what declines is the ability to 'step up' a gear. For example, as we get older, there is little change in the performance of our heart when resting, but the maximum output that can be achieved during exercise declines. This reserve is the same reserve we need to call on for activities of daily living as we get older. One thing we know about ageing is that we increasingly depend on our reserves, while at the same time these reserves can become more depleted. This is not just a physical phenomenon. Psychological and social reserves are equally important as we get older. The reserve will determine the threshold for, and impact of, illness and other challenges that befall us as we age. Diminished reserves in key tissues are a key factor in many age-related diseases, including dementia, osteoporosis and heart disease. A deliberate attempt to build and maintain these reserves can make the threshold of dependence recede, and ageing seem to slow.

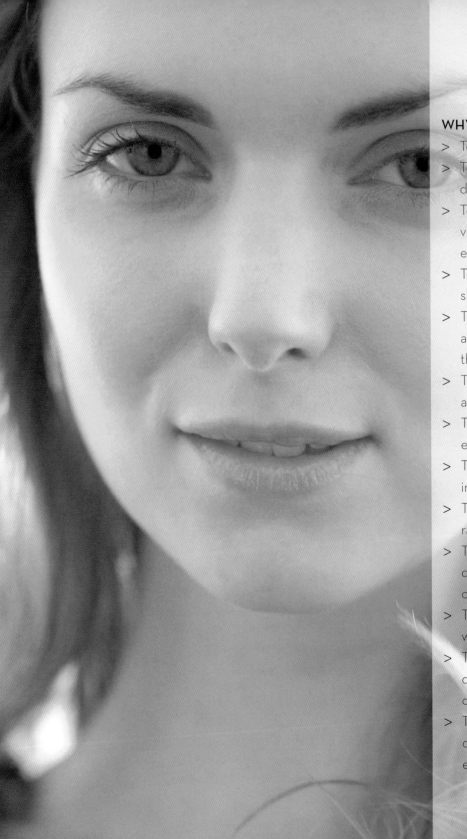

WHY SLOW AGEING?

> To enjoy life for longer
> To increase our satisfaction in day-to-day life
> To get more from life; increased vitality leads to increased capacity for engagement
> To prolong our ability to gather and share life wisdom
> To enjoy sustainable healthful living and feel consistently well (for most of the time)
> To enjoy a deeper experience of life as we worry less over our 'limited' time
> To have a longer period in which to experience personal growth
> To enjoy increased productivity as an individual
> To have more time to enjoy a greater range of experiences
> To reduce cell and system deterioration and so prevent the onset of common, lifestyle related diseases
> To help prevent any diseases to which we are genetically predisposed
> To prevent the decrepitude and dependencies that accompany rapid or even normal ageing
> To optimise our chances of ultimately dying in good health, with the ideal endpoint a painless death in our sleep

AGEING AS A DISEASE

Given the high prevalence of chronic disease as we get older and the fact that ageing is a key risk factor for many diseases, is it really possible to distinguish ageing from the changes caused by disease? Ageing can alter the onset, manifestation and severity of almost any disease. Yet most people achieve 'old age' without evidence of the diseases associated with ageing.

From about 20 years of age, the density of our bones slowly declines. At some point, thinning bones become so significant that the risk of fractures is increased. While this effect might be connected with ageing, a number of other factors, such as smoking, inactivity and poor diet, can also contribute to bone loss and therefore osteoporosis. Ageing just shifts the threshold in a way that makes it easier for other factors to push us over the edge.

WHEN I AM OLD

This is what ageing has in store for us. There will be positives and negatives. We will have losses and gains, compensations and vulnerability. We may also face disease. But like most experiences, we shouldn't just let ourselves be taken along for the ride. Ageing is something we have some control over. Quality is something we create, it is the manifestation of the many choices we make. Recognising what ageing is, and how we want to age, is the best basis to move forward. But with more control over the pace!

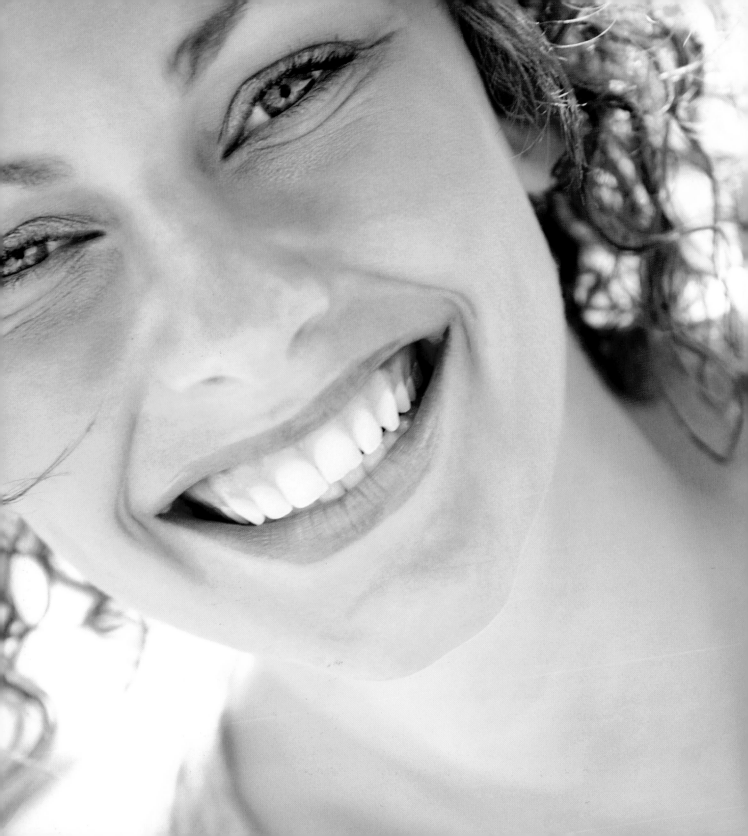

CHAPTER 02

THE PRINCIPLES OF SLOW AGEING

There is much to be said for taking it slow. The Slow movement has developed as a counter to the amoral culture of fast food and mass production. This culture sees food, clothing, travel or even sex as an end in itself, with no additional function (ie. it's just sex, it's just a pair of shoes). Slow is about finding the connections in any experience to allow us to savour its qualities. Different groups have used the SLOW acronym to highlight different issues.

For example, the slow food movement has used it to mean:

S = Sustainable (not having an impact)
L = Local (not someone else's patch)
O = Organic (not mass produced)
W = Whole (not processed)

WHAT IS SLOW?

Each of the S.L.O.W concepts is a practical way to foster connectedness between what is being produced and what we are eating. However, the same principles can also be applied to our own lives. It is very easy to feel that our choices have no importance. Like flying in a plane, time seems to melt away until suddenly we're a long way from where we started. We don't expect time to stand still, but we know time can get away on us. Slow is about taking our time (back).

We cannot expect that enjoyable and fulfilling lives will simply come from longer ones. Slow ageing therefore has the complementary goals of disease prevention and maintaining structure, function and quality of life. These aims are distinct from anti-ageing practices, which propose to intervene in the processes of ageing, with the goal of extending lifespan. It is reasonable to have expectations of technology and medicine. Over the last hundred years, lives have become healthier and longer, and more advances will be made in our lifetime. Yet the notion that ageing may be controlled by a single pill or diet is naive. Ageing is not even a wholly biological experience, but a complex change determined by environmental, behavioural, cultural, socioeconomic, as well as biological factors. As an analogy, it is now possible to contain the entire nutrient content of an apple in a tablet. While it may be chemically identical, it does not have the crunch of the first bite, the shine of the skin or the joy of picking it fresh from a tree. In the same way, health and ageing are much more than biology or chemistry.

A deeper understanding of health, disease and ageing allows us to take rational steps to better support structure and function and maintain quality. Rather than simply being passengers in our bodies, we can engage in our lives and our environment, and start to make positive and informed choices about things they can do today with tomorrow in mind.

HOW CAN I SLOW DOWN?

We all want to delay the onset of age-related decline and disease. So did Faust and Dorian Grey. But as each found out, the ends do not justify the means. Slow means not giving control over to anyone else, whether that be the devil, professional experts or large corporations. Slow puts you in control of your choices and their consequences.

There are many different ways to slow down. They will be intrinsically different for different people with different needs and in different settings. However, in common to them all are seven principles. In this book we will use these principles to illustrate some of the opportunities to slow ageing and extend our healthspan. These principles are also starting point to guide policy makers, funders and the healthcare system.

STEP 1: SLOW SOLUTIONS INVOLVE AWARENESS AND ENGAGEMENT

In this busy world, it is easy to fall asleep at the wheel and find ourselves somewhere we didn't want to be, like in a ditch! We have to take the time to change bad habits if we choose to notice. Slow is for people who are 'awake' to the benefits of choosing wisely and living in a state of wellbeing. This means assuming a degree of self-awareness and making some effort to remain vigilant. It means taking a closer look inside our biology, as well as outside to the world we live in, to identify risks and strengths. It means taking a close look at what we eat and drink, our work, stress and activity, as though our choices will have a significant bearing on our future. Much of the discomfort and disease associated with ageing are the result of choices we make or fail to make in earlier phases of our lives. Slow is about finding these connections and finding opportunities for every individual to merge understanding and awareness with a willingness to do what it takes to age well and keep at it for life.

The slow approach also seeks to educate - what, how, why and when. It helps to know more about the challenges we will face on the road (and there will be many over the journey of our lifetime). It means understanding the risks, options and possible results of different pathways. There is a lot to think about, which is why we have written this book and hopefully why you are reading it. Unfortunately, this book will only take you part of the way there; the rest must come from you. Only you can recognise your own skills, enjoyments, appetite for change and commitment to the road ahead.

> WE DON'T HAVE TO AGE
> AT OUR CURRENT RATE
> DON'T ACCEPT
> DECLINE AS INEVITABLE
> WE HAVE A CHOICE

STEP 2: SLOW SOLUTIONS HAVE CLEAR AND REALISTIC GOALS

Taking the long way home doesn't mean you don't know where you're going, an aimless meander. Slow is not the easy option. It takes a good deal of strength and commitment.

It is not enough to simply want quality of life or longevity as we age. We need to be clear about what we're prepared to do, when and how, and understand that the choices we make really matter. Slow solutions set objectives that match our personal goals and capabilities, goals that reinforce our actions. It is about taking stock of where we are now and being realistic about the health planning process. This takes organisation, as much as execution. In fact, the acronym could equally be used to describe planning that is:

S = Strategic - becoming aware, investing time in planning
and making the critical decisions required for us as
individuals to slow the ageing process.

L = Long-term - to persist for a lifetime.

O = Organised - implementing our plan against measurable
objectives and investing effort into interventions that work for us.

W = Wilful - unhurried actions are undertaken and choices
are made with full consciousness of their nature and effects.

STEP 3: SLOW SOLUTIONS ELIMINATE THE NEGATIVE

Slow ageing seeks to redefine ageing as a positive growth experience, rather than one inexorably linked with decrepitude, degeneration and decline. The anti-ageing movement generally seeks to position 'getting old' as something to be avoided at all costs. It feeds on people's fears and typically doesn't provide real solutions. This is unrealistic and unnecessary. We want to slow ageing, not fear it. Attitude is the single most important factor in healthy ageing. A positive attitude drives healthy behaviour and gives us control over our lives. It can more than compensate for a number of other things that may be failing. Ageing needs to be re-positioned as an experience of value, not only for ourselves as individuals, and our society. It is possible to LOVE the ageing process, to re-frame ageing as a positive experience and take control so we age with pleasure, resilience and growth.

There is always a certain guilt associated with poor health and disease. Did we cause this by something we did or didn't do? Equally, in considering steps to prevent illness or ageing, it is easy to fall into the trap of believing that some suffering is the price of good health, the distasteful medicine we must swallow to get well. However, slow solutions are not punitive, they are a positive experience. For example, for a weight-loss diet to be successful in the long-term, it cannot be a punishment, it must be intrinsically rewarding. Similarly, good sleep, hygiene and exercise will effortlessly find their way into daily life when they come with their own rewards, such as the kick we get from waking up revitalised and refreshed. Additional reward comes from achieving control and related feedback. It is important for each individual to find their own incentives and rewards for any activity to be continued and its full benefits revealed. Slow ageing means we are equipped to savour our life's journey, stay on track and find the best way home.

STEP 4: SLOW SOLUTIONS ARE SUSTAINABLE IN THE LONG-TERM

Slow solutions are long-term solutions for long-term problems. They are never a quick fix. They can be distinguished from fads that claim to achieve miracles in only six weeks! There is no point buying into diets, or joining a gym but rarely going, or getting good medical advice but only following part of it. We will only rebound and be left feeling less in control than ever. We're in this life for the long-term. So whatever we do to slow the ageing process, it must be something we can incorporate into our lives on an ongoing basis. Slow solutions are seldom more than good habits. That's what makes them work so well! The desire and momentum to keep habits in place usually comes from the individual. Of course, it helps if you like it, you know why you are doing it, and it realistically fits in with your personal goals, your lifestyle and your environment. This makes it easy to keep at it until it simply becomes a good habit. This does not mean becoming angels or fanatics who do everything correctly all of the time. This will never be sustainable. Ultimately, practice makes perfect most of the time.

STEP 5: SLOW SOLUTIONS ARE NOT EXCLUSIVE

The complex challenges that face the ageing body and mind require complex multimodal solutions that are most effective when used in combination. The key to slow ageing is not an individual antioxidant, an exercise regime or eating five fruits and vegetables every day (although each may help). It is having a focus and understanding of the whole process and the options available. This leads to awareness and rational choices that sit right for each of us. This cannot be mass-produced. Slow ageing covers all aspects of our health – physical, mental and spiritual. Each of us place a different emphasis on these elements and, over time, that emphasis may change. Slow practices don't mean you can't adjust. As new ideas and information emerges, some change (even a sea change) may be necessary. When you understand you are in control and have the knowledge to make the right decisions, then change is both transforming and invigorating.

THERE IS ALWAYS A CERTAIN GUILT ASSOCIATED WITH POOR HEALTH AND DISEASE. DID WE CAUSE THIS BY SOMETHING WE DID OR DIDN'T DO?

STEP 6: SLOW SOLUTIONS NEED SUPPORT

A central theme to slow is that the individual must be at the core of the process, controlling key decisions. But even while we sit in the driver's seat, it helps to have a navigator. This is one reason we have written this book – to provide our experiences of the roads, the potholes and the downhills. There are also many good practitioners available and the best of them are willing to act as health 'coaches', rather than simply demanding allegiance to their therapeutic strategies. It is valuable to use them to organise our thinking and explore the many options available to achieve our objectives. Don't be afraid to look for knowledge from friends and family too. Sometimes they also want to know (and participate). Ultimately, the most successful program involves a strong relationship between the driver and navigator, whether they are a doctor, dietician, trainer, motivator, friend or family member.

STEP 7: SLOW SOLUTIONS DO WHAT'S RIGHT FOR YOU, GOLDILOCKS

Once upon a time, there was young girl called Goldilocks. When approached with a challenge, she resolved to explore the alternatives, ultimately choosing the one that best suited her needs. When considering the many options available, it's a good idea to take a leaf out of Goldilocks' book. There is no one answer to ageing. Some options may not work, but there will always be one that is right for us. A slow solution means choosing the RIGHT approach for ourselves in the RIGHT doses and at the RIGHT pace for your life, and sticking to it. It is about ageing at the right speed for us as individuals.

Matching our needs to potential slow solutions occurs on many levels. Some of this comes from an awareness and understanding of our needs, skills and capabilities. If we don't enjoy it, or if we feel it's too risky for us, we'll never keep at it. Another way to 'match up' is through the new technologies that help us target what is right for us. Many of these will be discussed in this book.

Finally, getting the choices right also means getting FEEDBACK to provide some indication that we're heading in the right direction. Is the way we're ageing now truly supporting us to be happy? Successes and failures in the course of any activity can be used to keep us on the right track and to set personal benchmarks. The more we understand ourselves, the easier it is to make the best decisions. Little bears need little bowls. Big bears need big beds. One size never fits all!

TAKING IT SLOW

There are many opportunities to slow our lives. In this book we use these seven principles to illustrate only some of these opportunities. There is not enough room to cover them all. However, these 'AGELESS' slow principles apply equally to a range of different interventions. As you read this book, take the time to look through your own pages. What are you are doing today for tomorrow (apart from reading this book)? Can you say that these are slow solutions? Can you use the principles of slow to make them more beneficial, more sustainable and more enjoyable? Often it doesn't take much to make a real difference, just the awareness that we can.

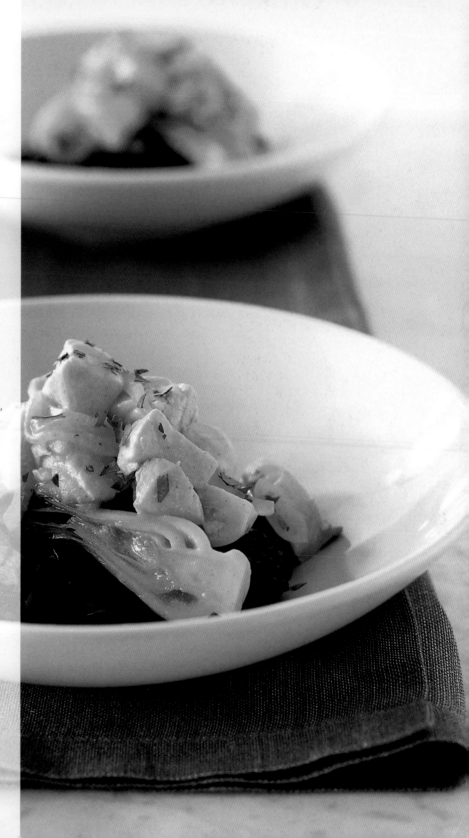

AGELESS

THE 7 PRINCIPLES
of SLOW AGEING

1 AWARENESS AND ENGAGEMENT IN THE AGEING PROCESS.

2 STRATEGIC PLANNING AND TARGETING OF APPROPRIATE GOALS.

3 ACCENT THE POSITIVE, ELIMINATE THE NEGATIVE.

4 MAKING CHOICES THAT ARE SUSTAINABLE IN THE LONG-TERM.

5 DON'T BE EXCLUSIVE. COMPLEX PROBLEMS REQUIRE COMPLEX SOLUTIONS.

6 SUPPORT IS OUT THERE, SO GET HELP.

7 BE SELECTIVE. LIKE GOLDILOCKS, DO WHAT'S RIGHT FOR YOU.

CHAPTER 03

HOW DO WE AGE?

A number of factors act in concert to produce the signs and symptoms we know as 'getting old'. In this chapter, we will look at some of the important drivers. It is important to note there are many different components and we need to address more than just one if we wish to modify the ageing process. In fact, addressing only one factor may cause more harm than good! For example, if you give a cell limitless regenerative abilities, you may create one that just keeps on growing, like a cancer.

IT'S NOT THE YEARS, IT'S THE MILEAGE

Our ageing body can be compared to our car. If we drive it every day for long distances, it will wear out faster, even more so if we don't maintain it. However, if we keep it well maintained with regular services, it will continue to run smoothly for a very long time. To some extent, the same can be said for our body. The mileage we get from it is largely dependant on how well it is maintained and serviced!

Like our car, our body accumulates a lot of 'natural shocks' over a lifetime. These may be large and infrequent (like accidents) or low-grade, chronic or persistent damage (like the elements). The four most important of these elements for ageing will be discussed in chapters 8 -11. Unless prevented or repaired, the damage accumulates and has a large effect on how we age. A good example of this is the damage to our cell's genetic code, known as mutations. Many cancer cells have accumulated mutations in their genes which result in their uncontrolled and unruly growth.

GENETIC PROGRAMMING AND REPROGRAMMING

It is often suggested that longevity is 'all in your genes'. Many people feel reassured if they have a relative who has lived to be one hundred years old. Certainly some genes have been shown to affect lifespan or predispose us to some diseases. However, less than a third of variability in human lifespan is due to inherited differences in our DNA. This is why there will never be a genetic test for ageing.

Moreover, our genes are far more plastic than a fixed DNA blueprint. As every cell respond and adapt to their environment, (epigenetic) mechanisms determine which genes are expressed. Our lifestyle, diet, activity, stress, ageing and numerous other factors can impact our DNA and the way it functions. For example, although identical twins have exactly the same DNA they become easier to tell apart as they get older. By the time they are ready to retire, the expression of their genes may be four or five times different. Ageing is really a form of memory, where our accumulated experiences and exposure are cemented within our chemistry.

TOO CLOSE TO THE EDGE

We sometimes describe the likelihood of an accident happening as 'only a matter of time'. Consider the man who walks towards a cliff. It is not just time that determines the likelihood of him falling, but also his proximity to the edge. This is partly how we age. Although youth is not free from harm, the likelihood of impairment becomes greater as we get older. Small accidents can therefore have more important consequences as we age due to the decline in redundancy, adaptability, reserve function and repair mechanisms.

When we look in the mirror, many of the features we identify as 'old' are a threshold. The time that it takes to reach this threshold is 'ageing' and many factors affect the speed at which this happens. For example, ageing is only one factor involved in going grey. Smoking, UV exposure, stress and other factors all shorten the time it takes for the grey to take over. This is how we can appear to get older faster. Equally, by preventing this damage, we can appear to age more slowly. Slowing ageing does not mean stopping time, but modifying the risks and stepping back from the edge so time is no longer the enemy.

DEFENCE, REPAIR AND MAINTENANCE

Damage (ageing) accumulates when defence, repair and maintenance mechanisms become inadequate to cope. Many of the interventions currently available to modify ageing focus on supporting and augmenting these mechanisms for as long as possible.

The human body has a number of mechanisms to defend against the ravages of time. For example, certain cells generate their own antioxidants. Our immune system is also on the constant look out for threats. Decline in both these important defence systems is thought to significantly contribute to ageing.

But if you can't defend, another way to help keep your castle intact is to repair the damage, where it occurs, when it occurs. For example, in order to limit mutations, there are hundreds of different proteins that recognise and repair any damage to our DNA. However, as we age, these DNA repair mechanisms can become defective. The importance of this change is illustrated by the fact that diseases that cause the DNA repair mechanisms to fail also lead to accelerated ageing.

Many of the maintenance and repair tasks in the human body are performed by stem cells. These cells have the ability to repopulate damaged tissues or organs with healthy new cells and contribute significantly to the regenerative process. However, as we get older, the number of stem cells in our body declines, so regeneration and ultimately function becomes compromised.

The failure of defence and repair is often cited as the key reason for ageing, yet one of the most important factors that is overlooked is maintenance. Just like our cars, regularly doing the simple things help to keep things running smoothly and healthy. A simple example is taking out the garbage. As part of our normal function, broken parts are regularly removed, destroyed or recycled. But in the ageing body, abnormal proteins accumulate, so you end up with a backyard full of old cars and other garbage! In many studies, the efficiency of this kind of maintenance has been directly related to longevity.

AGEING AND THE BIOLOGICAL CLOCK

Many cells in the body can divide and replace losses that occur naturally over time. However, there may be a limit to this regenerative capacity. This phenomenon is known as the Hayflick limit (after Dr Leonard Hayflick, who described how cells lose their ability to divide after a certain number of divisions). For example, fibroblast cells from babies can undergo about 50 divisions before they become exhausted. The same adult cells last half as long. Like a cat with nine lives, the capacity for regeneration is finite and eventually life runs out. This also means there must be a 'biological clock' that knows how far we've travelled and when our time is up.

An example of our body's timer is telomeres. These are bits of DNA that sit at the end of each chromosome, like the plastic ends of a shoelace that protect it from fraying and make it easier to thread the lace through the eyelets of our shoes. Every time a cell divides, our telomeres get shorter. Eventually they become so short that they can no longer protect the adjacent DNA. This triggers a break that stops further cell division and leads to the death of that cell. However, it's not only time that can shorten our telomeres. Because of their exposed position, telomeres are also vulnerable to damage by the elements which act in concert to run down the clock (see chapters 8-11).

SOME PARTS SIMPLY CANNOT BE REPLACED

We have a complement of specialised cells that are so caught up in their jobs, they have little or no capacity to divide. Examples include the nerve cells in our brain, the beating muscle of our heart and the insulin- producing cells of our pancreas. These cells are designed to last a lifetime and cannot be replaced if lost. When we are born, we have as many as we will ever have. As the years go by, our stocks are irreversibly depleted. This is why the effects of ageing are potentially more important in these cells and why our endowment at birth is one of the most important predictors of outcomes in adult life. The number of 'filter units' we are born with in each kidney varies from 150,000 to 500,000. If we lose 100,000 through normal attrition by the time we are 60, it's not such a problem if we started with 500,000, but if we started with fewer then the loss of 100,000 may put a lot of stress on our kidneys.

USE IT OR LOSE IT

As we get older, if we don't use it, we lose it. All cells require stimulation for healthy growth and activity. Being deprived of stimulation, like hearing or visual loss, seems to speed up ageing. By contrast, those who continue to be active - physically, mentally, socially, sexually and spiritually - not only retain a greater quality of life, they tend to age more slowly in key areas. Ageing can be a positive process, where health feeds into activity and stimulation, and ultimately more health and quality of life result.

Ageing is not a single factor, but rather the sum of many factors - some damaging, some protective. In our youth, these forces are kept in balance, but with the passage of time, there is accrual of injury and the 'memories' of the injury's effects. Although the makeup of our bodies is incompatible with indefinite survival, we can still change the odds in our favour. A better understanding of the factors and pathways involved in ageing allows us to explore ways to slow ageing. In the following chapters, we examine some specific interventions and how they can modify the rate and reasons for ageing.

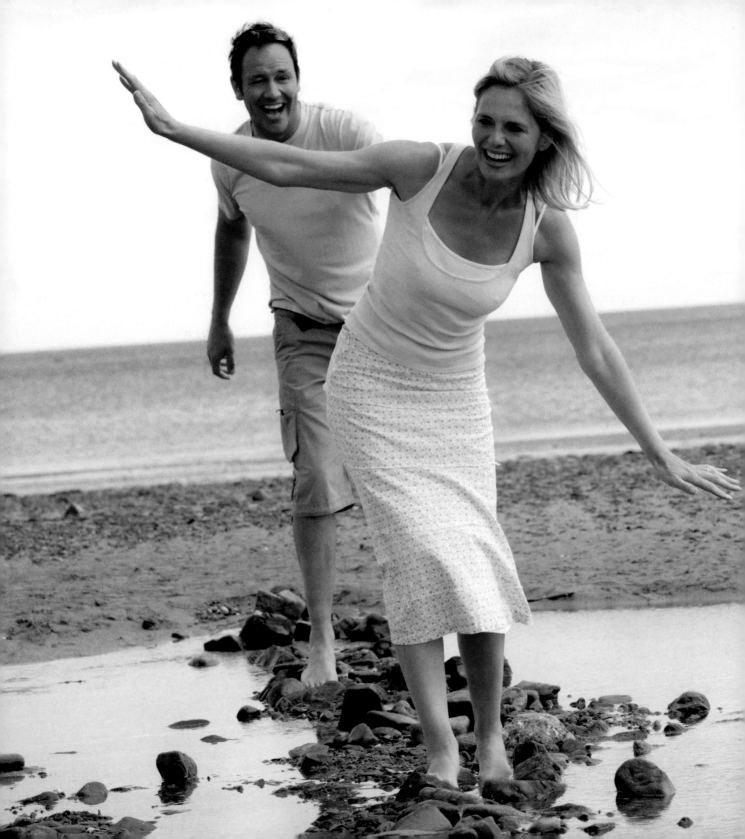

CHAPTER 04
MAKING HEALTHY LIFESTYLE CHANGES
[HOW DO WE DO IT?]

Changing lifestyle can take time and effort but the rewards are great - a healthier and longer life!

While some things in life are easy to change, others can be extremely challenging. The fact is our brains are hardwired to resist change, preferring the comfort and status quo of old habits, be they healthy or toxic. The thought of replacing bad with good habits, while exciting to our rational brain, can upset our emotional brain which is attached to those habits.

This chapter will help you understand the steps you can take to align your rational and emotional brain so they can work together and achieve your goals.

STEPS TO MAKING HEALTHY LIFESTYLE CHANGES

The first step to getting your emotional brain excited about a healthier lifestyle is to create your vision for a healthy fulfilled life. Next, you develop a logical plan of action which will satisfy your rational brain. As you execute your plan, it is important to start with small actions that you are confident of achieving, so your emotional and logical brain work together. If you take on lifestyle changes that are too numerous or too difficult, this can trigger a fight or flight (fear) response from your emotional brain which will ultimately undermine your confidence. However, if you take several small steps, that then elicit small wins, this will help bypass this fear and strengthen your confidence and capacity for change.

Long-term change doesn't happen overnight. Change is a process where you'll continuously move back and forth through different stages. You can expect good and bad days and indeed relapse is a part of the change process. Falling into old habits is part of the journey and an opportunity to further practice new skills so you can do things differently. It can be helpful to use the following model of the Stages of Change (by James Prochaska) and think about the questions you might ask yourself at each stage so you can move forward with ease.

PRE-CONTEMPLATION	CONTEMPLATION	PREPARATION	ACTION	MAINTENANCE
DENIAL: *"Who Me?"*	AMBIVALENCE: *"Maybe one day"*	YES!: *"Let's do it"*	DOING IT: *"I am"*	LIVING IT: *"I am still"*
You are unaware of the problem, resistant or disinterested in change.	You are possibly aware of the problem and risks, but not yet ready to change.	You are motivated to make changes and create a plan of action.	You are making changes, developing strategies and doing it!	You are living with change, determined to succeed and adjusting to change.
What are the risks of not changing? Who can I trust to speak openly about this with?	What is good about change? What stops me from taking steps towards making change?	What are the barriers? What can I do to overcome these?	What small steps will keep change happening? What has been good about change?	What's helped me be successful? What can help me maintain change?

PROGRESS ⟶

RELAPSE ⟵

OH NO! *"Time to start again"!* It is an opportunity for me to again practice developing skills in how to do things differently.	What would help me when I give it another try? What triggered my relapse? What can I do to avoid these triggers and whom can I talk to about this? How can I plan to better deal with future temptations?

The journey to keep yourself in peak condition mentally, physically and spiritually is a precious one. Take it slowly, one step at a time. Be patient and remember - you have time... A full life ahead!

CREATING YOUR SLOW AGEING PLAN

A. CREATE YOUR VISION

Your vision acts as a compass, guiding you on the path to wellness. It is vitally important to spend plenty of time on this essential first step.

Here are some questions to start the visioning process:

> WHAT do I want to create for myself in the coming years?

> WHY do I want it?

> How will I FEEL when I have it?

> WHICH elements would contribute to my state of wellbeing (e.g.: physical, emotional, social, spiritual, creative, intellectual, contribution, community)

Here are some guidelines for creating a written vision:

> PRESENT: describe your vision in the present tense, as if it is already happening (I am…)

> POWERFUL: develop a strong statement of actions and values that describe who you plan to be!

> POSITIVE: focus on your strengths and on what you want, not on what you don't want or have.

> PUT IT OUT THERE: place your vision where you can read it daily.

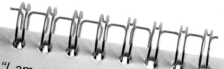

"I am active and energetic. I dance to music or walk each day. I nurture myself through eating wholefoods and drinking clean water. I am connected to people with similar values where we can support each other.. I am an inspiring role model for my kids by living with appreciation, determination and calmness. I accept the limitations of myself and others.

Use the following steps to move your vision toward actions and ultimately towards reaching your goals.

> TICK the options in the boxes at the end of each chapter of changes you want to make that are aligned to your vision.

> ADD your own ideas at the end of each chapter (so all your options are in one place).

> CATEGORISE your actions. Put your actions into lists under the following three categories.

1. SIMPLE ACTION LISTS

These are simple steps that are completed with one action, such as a phone call or a purchase. The first step toward building confidence is completing simple actions.

> Put actions into clusters as this will make it easier for you to complete them:

> TO BUY: shopping lists of foods, nutrients or supplements you want to buy

> TO CALL: list appointments with health practitioners or for tests or assessments

> TO ORGANISE: changes in your home or office to support better lifestyle

> Diarise times to do them so you are planning ahead

> Start with the most important actions first

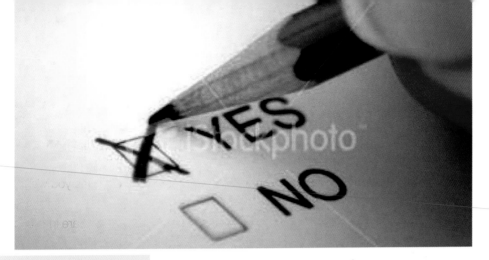

2. RESEARCH TIME

We hope that reading this book will stimulate your curiosity and encourage you to further explore the things you find most relevant or interesting. Research Time means taking time out so you can research the many and varied options – talking to a health professional, watching a documentary, going online or reading a book. This is a very important step as it will set you up to make an informed choice; one that is aligned with your values, rather than just acting on the first thing that comes along. Finding a great doctor, physiotherapist, home exercise machine or exercise buddy can take time, but might be key in motivating you and building the foundations of your future wellbeing.

It will help to schedule Research Time in your diary - whether once a week, once a month, or for a full day. Ensure you are taking time to move forward, but in small enough chunks so you don't feel overwhelmed.

3. SMART BEHAVIOUR CHANGE

Behaviour changes are the most challenging of changes to make. SMART changes are **Specific, Measurable, Attractive, Realistic and Time Bound.**

Here is a checklist of habits you might want to change. Tick the ones of interest and number them in terms of importance from 1 - 10 (10 being most important).

General behaviour change checklist:

/10	Reduce weight	/10	More & regular exercise	/10	Drink more water
/10	Reduce alcohol	/10	Stop smoking	/10	Increase hobbies
/10	Reduce stress	/10	Reduce junk food intake	/10	Improve sleep

Start with ONE that is important to you (> 7/10 in importance) AND that you feel CONFIDENT you can take some steps forward with.

Now use the following Smart Behaviour Change Steps to develop a plan.

SMART BEHAVIOUR CHANGE STEPS OPTIMISING SUCCESS

	ASK YOURSELF	EXAMPLE ONE	EXAMPLE TWO
1	What change in behavior do I want?	*More & regular exercise*	*Improve my sleep*
2	Why is this important to me?	*Reduce risk of cancer Reduce risk of heart disease*	*Reduce my stress levels Create more energy*
3	How will I do it? Brainstorm alone or get help and then make a list of as many options you can think of	*Dancing, walking, yoga, join gym, mat exercises, swimming, Pilates class*	Go to bed earlier, *use Melatonin, meditation, relaxation CDs, herbal tea*
4	Choose one or two options you feel most confident about taking	*Dancing & walking regularly*	*Start meditating*
5	Write this option as a SMART goal using the 5 guidelines below	*"I will dance or walk twice a day for 10 -15 minutes during work breaks 3x/week starting Monday. I will keep a diary on my fridge to track this."*	*"I will meditate for 10 minutes each night before I sleep. I will track this using the phone app Insight Timer."*
S	**Specific =** Well-defined goal including how much or what	*30 min walk or dance / day*	*Meditation just before sleeping*
M	**Measurable =** Measurable outcome that indicates success	*2 x 15 minutes/day*	*10 minutes/day*
A	**Attractive =** Something you will actually do which is connected to your vision	*Walk fast and dance*	*Will calm me down and teach me mindfulness*
R	**Realistic =** Realistic given your situation, resources and available time!	*At least 3 days a week*	*7 days a week*
T	**Time Bound =** Have realistic and specific timeframes	Starting tomorrow morning for 6 weeks	Starting tomorrow morning for one month
6	How will I monitor my progress positively?	*Keep a checklist on the fridge that I use daily*	*I will track this using the phone app Insight Timer*
7	How will I celebrate success? Reward yourself for achieving your goals	*Buy a new dress*	*Have a massage once I have done each day for a month*

OPTIMISING SUCCESS

Simple things can add to your chance of success so consider doing the following:

THE POWER OF POSITIVITY

Remember to appreciate what is working well rather than not working. Make a list of your strengths and the strengths of those around you.

THE POWER OF PEOPLE

Choose to be with people who support you. Avoid people and situations that trigger habits you are trying to change! Make a list of people and places where you feel affirmed in your life and spend time with those people and at those places.

THE POWER OF YOUR ENVIRONMENT

Look at whether your home or workplace reflects and supports your goals. Discuss with others or those who share your space about how you can create a space to support your new direction.

RESOURCES FOR CHANGE

There are many fantastic resources that can support and motivate you and provide you with the knowledge and skills so you can make your desired changes. Find a solution that is right for you. You are an individual, so you need to be aware of your strengths and weaknesses and plan actions that suit you, not those that suit a friend or someone you've read about in a weight loss magazine!

GET EXPERT GUIDANCE TO MAKE CHANGE EASIER

Check out www.slowageingcoach.com where you can download a workbook that provides greater detail on making change and which will help you navigate the stages above, with space for you to develop your Master Action Plan.

Get a wellness coach. If at first you don't succeed, don't give up. Go to www.slowageingcoach.com to find a wellness coach who can support you to achieve your goals via phone or Skype.

And finally, don't forget to celebrate each success by doing things that make you feel great!

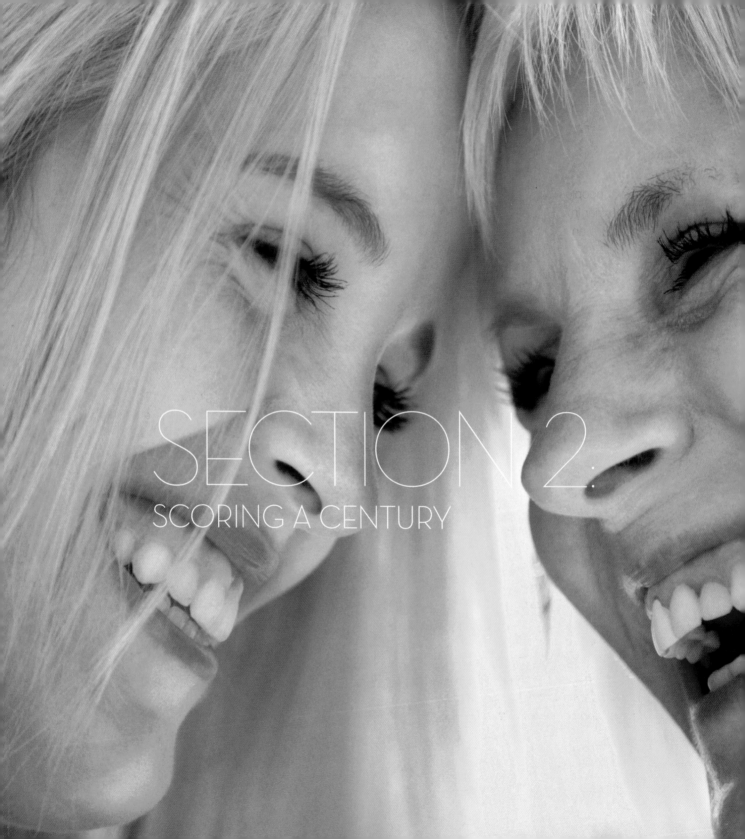

SECTION 2.

SCORING A CENTURY

CHAPTER 5: AVOIDING HEARTACHE
CHAPTER 6: SWEET & SOUR
CHAPTER 7: THE TOPIC OF CANCER

Most people who live to 100 do so by escaping the diseases that often kill people far earlier in life. Although healthy ageing is more than the absence of disease, any effective anti-ageing strategy must also include participation in disease prevention programs and compliance with effective disease management. In this section, we look at practical ways to avoid the four major killers: heart disease, stroke, diabetes and cancer. It has been estimated that prevention of these four diseases could see average life expectancy reach towards 100. Who wouldn't want to bat with that kind of average?

KATE'S EXPERIENCE

There is no point trying to fix the factors that contribute to ageing, or its manifestations, if you never live to old age. When I started this process, I found I knew very little about what was potentially in store for me in the years ahead. I got quite a shock when I researched my full family history. I learnt that my family was riddled with cardiac disease and suffered our fair share of cancers. Having spent time as a nurse and seeing what these illnesses can do, I made a conscious decision that I didn't want disease as part of my life. Yes, the family health discoveries were a shock, but they certainly motivated me to make positive choices regarding my health and the way I choose to age.

The human body is extremely resilient and can live with an enormous amount of debilitation before finally collapsing! As a result of early exposure to ageing and sick people, I knew I never wanted to contract any of these diseases, then have to try to cure them. I was going to prevent them, whatever it took. I now make it a point to get a regular cancer screening and I don't care what it costs. I don't wait for my doctor to remind me when to test for things as I want to protect my investment in my health. I'm also clear on what I put in my mouth as I understand the link between diet and my risk. My health is my most valuable asset and I choose to invest in it wisely!

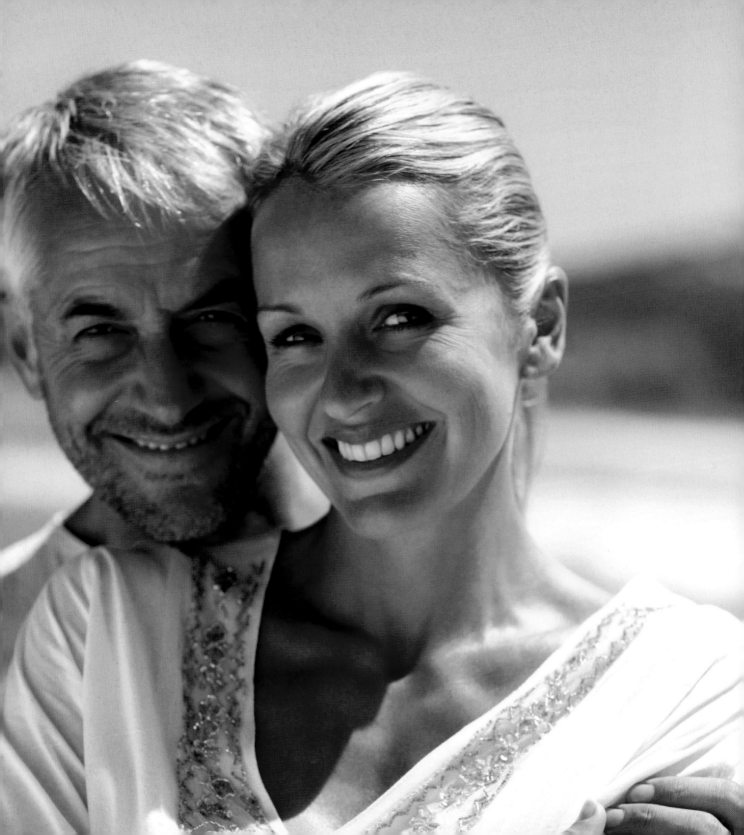

CHAPTER 05
AVOIDING HEARTACHE
[HEART DISEASE, STROKE & AGEING]

Every cell in our body depends on the flow of blood for survival. If this is compromised, even for a brief period, the cells and tissues downstream suffer and eventually die. When this occurs in the heart, it is called a heart attack or myocardial infarction (MI). When a severe reduction in blood flow occurs to the brain, it is called a stroke or cerebrovascular accident (CVA). Together, heart attack and stroke are the major killers in the Western world. Quality of life for survivors is also greatly reduced. Finding ways to prevent or reverse these diseases is an integral part of any slow ageing strategy.

POTHOLES AND ACCIDENTS (HEART DISEASE AND STROKE)

Think of the arteries of the heart and brain as a major freeway that handles heavy traffic. Over time, a number of changes occur under the surface, causing it to thicken and soften. Still the traffic drives over the road, but the pressure of the heavy trucks has a greater effect as the sub-structure is less resilient. Years may go by and the sub-structure gets weaker and weaker. It may start to bulge a little bit, but still the seal remains intact and the traffic flows. Then one fateful day, usually after a large stress, the surface cracks and erodes, and a pothole occurs. The next car hits the hole and flips. The car behind it hits the first car and a major pileup ensues, completely blocking the road. This is what happens when we have a heart attack or stroke. In at least half of men and women, this is the first sign of problems with their blood vessels. For many, it is also their last. If the blockage is not quickly cleared, everything downstream eventually dies.

THE BEST PREVENTION BEGINS EARLY WITH THE CHOICES WE MAKE IN OUR LIFESTYLE, DIET AND OTHER AREAS.

The cells of the heart and brain cannot grow back. Any loss of cells means some permanent loss of function. But if blood flow can be rapidly restored, the traffic flow can return to normal, at least until the next pothole forms in the weakened surface. However, repeated small surface erosions and ruptures eventually lead to narrowing of the road. This scenario is preventable on a number of levels. The best prevention begins early with the choices we make in our lifestyle, diet and other areas. The combination of these measures will reduce the chances of crashing in a pothole and keep us safely on the road for many years to come.

OPTIONS TO PREVENT HEART ATTACKS AND STROKES

☑ Stop smoking
> Call Quitline, contactable on 131 848 or 13 7848
> Get a buddy – when about to reach for a cigarette call them
> Visit non-smoking venues such as cinemas, museums, libraries and cafes
> Make a change in your routine – get up earlier and go for a walk
> Chew gum
> Have a pen and paper handy to you can doodle when you have time on your hands and nothing to do!

OPTIONS TO PREVENT HEART ATTACKS AND STROKES

☑ Increase physical activity - increasing your physical activity has a range of positive effects on the body, reducing stress on arteries, preventing clogging, improving glucose and blood pressure control, and helping us maintain a healthy weight. A combination of cardio and weight bearing exercise is best. At the start, aim for 30 minutes daily achieving a minimum heart rate of 65% of your maximum (see chapter 22)
  > Have a fitness assessment and find out what you really need to do to meet your goals
  > Find an exercise buddy to work out or walk with
  > Buy a pedometer and join the 10,000 steps program (www.10000steps org.au)
  > Find out about classes run at your local community centre. Aerobics, yoga or dancing may be options
  > Try karate or another martial art

☑ Reduce calorie intake
  > See a dietician or nutritionist for a dietary program that suits your needs
  > Clear out your pantry – bin all the lollies, chips, snacks, biscuits and 'empty calorie' foods
  > Figure out your caloric intake needs and then reduce by 20%. If you are unsure what your caloric needs are see a nutritionist or dietician to guide you

☑ Prevent diabetes
  Excessive levels of sugar damage blood vessels, like the baking sun causes a road's surface to become brittle and damage more easily when exposed to stress. The presence of diabetes at least doubles the risk of heart disease. Measures to prevent diabetes are more effective than anything else in reducing heart disease:

  > Eat more fibre by increasing wholegrains and eating 3 serves of fruit and 5 serves of vegies each day
  > Reduce your total fat and saturated intake by trimming meat, choosing lean cuts and substituting full fat dairy with low fat alternatives
  > Avoid trans fats by reducing fried foods, use olive or rice bran oil for cooking and avoiding processed and packaged foods
  > Increase resistance exercises (see chapter 22). Try including weights in your program

OPTIONS TO PREVENT HEART ATTACKS AND STROKES

☑ Lower your blood pressure

Blood pressure is the stress placed on our arteries. If we can find ways to lower it and keep it low, just like reducing the number of heavy vehicles, it will keep a road in better shape for longer. For every 1 mm Hg decrease in systolic blood presure, the long-term risk of a heart attack is reduced by 2% to 3%. Regular exercise, staying in a healthy weight range and eating a diet low in salt (<6g/day) and fat can reduce systolic blood pressure by 10-20mm Hg and therefore the risk of heart attack or stroke by 20% to 50%.

> Start with 10 minutes walking per day of exercise and slowly build up to half an hour
> Try resistance training with a Thera-band. An exercise physiologist can write you a home program
> Reduce your intake of meat and thereby saturated fat by increasing portion sizes of ve etables, rice and dry beans in meals
> Try casseroles or stir-fry dishes, which have less meat, more vegetables and beans
> Include two or more meat-free or vegetarian-type meals in your weekly diet
> Use herbs and spices to flavor food rather than salt
> Limit the amount of salt used in cooking, and do not add salt to food at the table
> Choose foods labeled 'no added salt'
> Avoid canned, fast and processed foods as much as possible as they tend to be higher in salt

☑ Increase your antioxidant defences

Oxidative stress is bad for blood vessels and their function. You can increase your antioxidant defences by choosing foods that are naturally high in antioxidants, especially the richly coloured (rainbow) foods (see chapter 8). The more naturally coloured fresh fruit and vegetables the better. Other useful sources of antioxidants with a range of bonus benefits include:

> Red wine – contains the antioxidant resveratrol, as well as a host of other useful compounds
> Green tea – contains catechins; epigallocatechin gallate (EGCG) one of the most efficient antioxidants
> Garlic – has many positive effects on the heart including lowering blood pressure and cholesterol levels, blood thinning, as well as antioxidant effects
> Turmeric – is both antioxidant and anti-inflammatory. It also lowers LDL cholesterol. Team it up with your antioxidant vegetables, like brassicas and legumes; a quarter of a teaspoon a day

☑ Lower your LDL cholesterol levels

LDL cholesterol is the badcholesterol that deposits its cargo under the surface of blood vessels. If we reduce our LDL cholesterol, our risk of death from a heart attack or stroke risk is also reduced. We can reduce our LDL cholesterol through exercise and choosing foods that low in saturated fat and cholesterol

> Reduce your intake of saturated fats from dairy products (especially whole milk, cream cheese and ice cream), coconut, palm oils, fatty meat
> Include phytosterols/stanols in your diet that reduce cholesterol absorption

OPTIONS TO PREVENT HEART ATTACKS AND STROKES

> Include soy, nuts and whole grains on a daily basis. Use them to replace other calories (like dessert) not to add even more energy to our diet. ¼ cup(30g)nuts or seeds is a perfect snack size
> Get help from your doctor if your cholesterol levels are too high (LDL > 3.5mmol/L) or your risk of heart disease is too great (high blood pressure, diabetes, family history, etc)

☑ Increase your omega-3 fats - Omega-3s can reduce cardiovascular disease, partly by reducing cholesterol and inflammation, as well as thinning the blood.
> Eat cold-water oily fish (such as salmon, herring, mackerel, anchovies, sardines and tuna) three times a week or meat from grass eating animals, such as lamb or kangaroo.
> Choose fruit and vegetables high in omega-3 fat like flax seed (linseed), purslane, kiwifruit, lignon berries and walnuts

☑ Consider omega-3 supplements (fish oils, flax or linseed oil); about a gram per day of combined EPA and DH or 4-5 grams of alpha linolenic acid

☑ Include half a handful (1/4 cup) of nuts and seeds in your diet daily. Eat them raw, avoiding salted and roasted varieties

☑ Eat more whole grains and dietary fibre - Aim for 30g of fibre each day.
> Sustitute refined products with wholegrain equivalents.
> Substitute fibre for animal protein.
> Consider fibre-rich legumes instead of steak mince

☑ Use wholegrain pasta, bread and brown or wild rice

☑ Have 5 serves of vegetables per day

☑ Include legumes such as red kidney beans, lima beans, broad beans or lentils in your diet 2 - 3 times a week

☑ Check your risk factors regularly:
> Systolic blood pressure
> Bad (LDL) pressure cholesterol and Good (HDL) cholesterol
> Triglycerides and Homocysteine
> Waist circumference (see chapter 6)
> Markers of inflammation including hsCRP and fibrinogen (see chapter 11)

SWEET & SOUR
[DIABETES]

In the healthy body, our glucose (sugar) levels are kept constant. If we eat a chocolate cake, the body simply puts out hormones, including insulin, that tell the body to start using glucose at the same rate as it is absorbed from food, so the glucose levels in our blood stay the same. When we're not eating, the body slowly releases its glucose stores to drip-feed the brain at the same rate at which it uses glucose. The glucose levels in our blood thus stay in balance. Diabetes is the state in which this balance fails and sugar levels start to rise.

SWEET AND SOUR (DIABETES)

Diabetes occurs when there is damage to the insulin-producing cells of the pancreas. In children and adolescents, the immune system can inadvertently destroy these cells. This is called type 1 diabetes, or insulin dependent diabetes (IDDM), because insulin injections are needed to survive. Insulin-producing cells can also become burnt out in ageing adults by too many years or too many calories. This is called type 2 diabetes, or non-insulin dependent diabetes (NIDDM), because the body retains the ability to produce a little insulin, at least initially. This may be enough to cope with small meals, but there is inadequate reserve to deal with additional demands. So the first sign of trouble may be when glucose levels rise after a big meal. This is called impaired glucose tolerance (also known as pre-diabetes) and is detected by observing a rise in glucose levels within two hours of eating sugar.

> DIABETES OCCURS WHEN THERE IS DAMAGE TO THE INSULIN-PRODUCING CELLS OF THE PANCREAS.

TESTING FOR DIABETES

It is possible to detect any loss of function with a glucose tolerance test (GTT). For this simple, non-invasive test, a large amount of sugar is taken orally or injected. If your pancreas can't handle it, your blood sugar levels rise, indicating the presence of diabetes.

	CONSIDER GETTING CHECKED FOR TYPE 2 DIABETES IF:	
MEASUREMENT	You have too much around your middle: Find the mid-point between your bottom rib and the top of your hip bone. Breathe out normally and measure your circumference with a tape measure across this point. (This may not be the narrowest part of your waist, or exactly in line with your belly button).	
MEN	94cm (37 inches) or more 102cm (40 inches) or more	= increased risk = substantially increased risk
WOMEN	80cm (32 inches) or more 88cm (35 inches) or more	= increased risk = substantially increased risk

Diabetes is worth preventing, especially if we want to live long and prosper. For every year we have type 2 diabetes, we can effectively add a year to our age, so a 60-year-old who has had diabetes for 10 years has, on average, the life expectancy of a 70-year-old. If we have diabetes, all the elements of ageing (calories, oxidative stress, AGEs, inflammation – see chapters 8 to 11) are enhanced and all the diseases of ageing happen at an earlier age, including Alzheimer's, heart disease, stroke, hypertension, kidney failure, vision loss, arthritis, impotence, some cancers and even grey hair. One way we can slow ageing is by not allowing it to speed up.

OPTIONS TO PREVENT TYPE 2 DIABETES

☑ Increase physical activity.

As adults, regular physical activity is the best way to keep our pancreas working effectively into old age.

Exercise acts to reduce insulin resistance, which, like leaving the hand break partly on while driving, asks for even more work from the pancreas in order to climb over the same hill. A combination of cardio and weight bearing exercise is best. Initially aim for at least 30 minutes daily achieving a minimum heart rate of 65% of your maximum (see chapter 21)

> Try interval training – walk briskly for 100 metres then jog for 100 metres or ramp it up and jog for 100 metres then run for 100 metres. Ensure your heartbeat is raised. Remember you must be huffing and puffing

> Build lean muscle mass — try a weight training session with an experienced trainer. Increased lean muscle mass is associated with decreased insulin resistance

☑ Reduce your energy intake. Excess calories are the main reason why the pancreas wears out as we get older. There are many different ways to reduce the amount we eat. These are discussed in chapter 9

☑ Instead of 3 main meals, include 3 meals and 2-3 small snacks spread over the day. Evenly distributed meals will help with sustained energy and stable blood sugar levels. The bigger the meal, the harder your pancreas has to work to produce insulin

☑ Eat food with a low Glycaemic Index

Low-GI foods break down to form sugar in your blood more slowly, so the demands on the pancreas are not so great

> Choose high fibre options such as whole grain bread, oat based cereals, legumes

> Substitute white potato for sweet potato

> Substitute white rice for Basmati rice, pasta, barley or noodles

> Eat 3 serves of fruit and 5 of vegetables every day

OPTIONS TO PREVENT TYPE 2 DIABETES

☑ Eat foods that are high in antioxidants
   Especially the richly coloured (rainbow) foods. Think red - tomatoes, orange - sweet potato, yellow -corn, green - spinach, blue - berries and purple - onion

☑ Eat foods low in saturated fat
   Not only does fat increase your waistline faster, it increases your risk of diabetes. Substitute monounsaturated fat, like olive or nut oil for saturated fat like butter

☑ Substitute whole grains and dietary fibre for processed starch
   All the good bits are in the germ or bran, while the added fibre makes you full without adding to your calories (see chapter 14)

☑ Eat fresh foods and reduce exposure to AGEs and other toxic products generated during processing (see chapter 10)
   > Shop at your local fruit and vege shop or weekly markets for fresh produce
   > Buy from your local butcher for prime, lean and fresh cuts of meat
   > Keep chickens for a steady supply of fresh eggs
   > Start a vegetable patch or even a windowsill herb garden
   > Plant fruit trees
   > Do a cooking class or buy a recipe book for inspiration
   > Make cooking a family or friend affair and share your fresh produce
   > Order from an online organic supplier
   > Challenge yourself – how many different vegetables can you eat in one meal or one day
   > See how many colours you can create on your plate
   > Have at least one vegetarian day each week
   > Try a new vegetarian recipe each week
   > Try new foods - have spelt instead of wheat, quinoa instead of rice, soy or rice milk instead of cows milk, sheep's fetta instead of soft cheeses, 70% dark chocolate instead of a chocolate bar and dark grape juice instead of red wine
   > Join a fresh food co-op

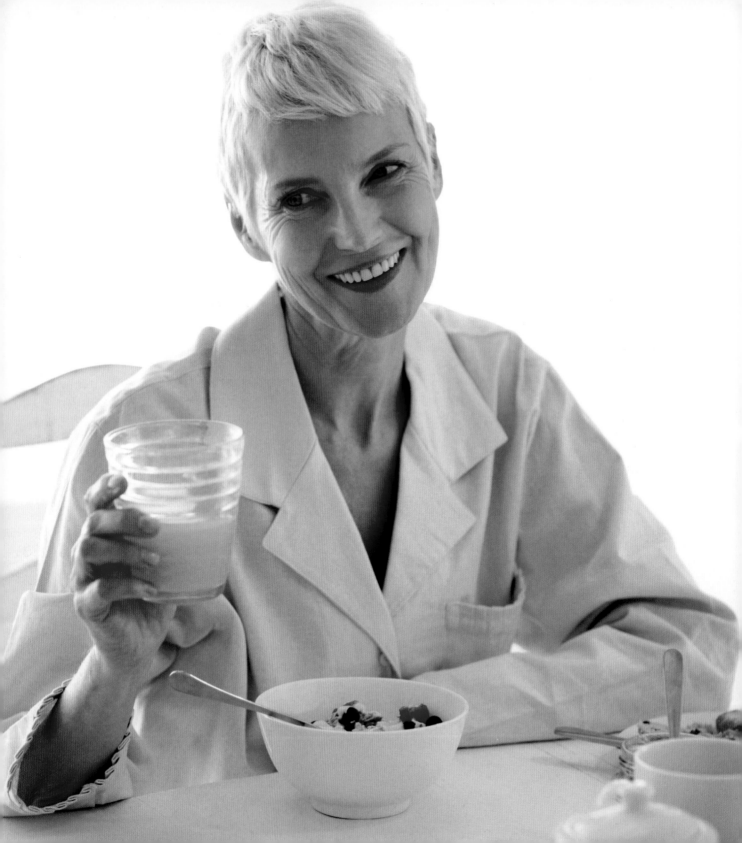

CHAPTER 07

THE TOPIC OF CANCER

People who live to 100 do so by avoiding the common diseases that cause death, including cancer. At least a third of us will face cancer during the course of our lives, mostly after the age of 64. When considering strategies to improve our chances for continued health and longevity, we need to understand what cancer is and what we can practically do about it as we get older.

OFF THE RAILS

In a healthy human body, different cells pull together for the common good. In its simplest terms, cancer is a disease that develops when this cooperation breaks down. Instead of being team players, some cells go their own way, leading to uncontrolled growth. They intrude on and destroy adjacent cells and tissues. Sometimes these unregulated cells spread to distant parts of the body (metastasis), where they intrude on and destroy other cells and organs.

In most cases, what transforms healthy, cooperative cells into unconstrained cancer cells are changes in their DNA programming. Alterations (hits) at several different points over a cell's lifetime are required to knock it off the rails, which is why time is ultimately the greatest enemy. These changes may occur as random errors as cells duplicate. A number of external factors (carcinogens) may also damage the DNA sequence and generate a cancer. Common factors include tobacco smoke, radiation, oxidative stress, dietary toxins, pollution and infections. There are many factors that normally act to prevent DNA damage. If these are also deficient, as happens when we age, cancers are more likely to occur.

PREVENTING MELANOMA

Most deaths from skin cancer are due to melanoma, which is when a skin cell that normally confers pigment to the hair and skin (melanocyte) becomes derailed and starts to grow autonomously. To become a melanoma, cells must go through a number of steps, usually beginning with the formation of a mole. Moles are limited growths that remain static, unless triggered to become malignant by additional DNA damage.

PREVENTING LUNG CANCER

Lung cancer is the most common cause of cancer-related deaths in men and it is on the increase for women. Like the skin, the surface of the lungs has a high degree of exposure to the outside environment, so it is highly susceptible to inhaled carcinogens. By far the most damaging carcinogens are those in cigarette smoke, whether inhaled from smoking or passive smoking. Avoiding cigarette smoke is the only effective way to prevent lung cancer. Encourage others around you to do the same.

PREVENTING BREAST CANCER

For women, breast cancer is the leading cause of cancer deaths. One in eight women will develop breast cancer at some time in their life, most often after the age of 60. However, prevention is possible. Increased awareness, earlier detection and improved treatment have resulted in declining death rates from breast cancer.

AT LEAST A THIRD OF US WILL FACE CANCER DURING THE COURSE OF OUR LIVES, MOSTLY AFTER THE AGE OF 64.

One important action a woman can take to prevent breast cancer is to perform regular screening to facilitate early detection of lesions. The most widely used test is mammography, where close-up x-ray pictures are taken of each breast from several angles while it is gently compressed onto a flat surface. Most cancers can be detected in this way. It is recommended that all women over the age of 40 undergo a yearly mammogram and continue to do so for as long as they are in good health. In the absence of a strong family history, women under this age have lower rates of breast cancer, making screening less valuable. Women who have a family history or are at a higher risk of breast cancer should consider magnetic resonance imaging (MRI). This is a more detailed procedure and can detect cancers at an even earlier stage. While regular self-examination is not a substitute for mammography or other screening tests, it is valuable in detecting some types of breast cancer and it also helps foster awareness.

ACTIONS AND OPTIONS TO PREVENT MELANOMA

☑ Keep a close eye on your moles

☑ By closely monitoring any moles, you can identify if growth is no longer restricted and a cancer may be forming. If you have a mole or unusual freckle that is new or has changed in shape, size or colour (e.g. dark brown to black, blue-black or red), you should get it checked. The earlier a cancer is identified and treated, the better your chance of avoiding surgery, disfigurement or death. Early detection is good protection

☑ Get an annual total-body examination of your skin

☑ It's hard to keep an eye on everything. You should make sure you get checked all over every year

☑ Protect yourself against solar damage

☑ Ultraviolet and infrared light are the most important causes of DNA damage in the skin. Do what you can to limit your exposure to harmful rays:
  > Wear hats and protective clothing (even on cloudy days)
  > Use broad spectrum SPF 30+ sunscreen (apply every 2 hours when exposed). Make sure it is protective against UVA rays as well
  > Avoid unprotected sun exposure (especially 11am to 2pm)
  > Don't use tanning salons

ACTIONS AND OPTIONS TO PREVENT BREAST CANCER

☑ Get an annual mammogram

Screening should be performed annually from the age of 40 years or earlier if you have a family history of breast cancer

☑ Perform a monthly breast self-examination:

Just after the end of a period is best, when your breasts are least likely to be swollen and tender. If you do it regularly and become familiar with the feel of the breast tissue you can recognise any changes

Things you should bring to your doctor's attention include:

> Dimpling, puckering, or bulging of the skin

> A nipple that has changed position or an inverted nipple

> Redness, soreness, rash, or swelling

> Fluid coming out of one or both nipples

> Distortions, lump or swelling, especially if they are new

☑ Actively prevent weight gain, especially after the menopause

> Get fit – see how in chapter 21

> Reduce your intake of empty calories (see the end of chapter 9 for options)

☑ Give up smoking—encourage others to give up too as passive smoking will still affect your risk of breast cancer

> Log onto www.quitnow.info.au for tips and information

> Get a quit coach — someone who can help you plan quitting and stay off cigarettes

> Write a smoking diary to identify times that you may be tempted and learn about your behaviour associated with smoking and cravings

> Make an appointment to see your doctor to look at available medical options

> Investigate hypnotherapy — it works for some people

ACTIONS AND OPTIONS TO PREVENT BREAST CANCER

☑ Eat a low fat diet naturally high in antioxidants
  > Include at least 4 vegetables or 'colours' on your plate with your main meal. Colour = antioxidants
  > Have half a cup of berries 3 or 4 times per week. Fresh or frozen are suitable. Add them into cereal, a smoothie or fruit salad
  > Have ½ cup of broccoli, cabbage or cauliflower daily as they have a chemical component called indole-3-carbinol that can combat breast cancer
  > Choose low fat dairy options such as 2% milk, fetta or ricotta cheese and low fat yoghurt
  > Ensure you choose trim cuts of red meat and remove the skin from poultry
  > Try pomegranate juice for an antioxidant hit

☑ Keep up your Vitamin D levels
  > Spend up to 20 minutes a day in the early morning or afternoon sun. Sun exposure to the back of the shoulders and the chest equates to the greatest level of vitamin D production
  > Get your vitamin D levels checked. The normal range of 25 Hydroxy Vit D is 50 to 150 nmol/L, however if you wish to obtain optimal levels for peak performance then you should aim for 115 to 128nmol/L
  > Take a vitamin D supplement if your levels are low

☑ Moderate your alcohol intake
  > Have at least 2 alcohol free days per week
  > Drink soda and lime without the vodka
  > Have a glass of water between each alcoholic drink
  > Try delay tactics – put off having a drink until later in the day or tomorrow
  > Distract yourself – do something to keep your mind off having an alcoholic drink, have a glass of water, go for a walk, have a piece of fruit or read a book
  > Deep breaths – take 3 deep breaths and see how you feel before you automatically pour a drink

ACTIONS AND OPTIONS TO PREVENT BREAST CANCER

☑ Get better sleep. Poor sleep, with disruption of circadian rhythms is associated with breast cancer, possibly because of low levels of melatonin (see chapter 26)

☑ Minimise your exposure to plastic products. Some studies have suggested bisphenol A from plastics and other environmental toxins may also contribute to breast cancer (see chapter 15)
  > Avoid bottled water. Buy a hard plastic, aluminium (lined) or stainless steel water bottle and take your own. It's cheaper too!
  > When renovating or redecorating consider non-toxic paints and woollen carpets or floorboards as they contain minimal bisphenol A and other plastic by-products

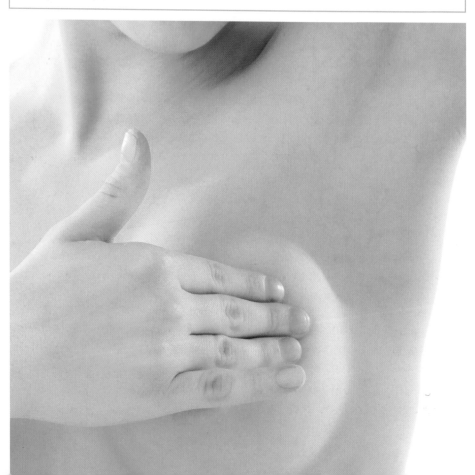

PREVENTING CERVICAL CANCER

Cervical cancer affects over half a million women around the world at any given time. In countries where screening programs exist, at least four out of every five deaths due to cervical cancer occur in women who have not had a Pap test in the past 10 years, or who have been inadequately screened. Currently the best way to prevent death from cervical cancer is regular screening with a Pap test (or cervical smear). This should be undertaken at least every 2 or 3 years, or more often if previous tests have been abnormal or there are particular risks (eg. HPV infection). Genital infection with the human papillomavirus (HPV) is responsible for most cervical cancers. HPV is a very common virus and four out of five sexually active men and women become infected with it at some point in their lives. Vaccination is effective in preventing infection from cancer-causing strains if performed before we first meet the virus during sex (eg. vaccination of girls aged 12 to 13).

ACTIONS TO PREVENT CERVICAL CANCER
☑ Get a regular PAP test; every 2-3 years from your twenties, or more often if previous tests have been abnormal or there are particular risks (e.g. HPV infection)
☑ Give up smoking > Delay – try to put off your first cigarette of the day as long as possible so that you gradually reduce your smoking hours > Distract – do something to take your mind off the cravings, have a glass of water, go for a walk, have a piece of fruit or read a book > Deep breaths – take 3 deep breaths and see how you feel before you automatically reach for a cigarette
☑ Eat a diet naturally high in antioxidants, especially lycopenes, CoQ10 and carotenoids (see chapter 8) > Include a tablespoon of tomato paste in your cooking each day as is a great source of lycopene > Have at least 4 rainbow foods on your plate each main meal. Choose in particular from red, orange and green foods such as capsicum, carrot, pumpkin, sweet potato and green leafies such as spinach, broccoli and rocket
☑ Protect against exposure to HPV and Chlamydia; use a condom and practice safe sex in general

ACTIONS AND OPTIONS TO PREVENT BREAST CANCER

☑ Screen for cancer with a digital rectal exam and a PSA blood test every year from the age of 50 if you are at risk. Ask your doctor about the risks and benefits for you

☑ Eat a diet naturally high in antioxidants
> Lycopenes (high in tomatoes, pink grapefruit, and watermelon)
> Isoflavones (in soy products)
> Sulforaphane and lutein and zeaxanthin (in cruciferous vegetables like broccoli, cauliflower, kale, Brussels sprouts, and cabbage)
> Selenium (in brazil nuts)

☑ Moderate your intake of animal fat (especially fried, roasted, broiled, grilled or barbecued meat). Diets rich in animal fats and red meat are associated with prostate cancer, possibly due to toxic chemicals generated when meat is cooked at high temperatures
> Rotate your animal products on a 4-day basis – one skin-free poultry day, one trim red meat day, one fish day and one vegetable day. Then repeat
> Grill rather than fry your meat to drain off the excess fat
> Boil chicken before browning and drain away the fat with the water

☑ Keep up your Vitamin D levels (sun exposure, oily fish, fortified foods or supplements)
> Choose from salmon, sardines, anchovies and tuna and have at least twice a week
> See other Vitamin options under breast cancer actions and options
> Take a walk in the early morning or late afternoon sun and expose your limbs to the sunshine

PREVENTING PROSTATE CANCER

The prostate is a small gland that sits under the bladder in men. The main function of the prostate is to make some of the fluid that protects and nourishes sperm. One in six men will develop cancer in their prostate during their life. Nearly 90% of new prostate cancers, and almost all deaths resulting from prostate cancer, are in men over the age of 60.

There are many things men can do today to lower their risk of prostate cancer. Diets rich in animal fats and red meat are associated with prostate cancer, possibly due to toxic chemicals generated when meat is cooked at high temperatures. By contrast, diets high in fruit and vegetables protect against prostate cancer.

The prostate is normally a rubbery, uniform structure. If a cancer forms, it often disrupts the architecture of the prostate. This can sometimes be felt as a lump or hardened area by placing a gloved finger in the rectum and pressing forward. Prostate cancer cells often produce increased amounts of prostate-specific antigen (PSA) that can also be detected via a simple blood test. It is controversial whether regularly performing either of these screening tests is able to prevent disability or death. This is because even though doctors can detect a few cases that kill, screening may result in some innocuous cancers being unnecessarily treated with major surgery. Men who have prostate cancer prevention high on their priority list should have both a digital rectal exam and a PSA blood test every year from the age of 50. This is a discussion worth having with your doctor.

NEARLY 90% OF NEW PROSTATE CANCERS AND ALMOST ALL DEATHS RESULTING IN PROSTATE CANCER ARE FOUND IN MEN OVER THE AGE OF 60

PREVENTING COLON CANCER

Cancer of the colon affects nearly one in 20 adults. Regular screening is the best way to prevent death from colon cancer. Most colon cancers arise from polyps, which are small outgrowths from the surface of the colon. Although the great majority of colon polyps are harmless, over time (at least 5 or 10 years) some may become cancerous. There are many different tests that can be used to screen for pre-cancerous polyps and cancers. If performed regularly every five years, these tests can prevent any new lesions from reaching an advanced or dangerous stage. Most guidelines recommend that from the age of 50, one of the following screening tests should be considered:

FLEXIBLE SIGMOIDOSCOPY > a flexible, lighted tube about the thickness of a finger with a small video camera on the end is inserted into the rectum to view the lower 60cm of the colon.

AIR CONTRAST BARIUM ENEMA > barium sulfate is pumped into the colon using a small, flexible tube inserted into the rectum. When the colon is half full, air is pumped into the colon through the same tube. The barium then coats the surface of the colon and any bumps or projections from the bowel surface can be easily identified.

CT COLONOGRAPHY (VIRTUAL COLONOSCOPY) > a CT scanner takes many pictures as it rotates around the body and a computer combines these pictures into detailed images of the inside of the colon and rectum to look for polyps or cancer.

Any suspicious or positive test result can then be followed up with a colonoscopy, where the whole colon can be visualised and, if necessary, a biopsy taken for further examination. For individuals with an increased risk, such as those with a strong family history, a regular colonoscopy should be considered as a first-line screening test.

Another approach to screening for colon cancer is based on the finding that polyps and colon cancers bleed easily, meaning that microscopic quantities of blood are lost into the stool. This is called occult blood loss, as it cannot be seen by the naked eye. However, occult blood loss can be detected by sensitive tests of stool samples. If stool tests are performed on multiple occasions (usually annually), they significantly reduce the rate of cancer deaths by facilitating early detection. The more compliant an individual is with testing and the more regularly they have the test done, the better the outcomes.

ACTIONS AND OPTIONS TO PREVENT COLON CANCER

☑ Talk to your GP about participating in a colon cancer screening program

☑ Fight weight gain (see chapter 9).
There are strong links between weight gain and colon cancer
- > Try to keep your stress levels under control so you are less likely to eat for emotional reasons. See chapter 25 for guidance on increasing stress resilience
- > Check the quality (eat whole foods, fruits and vegetables, whole grains and lean protein), quantity (when in doubt, eat half of it or less) and frequency of eating. You should eat often – eat healthy snacks such as fruit, vege sticks with low fat dips such as hummus or low fat yoghurt
- > Avoid processed foods
- > Be accountable for your calories. If you are female and in your 40s or 50s and exercising (not an athlete), then you'll need about 1,500 to 1,600 calories a day. A middle-aged man, average height and not an athlete but exercising, needs about 1,800 to 2,000

☑ Start a daily exercise regime
- > Take up weight training
- > Try out bootcamp with a personal trainer
- > Take the stairs rather than the lift
- > Walk to the shops rather than driving

☑ Moderate your intake of processed and cooked meats. Individuals whose diets are high in red meat or processed meats (e.g. sausages, bologna, luncheon) have an increased risk of colon cancer
- > Choose canned fish such as tuna or salmon instead of luncheon meats
- > Use avocado and hummus with freshly cooked skinless chicken
- > Talk to your local butcher about low fat sausage options

ACTIONS AND OPTIONS TO PREVENT COLON CANCER

☑ Choose a diet high in fruit and vegetables. These are linked with a decreased risk. Although the exact component that leads to protection (fibre, folate, antioxidants, certain types of fats) remain to be established, it works.
> Have 5 serves of vegetables and 3 serves of fruit daily as rich sources of fibre and antioxidants
> Drink green tea as a wonderful antioxidant source
> Eat green leafy vegetables. They are the richest dietary source of folate

☑ Eat more whole grains and other sources of soluble fibre (see chapter 14)
> Have rolled oats in winter (rather than instant or quick oats)
> Choose raw, untoasted muesli with fruit for summer
> Try wholegrain spelt or kamut instead of wheat bread for toast

☑ Moderate your alcohol intake. Heavy alcohol use has also been linked to colon cancer
> Try a 'mocktail' instead of a cocktail next time you are in a bar
> Choose mid-strength beer options rather than full strength
> Have 2 alcohol-free days per week
> Have one glass of wine in the evening instead of two

DON'T SEEK AND YOU WON'T FIND

These are things the average person can do: Slow ageing is not an alternative approach. Any effective anti-ageing strategy must also include participation in disease prevention programs. There is good evidence that regular screening significantly lowers your risk of cancer and cancer-related mortality. These tests are easier than many of the interventions in this book, and are worth the commitment. We have the choice to use technology in our favour, or let our futures unravel by themselves.

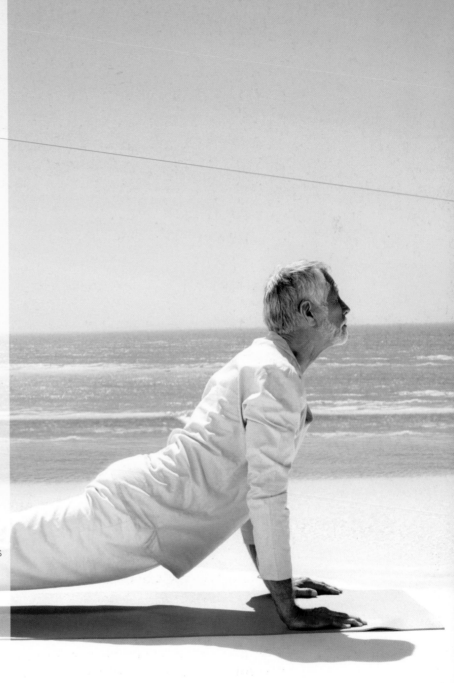

SCREENING FOR CANCER

> Melanoma – have your skin checked annually by a doctor or specialist, now*

> Breast – mammography every year from the age of 40*

> Cervical – PAP smear tests every two years from our early 20s*

> Bowel – sigmoidoscopy, barium enema or CT colonography every 5 years or

> Faecal occult blood test every year, starting at the age of 50*

> Prostate – PSA and prostate examination annually for men over the age of 50*

* More frequent or earlier screening may be appropriate for individuals at increased risk of cancer (e.g. those with a family history or specific risk factors). Ask your doctor if this applies to you.

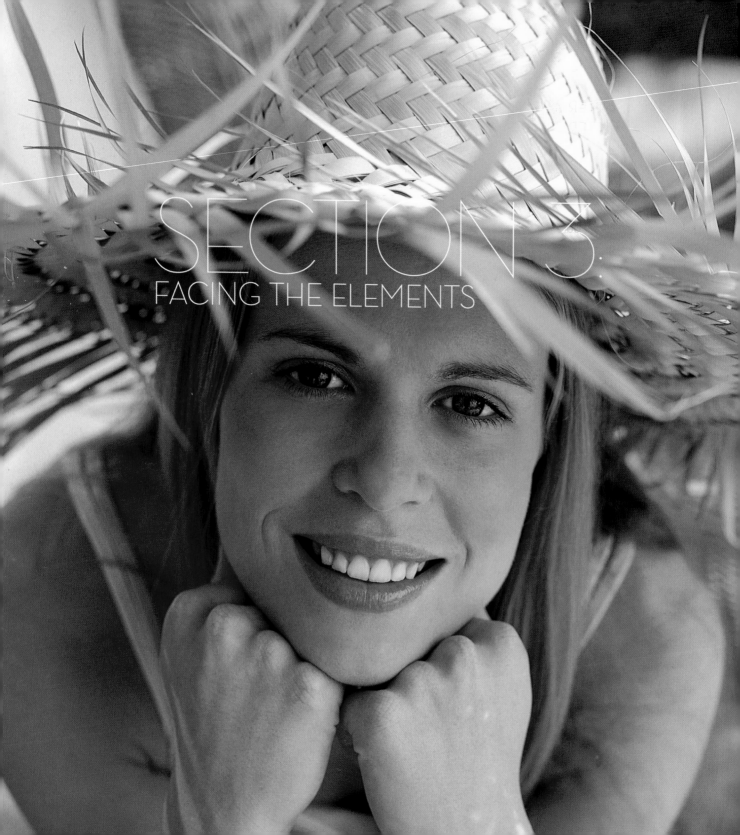

SECTION 3
FACING THE ELEMENTS

If we leave our things outside, unprotected from the elements, they will age and perish quicker. This also occurs with the human body. For example, chronic exposure to ultraviolet radiation leads to accelerated 'photoageing' of the skin. Inside the human body, there are also a number of factors that contribute to decline in structure and function. The most important of these we have called the four elements of ageing: oxidative stress, calories, advanced glycation and inflammation, which we will explore in this section. These elements are important because interventions to reduce our exposure to any or all of them are unequivocally associated with improved health and a longer life. There is quite a bit of science here, but knowledge is power.

KATE'S EXPERIENCE
Although reading the technical details can be challenging, it is important to take the time to read the science. I found that by understanding in detail how exposure to these elements influences how I age, some of the reasons for doing the things I do made a lot more sense. Otherwise it is easy to get sidetracked with fads and half-truths! Knowing what is going on under the covers, also makes it easier to stick to your long-term plans.

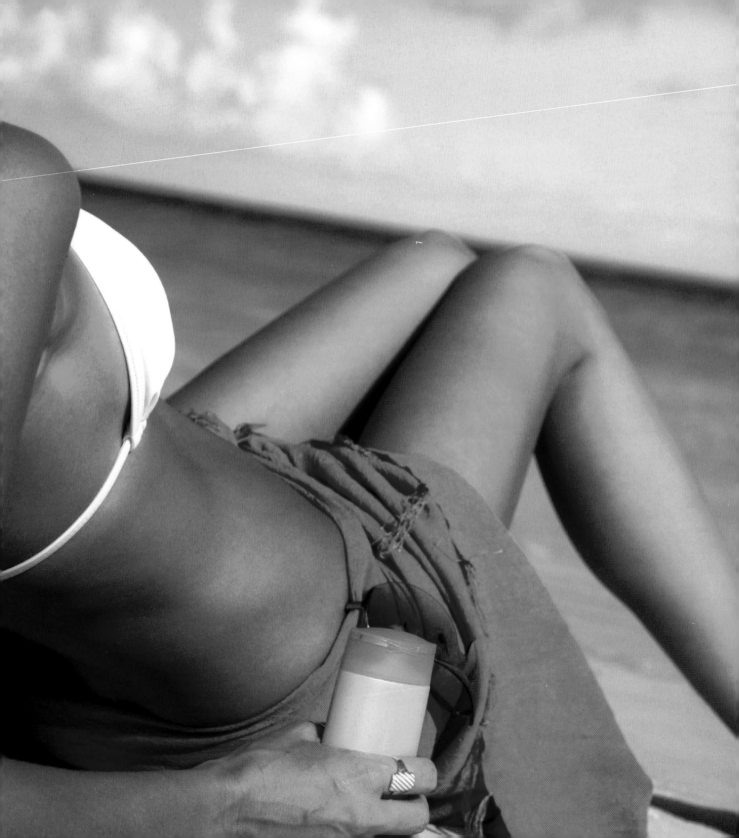

CHAPTER 08

THE ELEMENTS OF AGEING
[OXIDATIVE STRESS]

If we leave things outside, unprotected from the elements, they will age and perish quicker. This also occurs with the human body. For example, chronic exposure to ultraviolet radiation leads to accelerated 'photoageing' of the skin. Inside the human body, there are also a number of factors that contribute to decline in structure and function. The most important of these we have called the four elements of ageing: oxidative stress, calories, advanced glycation and inflammation. The pivotal importance of these four elements is that interventions to reduce our exposure to any or all of them are unequivocally associated with both increased health and a longer life. In this chapter we will look at oxidative stress.

FREEING THE RADICALS

Oxygen is the essence of the air that we breathe. It is vital for the creation of energy. Without it, we would die. But this dependence comes at a cost. During metabolism, a small proportion of oxygen is converted into toxic products collectively known as Reactive Oxygen Species (ROS) or free radicals. As we get older and our systems for metabolising oxygen become less efficient, production of free radicals increases. If the production of free radicals outstrips our antioxidant defence mechanisms, a state of oxidative stress is said to exist. This oxidative stress is one of the most important elements in the ageing process.

As their name suggests, Reactive Oxygen Species are highly reactive. In fact, they can react with almost anything with which they come in contact. When attacked by free radicals, proteins, DNA and lipids don't work as they should and the whole cell's function declines. The most common targets for free radicals are those closest to where they are generated, in the cell's powerhouse, the mitochondria. Damage to mitochondria means less efficient use of oxygen for energy production and a further increase in production of free radicals in a vicious cycle.

The accumulation of products modified by free radicals can be measured as biomarkers of oxidative stress. Many tests are now available both commercially and over the internet. Although each has been associated with poor health outcomes in different populations, none currently can tell us if we would benefit from treating them.

THE BEST PREVENTION BEGINS EARLY WITH THE CHOICES WE MAKE IN OUR LIFESTYLE, DIET AND OTHER AREAS.

Each cell and each tissue in our bodies has its own antioxidant defence systems to remove free radicals before they can do damage. These include enzymes that catalyse the destruction of free radicals, as well as antioxidant decoys that prevent damage by 'taking the bullet' themselves, thereby preventing other more important targets from becoming modified. There is good evidence that the effectiveness of these antioxidant defences correlates with lifespan. In general, the body's production of endogenous antioxidants declines as we grow older, while production of free radicals increases, leading to oxidative stress, as well as ageing itself.

SHOULD WE BE TAKING ANTIOXIDANT SUPPEMENTS?

Because of the strong association between oxidative stress and ageing, as well as a range of age-related diseases, it makes perfect sense to target free radicals as a means to slow ageing. Almost all anti-ageing strategies for the last 30 years have included high doses of antioxidants as a central ingredient. The problem is that although the idea of antioxidants is sound, the long-term effects on health and longevity are yet to be realised or understood. Unequivocally, diets naturally high in antioxidants can both prolong life and reduce the effects of ageing and have done so for centuries. More details on optimising our intake of dietary antioxidants can be found in chapter 17. However, with a few exceptions, clinical trials with antioxidant supplements have not demonstrated the advantages of dietary sources. Indeed some antioxidants have proven to be harmful to human health. So why the difference between antioxidants from supplements and antioxidants from food?

> Firstly, the antioxidants most commonly used in clinical trials (Vitamins A, C, E and carotene) are not very selective in their actions and have other effects on the human body, particularly in high doses. Some can actually generate free radicals!

> Secondly, most studies were not specifically performed in individuals with high levels of oxidative stress. It is possible that participants in these trials did not benefit simply because reduced antioxidant defence was not their problem.

> Thirdly, it may be that other components of a diet naturally rich in antioxidants

contribute to their benefits. These may include a range of polyphenols and pat way intermediates, such as lycopenes. It may also be that different dietary el ments have a greater effect when coupled together. Indeed, a basic principle of traditional medicine is that complex conditions are best managed by complex medicines. In order to capture the different defence and protective actions, a 'brew' often contained extracts from a range of different sources. In the same way, the health benefits of tomatoes are more than the sum of its lycopenes. Citrus is not just Vitamin C, but also rutin, other antioxidant bioflavonoids and a host of other ingredients.

> Finally, it may be too much to ask of a supplement to get into each cell, and especially each mitochondria of each cell, to reduce ROS levels. Neither Vitamin A, C or E actually inhibit production of ROS. They only clean up after the fact, by which time the damage may have already been done or molecules are generated that are immune to the scavenging effects of these antioxidants.

To this end, more specific interventions to reduce radical formation, like selenium supplements, may prove more useful than non-specific 'after the fact' scavengers. In the remainder of this chapter, we will look in detail at the most common antioxidants that are available as supplements and the evidence for and against their actions to slow ageing. There is no available data on which is the best of these many antioxidants when taken as supplements. Each of these will have their own supporters. It may be that, like the computer, we will kick ourselves for not investing earlier. Conversely, some may turn out to be a waste of money. The bottom line is we only know what we know, and this is the evidence so far:

VITAMIN A is a natural antioxidant found in both plant and animal products. In plants, it is present in richly coloured carotenoids, such as beta-carotene, which can be converted into Vitamin A during digestion.

Foods naturally high in Vitamin A are liver, beef, pork, chicken, turkey, fish, eggs and butter, as well a range of dark green and orange-yellow fruit and vegetables, including carrots, broccoli, kale, sweet potato, pumpkin, spinach, romaine lettuce, apricots and capsicum. Increased consumption of fruit and vegetables rich in carotenoids lowers oxidative damage. Fresh is best, as Vitamin A can be depleted from food during preparation, cooking or storage (by radicals produced by prolonged storage or high temperature).

In addition to being an antioxidant, Vitamin A maintains the production of cells that divide and regenerate repeatedly, such as those in skin, as well as the immune system. Vitamin A is also important for vision, particularly at night.

There are two kinds of beta-carotene supplements: those made from natural sources (e.g. palm oil, algae, D. salina) and those manufactured synthetically (all trans beta-carotene). The naturally-sourced carotenes appear to have better antioxidant activity and lower potential for side-effects. When used on its own in clinical trials, Vitamin A or beta-carotene did not significantly improve survival of its recipients, and had no significant effects on other age-related complications, including age-related blindness or cancer. In fact, recent studies have suggested that supplements containing beta-carotene (not dietary carotene) may act to promote cancer formation and liver damage in some circumstances, such as in smokers and alcoholics.

VITAMIN E is a natural antioxidant found in leafy green vegetables, nuts and seeds, whole grains, fortified cereals and some vegetable oils. However, many of the vegetable oils sold in supermarkets have had the Vitamin E removed during processing. As an antioxidant, it is particularly effective in preventing free radical damage to lipids in the cell membranes and circulating fats. In addition, Vitamin E also has significant effects on inflammation, immune function and fertility.

Vitamin E is available in both synthetic and natural sources. The natural form is more potent and better absorbed, and should be preferred over synthetic Vitamin E. Natural Vitamin E may be sold as alpha, beta, gamma, and delta tocopherol. In general, supplements that contain 'mixed tocopherols' with all these different components are emerging as the preferred form of Vitamin E supplements. Some manufacturers use this term to mean the synthetic dl-alpha-tocopherol, so we need to read the label closely. When used on its own in clinical trials, alpha tocopherol showed no beneficial effects in terms of heart attacks, strokes, cataracts, cancers or longevity.

VITAMIN C (ascorbate) is a natural antioxidant found in fruits such as citrus, currants, strawberries, tomatoes, and vegetables such as Brassica and peppers. It is also found in high levels in liver, brain and oysters. It is widely used as a food preservative, especially in processed juices.

Vitamin C is a non-specific antioxidant, with actions on a range of systems. Short-term supplementation with Vitamin C has been shown to have a number of useful antioxidant effects, including beneficial actions on vascular function, wound healing and immune function. High dose Vitamin C can also reduce the severity and duration of symptoms of cold and flu. However, high doses may cause increased bowel activity or diarrhoea. This can be lessened by using a buffered form of Vitamin C, such as calcium ascorbate, or a Vitamin C 'mix', which combines Vitamin C with chlorophyll, hesparin, rutin and other bioflavonoids.

Currently, there are no conclusive clinical trials showing Vitamin C in tablet form has benefits on longevity, cancer risk, heart disease or other age-related complications. However, intake of foods naturally rich in ascorbate, such as fruits and vegetables, are associated with reduced illness and longevity.

SELENIUM is a natural constituent of some of the body's enzymes, including the antioxidant defence enzymes, GPx and thioredoxin. Foods rich in selenium are meat, tuna and eggs. Plants grown in selenium-rich soils also contain increased levels of selenium, including wheat germ, nuts (particularly Brazil nuts), oats, whole wheat bread, bran, brown rice, turnips, garlic, barley and orange juice. Although most adults have sufficient selenium for their metabolic functions, additional supplementation with selenium increases natural antioxidant activity and boosts immunity and thyroid function. In clinical studies, selenium supplements have been shown to reduce the risk of some cancers and improve the chances for longevity.

LUTEIN is an antioxidant in the carotenoid family and is the primary carotenoid present in the central area of the retina, called the macula, where it protects from oxidative stress. Lutein levels are highest in green leafy vegetables, such as spinach, kale, collard greens and romaine lettuce, as well as leeks, peas and egg yolks. People who eat more lutein-containing foods appear to be at lower risk of age-related vision loss and cataracts. The benefit of lutein supplements on poor vision in humans is currently being studied. When taking a lutein supplement, take with food containing a healthy fat to improve its absorption.

COENZYME Q10 (also known as CoQ10) is a vitamin-like chemical whose job it is to help the mitochondria use oxygen efficiently. Reduced levels of CoQ10 leads to increased formation of free radicals. CoQ10 is synthesised in the human body with the assistance of numerous vitamins, including Vitamin C, Vitamins B2, B3, B5, B6, B12 and folic acid. Of these, Vitamin B6 has the biggest impact. One way to maintain CoQ10 levels is to have adequate intake of B vitamins.

As we get older, our ability to synthesise CoQ10 declines and we become more reliant on dietary sources of CoQ10. Foods containing the highest level of CoQ10 are those containing the highest levels of mitochondria, such as liver, kidney and heart tissue, fish and the germs of whole grains.

A number of CoQ10 supplements are now available providing significantly more CoQ10 than that obtained from food. CoQ10 supplements should be taken with meals to help absorption. Clinical trials have shown that these more selective antioxidants can reduce oxidative stress in a range of settings. In studies involving mice, CoQ10 has resulted in increased longevity. Whether this will translate into long-term benefits in humans is currently the matter of ongoing trials.

ALPHA-LIPOIC ACID is a potent antioxidant with additional actions to regenerate antioxidant defences. Foods rich in alpha-lipoic acid are potatoes, carrots, broccoli, beets and yams, as well as red meat.

In the body, alpha-lipoic acid occurs in two forms: R-lipoic acid and R-dihydro lipoic acid. R-dihydro-lipoic acid exerts a number of antioxidant and neuroprotective actions that are not seen with R-lipoic acid. In particular, R-dihydro-lipoic acid has been shown to improve mitochondrial function, reduce nerve damage in ageing and improve memory and performance. It may also reduce the formation of AGEs. When buying a supplement, look for the one that definitely contains the active component. When used as a supplement in high dose, generic alpha lipoic acid can produce side-effects, including skin rash, lowering of blood sugar and depletion of B group vitamins, especially B1.

CARNOSINE is a multifunctional antioxidant made up of beta-alanine and l-histidine. Found in meat, it is one of the most important antioxidants lacking in a vegetarian diet. Long-lived cells such as nerve cells (neurons) and muscle cells (myocytes) contain high levels of carnosine, where it functions both as a scavenger of free radicals, as well as AGEs. Carnosine also acts as an intracellular pH buffer, protecting the cell against damage under acidic conditions, such as after exercise. In animal studies, carnosine supplements delay the impairment of eyesight with ageing. Its long-term effects in human ageing are unclear, although it is widely touted as an effective anti-ageing therapy.

LYCOPENES are red pigments that are important intermediates in the synthesis of many carotenoids. Foods rich in lycopenes are red fruits such as tomatoes, watermelon, pink grapefruit, pink guava, papaya and rosehip. Unlike some compounds, cooking helps release more lycopenes from the plant fibre, so tomato paste has more lycopenes than fresh tomato (although less Vitamin C due to the processing). Invitro, lycopenes are more powerful quenchers of free radicals than Vitamin E. Diets high in lycopenes are associated with lower rates of prostate and gastrointestinal cancers, as well as a reduced risk of heart disease. Lycopene supplementation also boosts immune function and reduces systemic inflammation. The health benefits of lycopene supplements are currently being trialled in a range of clinical settings.

POLYPHENOLICS represent a range of plant chemicals including the flavonoids, which have potent antioxidant activities. They also have independent actions enhancing cell-protection mechanisms and reducing inflammation. Some of the best-known compounds from this group include the soy isoflavones, quercitin in onions, hesperidin and rutin from citrus, proanthocyanidin in grape seed extract and resveratrol. Each of these compounds, and others like them, have been shown to reduce levels of free radical damage in human studies. Supplements containing complex mixtures of bioflavonoids are now widely available and have been shown to be efficient antioxidant agents.

RESVERATROL is the most widely used polyphenolic antioxidant. It is produced in a range of plants, such as grapes, peanuts and knotweed, as part of their defence against fungal attack. Resveratrol is released from grape skin during fermentation, so red wine, which is fermented before the skin is removed, has higher levels than white wine. However, the amount obtained from red drinking wine is probably insufficient to explain the so-called French paradox (the fact that the people of southern France have low rates of heart disease, despite their high intake of fats). Higher and more consistent doses of resveratrol are available in health supplements. Most commercially available resveratrol is purified from Japanese knotweed or Hu Zhang root. In this purified form, it has proven to be a highly effective antioxidant. Apart from scavenging free radicals, resveratrol has been shown to have a number of beneficial effects on human health, including improved efficiency of energy production in mitochondria, activation of beneficial genes associated with longevity, and reduced oxidation of fats.

GREEN TEA is also high in polyphenols with antioxidant properties, including the catechin called epigallocatechin gallate (EGCG). Unlike black tea, which is oxidised before drying, green tea is made from leaves that have undergone minimal processing, so the antioxidants levels remain relatively intact. It must be noted that green tea still contains a lot of caffeine (see chapter 16). A number of studies have shown that a regular daily intake of green tea (at least three cups) is associated with reduced rates of some cancers, heart disease and cognitive decline with advancing age. Because not everyone likes the taste of green tea, or has time to drink three cups a day, extracts from green tea are available in pill form, standardised to contain 80% total polyphenols and 55% epigallocatechin gallate.

QUERCETIN is an antioxidant found in onions, apples, green tea and black tea. Smaller amounts are found in leafy green vegetables and beans. In addition to scavenging free radicals, quercitin has beneficial effects on mitochondrial function, thereby preventing radical formation. Quercetin has a range of other actions, including effects on clotting, inflammation and blood pressure. It also functions as a phytoestrogen (a plant substance with similar actions to the female sex hormone, oestrogen).

ELLAGIC ACID is a polyphenol antioxidant found in many red fruits and berries, including raspberries, strawberries, grapes, blackberries, cranberries, pomegranate and some nuts, including pecans and walnuts. Ellagic acid is effective at binding and quenching free radicals and preventing the consequences of oxidative stress in experimental models. It is also able to bind and neutralise a number of potent carcinogens and other harmful chemicals. In some trials, pomegranate juice, which is high in ellagic acid as well as other flavanoids, has shown some positive benefits on blood pressure and vascular function. Diets high in red fruits have been historically associated with lower rates of cancer and heart disease, although the role of ellagic acid in this benefit remains to be established.

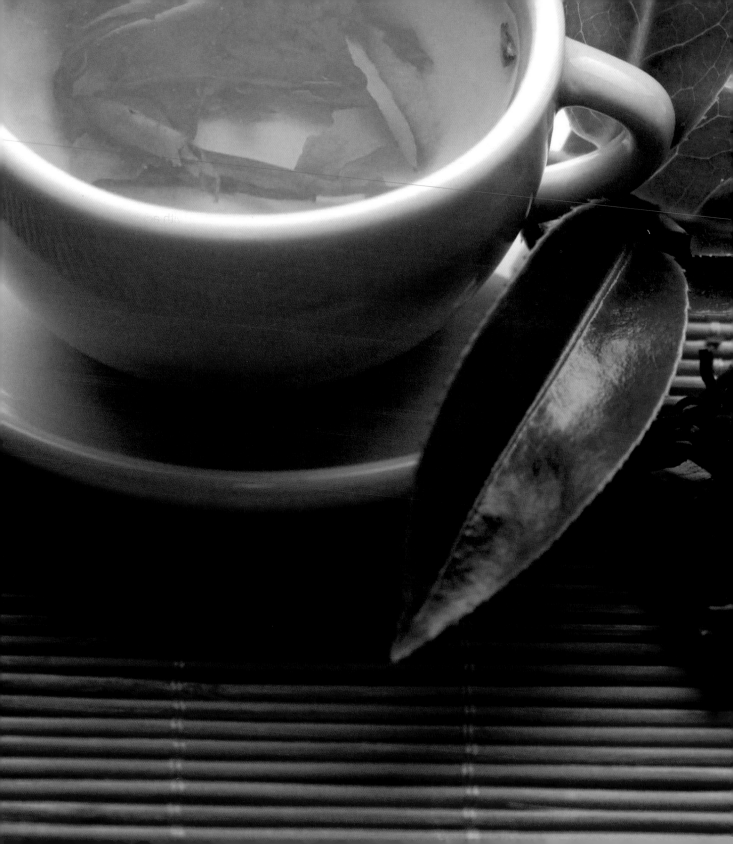

Sulphoraphane is an isothiocyanate antioxidant that is found in broccoli and other plants of the cabbage family. The highest levels are seen in broccoli and cauliflower sprouts (as opposed to the adult plants). In experimental studies, sulphoraphane has been shown to reduce oxidative stress, as well as prevent some cancers. It also stimulates the functions of the body's detoxification enzymes and may also be beneficial in treating the bacteria that causes stomach ulcers.

Indole-3-carbinol (I-3-C) is another antioxidant found in cruciferous vegetables (the cabbage family). I-3-C is released whenever these vegetables are crushed or cooked. I-3-C and diindolemethane (DIM), produced when I-3-C is digested, are widely available as supplements. In experimental studies, I-3-C has been shown to reduce oxidative stress, as well as slow the growth of some cancers. Sulphoraphane and I-3-C (along with other glucosinolates and isothiocyanates) associated with the consumption of cruciferous vegetables may contribute to lowered risk of prostate, cervical and breast cancer. It should also be noted that I-3-C is also able to modify levels of sex hormones, including oestrogens, which may contribute to both their anti-cancer activity and some of their side-effects.

LUTEOLIN is a plant flavonoid found in herbs and vegetables, including parsley, olive oil, basil, peppermint, capsicum, rosemary and celery. Luteolin is one of the more potent dietary flavonoids in preventing oxidative damage. Luteolin also has a range of effects beyond those of a simple antioxidant, including effects on clotting, inflammation and cancer growth.

Olive juice contains a rich mixture of antioxidant polyphenols, including the major olive oil antioxidant, hydroxytyrosol. Extra virgin olive oil contains more polyphenols than other olive oils, but concentrated olive polyphenols are also available as olive juice extracts. Previously discarded as a by-product of the process of extracting olive oil, olive polyphenols have a number of potential health benefits over and above their antioxidant activity.

Another food that is high in polyphenol flavonols is cocoa and dark chocolate (not milk chocolate or white chocolate, or those bars with caramel in the middle). These flavonols have been widely studied in a range of clinical settings. In general, these studies have demonstrated that chocolate flavanols are able to improve blood vessel function, reduce blood pressure and lower cholesterol - factors associated with slow ageing and improved longevity.

The extract of the Ginkgo leaves also contains a number of polyphenol flavonoids and other chemicals with antioxidant properties. Ginkgo leaf extracts are among the leading prescription medicines in both Germany and France. Apart from its antioxidant effect, Ginkgo has been shown to prevent clotting and improve regional blood flow, particularly in the brain and the heart, as well as the peripheries, where it helps cold hands and feet. Ginkgo also improves blood flow to the penis and can thus help to maintain erections. It is widely purported to have beneficial effects on memory and concentration, both in healthy subjects and those with cognitive decline. A number of supplements containing Ginkgo are available. Ideally look for a 'standardised extract' with 24% 'ginkgo flavonglycosides' as this is the form that has been tested in studies.

DIETARY ANTIOXIDANTS

Apart from taking pills or other supplements, a number of foods are naturally rich in antioxidants. These are discussed in detail in chapter 17. Those who have high levels of antioxidants in their diet also have better health outcomes. There a number of simple things we can do to make sure we are one of them.

OPTIONS FOR INCREASING YOUR INTAKE OF ANTIOXIDANTS

☑ Follow the rainbow to get important antioxidants via your food. For details on the actual actions of the following phytonutrients, go to chapter 18)
> Orange and deep yellow = beta-carotene. Try carrots and apricots, cataloupe, grapefruit, oranges, mangoes, papaya, pineapple, peaches, bananas, butternut squash and yellow peppers
> Red and pink = lycopenes and ellagic acid. Try raspberries, red grapes, blueberries, tomatoes, guava, apricots, watermelon, papaya and pink grapefruit
> Dark green = lutein and zeaxanthin. Try spinach, silverbeet, romaine lettuce, broccoli, zucchini, corn, green peas and Brussels sprouts
> Purple, dark red and blue = flavonoids. Flavonoids are the most abundant and powerful of all the phytochemicals contained in the foods we eat. Try blackberries, blueberries, dried plums/prunes, raisins, purple cabbage, eggplant and purple potatoes

OPTIONS FOR INCREASING YOUR INTAKE OF ANTIOXIDANTS

☑ Increase your intake of fresh fruit
  > Slice fresh fruit over porridge
  > Make delicious fruit-based desserts, such as fruit crumble with apple and rhubarb, baked apples or poached seasonal fruit such as pears or stone fruit
  > Dice fresh fruit and take to work as a quick convenient snack rather than eating a muesli bar
  > Make a delicious fresh fruit platter for breakfast, a snack or for dessert
  > Dice fresh fruit and keep in a container in the fridge so it is a quick convenient snack - this works well with fresh melon
  > Have a smoothie if you are on the run and tend to miss breakfast

☑ Increase your intake of vegetables
  > Serve chopped fresh vegetables with salsa or hummus for a healthy snack
  > Have vegetables at breakfast - add mushrooms, asparagus and tomatoes to omelettes
  > Ask for extra salad in a sandwich or roll for lunch or take a big fresh salad in a container to work for lunch
  > Grate vegetables into pasta sauces
  > Get a V-slicer and make interesting salads with zucchini and fennel
  > Get a juicer and if on the run make a vege juice. Combinations of carrot, apple, celery, beetroot and parsley are delicious and packed with antioxidants

☑ Eat raw or cook veges until 'just crisp and tender' to retain nutrients
  > Stir-fry, water fry or steam your vegetables instead of boiling in water or microwaving
  > Add fresh herbs at the last minute and stir through to retain the high antioxidant levels
  > Eat carrot, celery or capsicum sticks as snacks. Have with fresh yoghurt dip for extra taste

OPTIONS FOR INCREASING YOUR INTAKE OF ANTIOXIDANTS

☑ Eat fresh, whole food that retain their natural antioxidants
> Plant a vege garden. If you are in an apartment then plant one in a pot
> Check out your local farmer's market and shop there on the weekend
> Avoid anything in a sealed packet or tin
> Shop online and so avoid impulse purchases at the supermarket

☑ Increase your intake of herbs
> Buy parsley, chives, coriander, sage and thyme and other salad herbs and keep in a sealed container for daily use in salads, soups, curries and casseroles
> Plant some basil so you can easily make your own quick pesto sauce – blend pine nuts, garlic, basil and olive oil
> Reduce your intake of coffee and soft drinks and increase the intake of herbal teas such as lemongrass, camomile, or peppermint
> Try new salads that are predominately made from herbs such as tabbouli (parsley). Also Sabzi or herb salad is made from fresh spinach, rocket, celery, mint, parsley, basil, dill, spring onions, olive oil and lemon juice

☑ Increase your intake of spices
> Toss turmeric with fish or rice with steamed veges
> Have a curry meal once per week
> Stew apples, rhubarb or pears with cinnamon sticks and cloves; serve with yoghurt for a delicious dessert or breakfast
> Substitute your coffee for a chai latte
> Add chilli flakes to your spaghetti sauce
> Add turmeric to taste to scrambled eggs
> Sprinkle cinnamon on your porridge

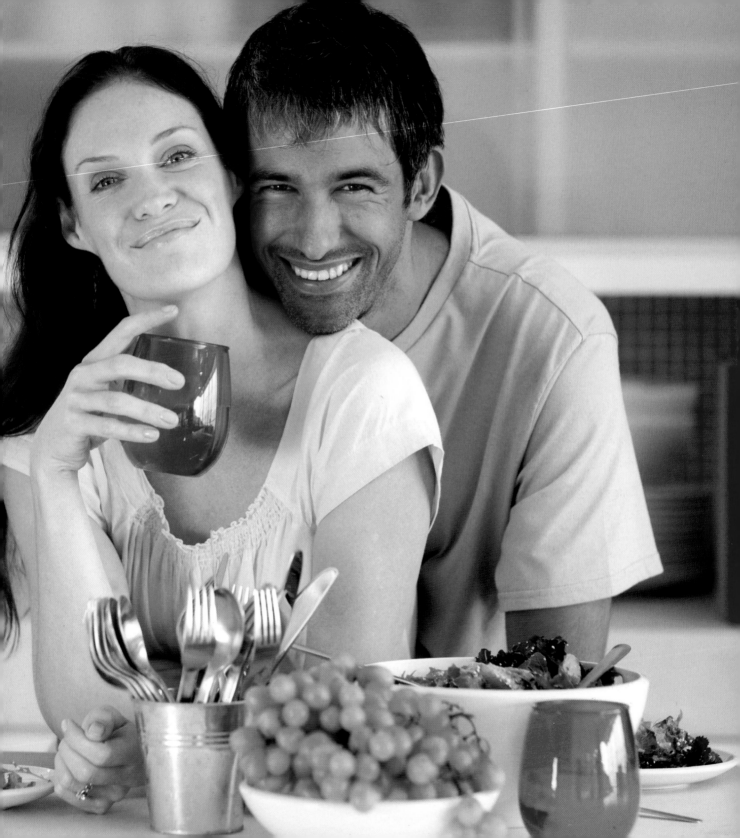

CHAPTER 09

THE ELEMENTS OF AGEING
[CALORIES]

The biggest health challenge we face as we get older is not so much cancer, heart attack or diabetes, but its direct antecedent - the accumulation of fat in our tissues. Obesity is responsible for up to 70% of chronic disease and is a major contributor to age-related decline. Despite this, at least every second adult will become obese in their lifetime. The main reason for this crisis is the combination of overeating and inactivity - an imbalance that tips the scales until overall health is compromised. In this chapter, we look at our exposure to one of the most important elements of ageing: the calories we eat.

THE CRISIS OF CALORIES

Food provides the body with energy in the form of calories. Some of this energy is used in metabolism. Any calories consumed that exceed our requirements are stored as fat. It is not only the fat we eat that is stored as fat, but also the excess energy from too much sugar and protein. If calories in whatever form exceed our needs, fat storage swells, particularly under the skin, and in the buttocks and breasts (peripheral fat). If this excess continues, our body creates additional storage capacity, particularly around the internal organs (visceral fat). Unlike peripheral fat, visceral fat is less efficient and far more dangerous to have around the waistline.

This is because fat cells are not simply lifeless lumps of lard, but dynamic regulators of health and well-being. All fat, but especially visceral fat, can cause a release of chemical factors that interfere with metabolism, the immune system and many other functions. Fat deposits can also have a direct physical effect. For example, fat around the organs can squeeze them, reducing their blood supply and raising our internal (core) temperature. Fat in the lining of our blood vessels can also serve to clog up, and ultimately block, the flow of blood.

Our fat deposits are neither the only consequence, nor the only part of the body, to be affected by overeating. In most cells, increased energy supply means faster growth and a shortening of the time between cell divisions (because it takes less time to build up the stores required to turn one cell into two). Since age is measured at the cellular level by the number of times a cell has divided, ageing is faster when calories are in excess. Conversely, when the intake of calories is limited, the time between cell divisions becomes longer, so when compared to the calendar, ageing appears to slow.

A SPOON LESS OF SUGAR KEEPS THE MEDICINES AWAY

Most Western diets contain more calories than required for our metabolism and daily energy expenditure. Consequently, if we eat fewer calories than we do now, while maintaining our supply of essential nutrients, we will improve many health-related indices in addition to our waistlines. In studies performed with animals, restricting calories eaten not only reduced the impact of ageing, it also significantly increased lifespan. But is this the same for humans?

IT IS NOT ONLY THE FAT WE EAT THAT IS STORED AS FAT BUT ALSO THE EXCESS ENERGY FROM TOO MUCH SUGAR AND PROTEIN.

We know that restricting energy intake is one way to reduce our visceral fat. And less fat means obesity-associated risks of heart disease, diabetes and cancer. Even non-obese people who limit the amount they eat show reduced body fat, beneficial changes in their metabolism and reduced risk factors for ageing and disease. However, reducing calorie intake on its own can reduce muscle mass and bone strength. Libido and energy levels may also decline in lean individuals. The balance of health benefits and risks is intrinsically different for different health and ageing outcomes. It is also different for each individual. While there is no 'one size fits all' approach, most of us consume far too many calories and get rounder as we get older. Consequently, almost any reduction in the amount we eat is a step toward a better balance.

SLOW SOLUTIONS FOR WEIGHT CONTROL

The most important way we can improve our chances of a healthy and long life is to achieve and maintain a healthy weight. If there was no obesity, our average life expectancy would increase by 10 to 20 years across the board, and our quality of life would improve substantially. Alongside an increase in our physical activity, there is a fundamental need to reduce our energy intake as we get older. But how can we fight weight gain as we age?

The average annual weight gain for most adults is equivalent to two bites of food every day. Consequently, a lifestyle that incorporates even a small change in consumption can ensure better outcomes in the years to come. Moreover, we can do it today.

It doesn't require a drastic change or a new fad. The best way to successfully combat over-eating is to take slow steps so they can become habit-forming and part of our lifestyle. If done regularly, it doesn't take much to cumulatively make a real difference. Following are seven simple steps to a healthier diet and consequently weight loss and maintenance:

1. ENGAGEMENT IN OUR DIET

We have a choice! There are many opportunities to exercise it and control our calorie intake. Instead of passively filling our trolleys, or our plates, the trick is to pay attention, engaging with our dietary choices. We can start to subtract calories by making small changes in our daily eating patterns.

One of the easiest ways to tip the scales is passive over-consumption. As consumers, we are attracted to energy-dense foods, typically those that are dry (e.g. chips, biscuits, confectionery and cereals) or high in fat or sugar. These foods often provide an appetising meal that can be quickly prepared (because heat transfer is quicker in the absence of water).

But if we aren't counting these calories, our waists certainly are! We can simply reduce our calorie intake by substituting foods that are less energy-dense (measured as kJ/g). Less energy-dense foods are usually low in fat and rich in water, such as fresh fruit and vegetables, as water provides weight and volume to food, but no calories. These foods often also have a low Glycemic Index (GI) on their label. Foods with a low energy density are still satisfying, yet they add less to our waistlines.

PAY ATTENTION, ADOPT A DIET

There are many 'diet' options out there, many more in total than the pages of this book! There is no shortage of people or books providing short-term dietary advice. One way to keep our weight under control is to follow a diet. It probably doesn't matter which one. Following any diet is a very useful way to focus our attention on what we are eating. The mere process of embracing any dietary limitations, thinking about and coordinating the foods we eat means we tend to consume less calories and eat better. In essence, if adopting a diet means we pay attention to what we eat and reduce our calorie intake, it will be successful.

How the composition of a diet affects weight control is controversial, and probably not as important as the fact that we have embraced it. Reducing or increasingour intake of fat, protein or carbohydrates will not lead to weight loss unless total calories are also reduced (and exceeded by our energy expenditure). Dieting is not the only way to pay attention to what we eat, but let's face it, some people need to be told what to do! The principle of weight control based on meal replacements is even easier, because if we eat their meals instead of our own, we eat fewer calories.

This is a temporary solution for many, but on its own it is not a slow solution because control is given over to others. And what happens when we stop?

PAY ATTENTION TO THE PORTIONS WE EAT

Even if we never change what we eat, or never follow a diet, it is still possible to lose weight by simply reducing the amount we eat. One simple rule is 'one on four'. For every four spoons of cereal we would consume, leave one behind. For every four potatoes we would eat, leave one behind. On its own, this technique can be challenging, as smaller portions can leave us feeling hungry and unsatisfied. The combination of reduced portion sizes and eating more filling (less energy-dense) foods is therefore better than either option alone.

PAY ATTENTION TO HOW OFTEN WE EAT

The more often we eat, the greater the chance we will take in calories in excess of our requirements. For most people, every calorie consumed outside of meal times is probably unnecessary. So find and fight the cues to snack. Skipping meals, like breakfast, is not a practical solution for weight control. Eating a regular breakfast helps control weight, especially when it includes whole-grain cereals. Put simply, breakfast gets us going and makes us feel nourished and satisfied, and less likely to overeat during the rest of the day. Missing breakfast means we have less energy and makes us more likely to crave snacks or larger portions at other meals.

THE BEST WAY TO SUCCESSFULLY COMBAT OVER-EATING IS TO TAKE SLOW STEPS SO THEY CAN BECOME HABIT-FORMING AND PART OF OUR LIFESTYLE

PAY ATTENTION TO THE CUES THAT MAKE US EAT

It is possible to change our environment to support weight management, just as it is possible to make things more difficult by leaving that packet of biscuits within arm's reach. We need to pay attention to what makes us eat and keep eating. As a start to noticing what you are eating, try keeping a 'diet diary'. Write down everything you eat and drink for a week.

Be honest. What caused you to eat? Was it walking past the bakery? The best way to avoid the apple, Adam, is to not sit under the tree. Was it because your plate was not yet empty? Try using smaller plates and bowls. Do we snack because we are depressed, strung-out or filled with other negative emotions? Are we looking to food for comfort? Sure it works, but only for a moment. What is important is to deal with the stress, not beat ourselves up over our diet.

2. PLANNING AND TARGETING CLEAR AND REALISTIC GOALS

There is no achieving the waifish standards of supermodels. Who would want to? They are no happier than the rest of us, nor healthier by all accounts. Successful weight control often comes when our expectations align with our goals. There is no value in a quick fix. It is best to initially aim for small, achievable targets. For those who are overweight, this might be 5% to10% of their current weight. But don't stop there, set a new target and begin again. Having a relevant target hardens our resolve and focuses our attention. It is more effective than just wanting to be thinner.

3. DIETING IS A POSITIVE EXPERIENCE

Dieting is not a punitive exercise, a punishment for the nutritionally wicked. If we take this view, we are doomed to failure. Success comes from the desire and momentum to keep new habits in place for a lifetime. Weight management can become a fun and conscious part of our lifestyle choices, because we are in control. When we shop, when we cook, when we consume, it is possible to have fun without excess calories. Finding these new experiences can be equally stimulating. Small changes on a daily basis can bring big results. The solutions that work should be incorporated into our life, not partitioned like a criminal record.

It is still possible to be satisfied by eating less. Our body tells us when we have had enough for one meal. When the intestines are distended, they send a message back to the brain indicating satiety. So eating foods that are high in volume, but low in calories, is a simple way to have satisfying meals and also reduce overeating. This can be readily achieved by substituting foods that have a high content of water or insoluble fibre, and avoiding those that are calorie-dense.

DIETING IS NOT A PUNITIVE EXERCISE, A PUNISHMENT FOR THE NUTRITIONALLY WICKED. IF WE TAKE THIS VIEW WE ARE DOOMED TO FAILURE.

4. SLOW SOLUTIONS ARE FOR THE LONG-TERM

Without noticing, excess can become a way of life. Old habits are hard to break once established, especially when they taste so good! Only later, when behaviours have become entrenched and their consequences are apparent, do we recognise the problem. But in the same way, good habits accumulate significant benefits in the long-term. All fads should be rejected, because our weight will return as soon as the enthusiasm fades. Find an approach that is sustainable and can be made a part of the person we already are. We don't need to become someone else to control our weight. The sooner and longer we keep our fat stores under control, the longer our survival. Waiting until we get fat before doing anything about our diets is not a smart option. Once we gain weight, the body resets its systems, so our attempts to reduce food intake by dieting are usually met by symptoms of hunger, even though there may be a billion calories still stored away in our fat.

This is because the large body thinks it needs a large amount of food, in the same way that big bears should appropriately have big bowls. As overweight adults, even if we can temporarily achieve weight loss, our brain and fat continue to signal their desire to get fat again. And so the vicious cycle of overeating continues. This is why the best way to deal with weight gain is to start before we get fat.

5. EXCLUSIVENESS SHOULD BE AVOIDED

One diet or one practice may have temporary benefits, but for weight control to be sustained, we need to combine diet with other interventions. Anyone who loses weight knows that without engaging in exercise, for example, any loss is quickly regained.

6. DON'T GO IT ALONE

Weight control is not easy at the best of times. It can be even harder on our own. There are many providers out there who offer advice and support. The most successful weight care programs involve a strong relationship and long-term interaction between provider and consumer, whether they are a dietitian, trainer, motivator or simply our friends and family.

7. THE GOLDILOCKS PRINCIPLE OF INDIVIDUAL

One of the keys to successful weight control is finding a plan that we like, and can adhere to, in the long-term. Many will not work, while others seem too costly or difficult. Like Goldilocks, it is important to try a number of different bowls and to find the one that best suits our individual needs. The correct bowl size for papa bear, mama bear and baby bear are different, reflecting their different body composition, daily energy expenditure and other metabolic needs. Our energy demands also depend on our genes, ethnic background and age.

IN THE END (AND OTHER PLACES)

There are many ways to slow ageing, some of which are contained in this book. But if we could reduce our exposure to only one thing, that element would be calories. If there was no obesity our average life expectancy would probably increase by 10-20 years across the board, and quality of life also improve substantially. In the end, we have are two basic options, reduce the number of calories we take and increase our physical activity, or get fat and die. To be successful slow steps, taken repeatedly and incorporated into daily activity can make real and quantifiable differences to our heath and prospects in our old age. It doesn't mean changing who we are. We can exert control over our diets and stop being a passenger in our own environment.

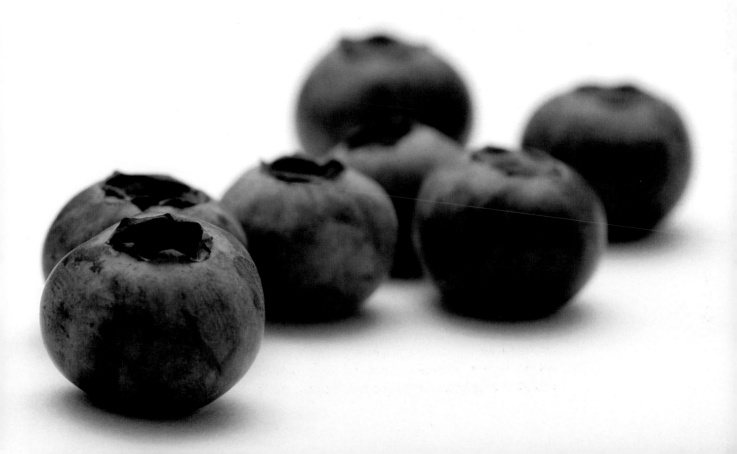

OPTIONS TO KEEP YOUR CALORIES UNDER CONTROL

☑ Pay attention to your eating patterns (WHEN, WHERE, WHAT AND WHY you eat)

☑ Keep a food diary to see what, when, where and why you eat

☑ Reduce size and number of portions:
> Put your fruit and nuts in small containers so you don't eat the whole bag
> Divide big bags of food into smaller bags
> Put leftovers in the fridge before you sit for dinner (so you don't go back for seconds)
> Buy smaller packet sizes at the supermarket
> Freeze extra food if portions are too large

☑ Have 3 dessert free evenings each week

☑ Eat fruit or a small handful of nuts for dessert
> Try interesting combinations – chopped mango and pineapple, blanched and sliced peaches or nectarines drizzled with Galliano then served with a good yoghurt, pears stewed in apple juice and cloves and cinnamon sticks and stewed rhubarb with strawberries

☑ Create a list of healthy snacks
> Fruit salad
> Vegetable sticks with preservative-free dip such as hummus, tsatsiki or baba ganoush
> Soy or rice milk smoothie with fresh fruit and natural yoghurt
> Tub of natural yoghurt with fresh fruit
> Half a handful of untoasted, unsalted nuts or seeds

☑ Address non-hungry eating – make sure you are not bored at night, think about something to do at night when at danger of eating

☑ Plan your weekly meals and only buy what you need

☑ Eliminate impulse shopping by taking a list with you

☑ Don't shop when hungry!

OPTIONS TO KEEP YOUR CALORIES UNDER CONTROL

☑ Reduce processed foods and those with added sugar

☑ Avoid the middle isles of the supermarket. The outer isles mostly contain fresh and unprocessed produce

☑ Eat foods that are:
> less energy dense (measured as kJ/g)
> low in saturated fat (but not high in carbs)
> have a low glycaemic index (low GI)
> served in smaller portions on smaller plates

☑ Stick with a diet. The process of embracing any dietary restrictions, thinking about and coordinating the foods you eat means you'll eat less (calories)

☑ Measure your waist circumference with a tape-measure:

Find the mid-point between your bottom rib and the top of your hip bone. Breathe out normally and measure your circumference with a tape measure across this point. This may not be the narrowest part of your waist or exactly in-line with your belly button. This risk of many health problems increases in proportion to your waistline

For men:
> 94 cm (37 inches) or more = increased risk
> 102 cm (40 inches) or more = substantially increased risk

For women:
> 80 cm (32 inches) or more = increased risk
> 88 cm (35 inches) or more = substantially increased risk

☑ Deal with other contributors to over eating (stress, bad habits, inattention)

☑ Make an appointment to see your doctor or weight management consultant

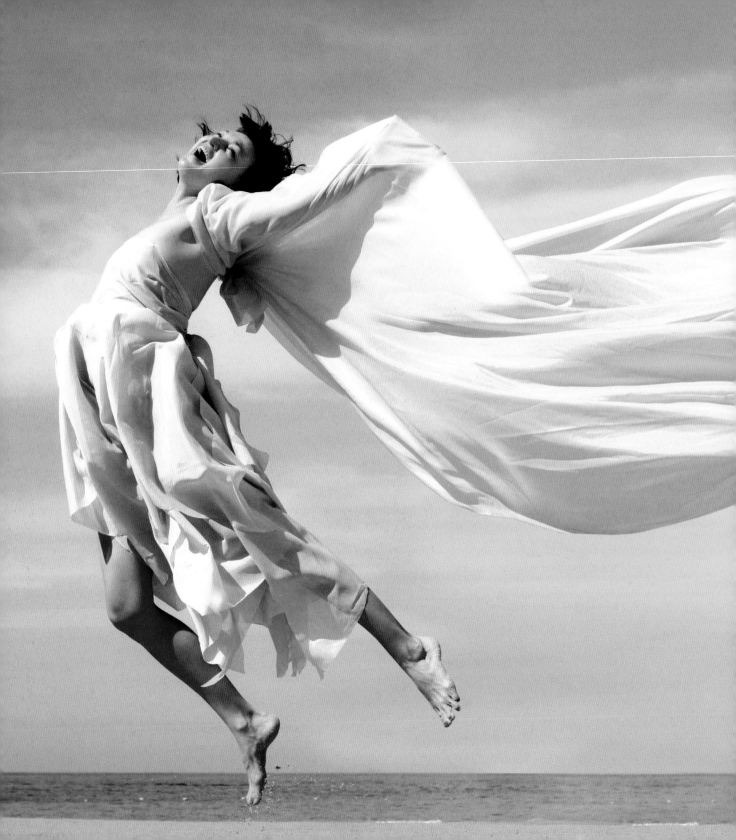

CHAPTER 10
THE ELEMENTS
OF AGEING [AGEs]

We are all made of sugar, protein and fat. What makes the recipe work is the combination of ingredients in the right amounts obtained from the right sources. These components interact in a magical, complex chemistry that contributes colour, texture and aroma to our lives. This chemistry is also an element of ageing.

SLOWLY TURNING BROWN

One of the most important interactions is browning, the reaction between sugars and protein that occurs during prolonged or high temperature cooking and fermentation. The brown hue of beer, the hard crust of bread and the stickiness of caramel result from the combination of sugars and proteins during processing. The curing and burning of tobacco also involves this chemistry. Cooking slowly away at 37°C, the same chemistry is also possible inside all of us, making us crusty!

Inside the body, the longer a protein lives, the greater the chance it will meet a sugar and become modified by it. The chemical products of these reactions are known as AGEs (Advanced Glycation End products) and they can be used as a marker of ageing. However, AGEs are more than just markers of the passage of time. In this chapter, we look at the ways that AGEs are a key element of the ageing process.

THE IMPACT OF AGEs

Over a lifetime of cooking, the amount and variety of AGE-modified tissue progressively increases. High sugar levels, elevated fats and increased oxidative stress all act to hasten the formation of AGEs, and with it the ageing process. These AGE-modifications interfere with the functions of anything they stick to. AGE-modification can also lead to the formation of cross-links that reduce the flexibility of structures, tying and fixing molecules in certain shapes. This is another reason why our blood vessels become stiff with age.

The human body has many devices to cope with ageing. One is the ability to identify those parts that are old and replace them with new. But how do you tell an old protein from one you made yesterday? On a tree, how do you spot an old leaf? Of course, it's the brown one that is likely to be older. Likewise in the human body - browning is one way to tell how long each part has been around and when its time is up.

Sensing the type and quantity of AGE-modification is the job of the AGE-receptors. Over recent years, a number of AGE-receptors have been identified. Some of these are (good) receptors, whose job it is to remove AGEs from the body. Other (bad) receptors are activated by AGEs, triggering a cascade of pathways that lead to ageing and disease. The best known of these is appropriately known as RAGE (Receptor for Advanced Glycation End-products). Atherosclerosis, cancer, Alzheimer's and diabetes are all influenced by activation of RAGE.

> HIGH SUGAR LEVELS, ELEVATED FATS AND INCREASED OXIDATIVE STRESS ALL ACT TO HASTEN THE AGEING PROCESS.

HOW DO I SLOW AGE?

The browning of proteins by sugars is not the only element that leads to ageing. But it is one that we can do something about. Preventing diabetes is the most straightforward way (see chapter 6). A number of widely available supplements have also been shown to reduce the accumulation of AGEs. Most antioxidants (see chapter 8) have significant AGE-inhibitory activity. However, some have important additional effects.

Thiamine (Vitamin B1) can reduce the AGE generation inside the body. Diets high in fibre often contain useful amounts of thiamine. Our thiamine reserves can be deleted by chronic alcohol consumption, which is best avoided on many fronts. The best way to get thiamine is to take special forms that have improved absorption properties. These are naturally found in garlic and onions. Botanically, these plants are of the allum family. These chemicals are called allithiamines, the best studied of which is benfotiamine.

Pyridoxamine (a derivative of Vitamin B6) is able to reduce the formation of AGEs, particularly those derived from fats. Pyridoxamine is safe and well tolerated as a supplement, and has been shown to be effective in reducing AGE levels and in preventing some of the complications of ageing and diabetes in animals.

Rytine, a natural flavonoid found in high concentration in tomato juice, has the ability to inhibit AGE formation.

Carnosine (an antioxidant from meat, typically lacking in a vegetarian diets) inhibits AGE formation and prevents protein modification by acting as a scavenger.

Alpha-lipoic acid (highest in foods such as potatoes, carrots, broccoli, beets and yams) can prevent AGE-modification.

REDUCING YOUR INTAKE OF AGEs

Another way to limit our burden of AGEs is to prevent any unnecessary intake. Many of the foods we eat contain AGEs. This has a number of consequences, both positive and negative. For example, browning produces flavours, textures and aromas that give many foods their appeal. Incorporating AGEs into foods and their processing helps boost flavour. For example, the crunch of crisps is conveyed by cooking at very high temperature and low humidity. Equally, the delicious smell and taste of pork crackling comes from cooking fat at high heat. Sure the chips taste better, not to mention that extra crunch, but at what cost?

There is a strong relationship between the levels of AGEs in our blood and the amount of AGEs consumed in our diets. Essentially, eating AGE-modified food means we gain some of these AGE modifications. It could be said that you are only as old as what you eat. A number of studies have shown a relationship between high dietary intake of AGEs and development of age-related problems. It is possible to significantly lengthen the lives of mice by restricting the amount of AGEs they eat, even if they are allowed to eat as much and as often as they like. So if we were mice, there would be two good options to slow ageing: eat significantly less processed food, or eat as much fresh, unprocessed food as you like. This approach may not be far off the mark for humans either.

OPTIONS TO REDUCE AGEs

☑ Eat fresh and unprocessed foods - these always have the lowest levels of AGEs

☑ Eat more raw vegetables

☑ Eat foods low in fat, especially for cooking
  > Use ricotta instead of yellow cheese
  > Use yoghurt as a cream or sour cream substitute
  > Choose low fat coconut milk instead of coconut cream
  > Choose trim cuts of meat and remove the skin from poultry
  > Cook with a grill instead of frying or baking to reduce retained animal fat

☑ Cooking on a low heat (<250C) over long periods of time and in the presence of excess humidity (boiling, poaching, stewing, steaming, or using a slow cooker)

☑ Marinate or use garlic and spices to flavour food rather than browning meat

☑ Eat foods naturally high in antioxidants, especially garlic, onions, tomatoes, broccoli, beets and yams

☑ Moderate your drinking habits
  > Have 3 alcohol-free days per week
  > Substitute bitters lime and soda for every second drink
  > Drink water after each alcoholic beverage

☑ Avoid foods rich in fat particularly trans and saturated fats
  > Read food labels to check for trans fat content (there should be none!)
  > Check the fat content of processed foods
  > Choose low fat options

OPTIONS TO REDUCE AGEs

☑ Choose a low GI diet
> Buy a small reference book with a list of foods with their Glycemic Index so you can more easily choose low over high GI foods
> Check out the official GI website: www.glycemicindex.com
> Avoid 'white' food – high GI foods are typically pasta, potatoes, white sugar and rice
> Eat more beans and legumes
> Have a daily serve of nuts
> Eat a predominately fruit and vegetable-based diet
> Eat lots of whole grains – choose brown rice over white, wholemeal bread or bread made using whole grains over white bread, whole wheat products over refined wheat foods
> Avoid bottled dressings
> If you eat high GI foods, then combine with low GI foods. For example, eat jasmine rice with dhal (lentils)
> Use vinegar as a vinaigrette as this will lower the GI of foods

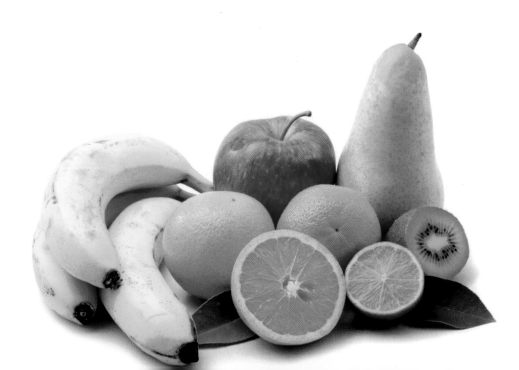

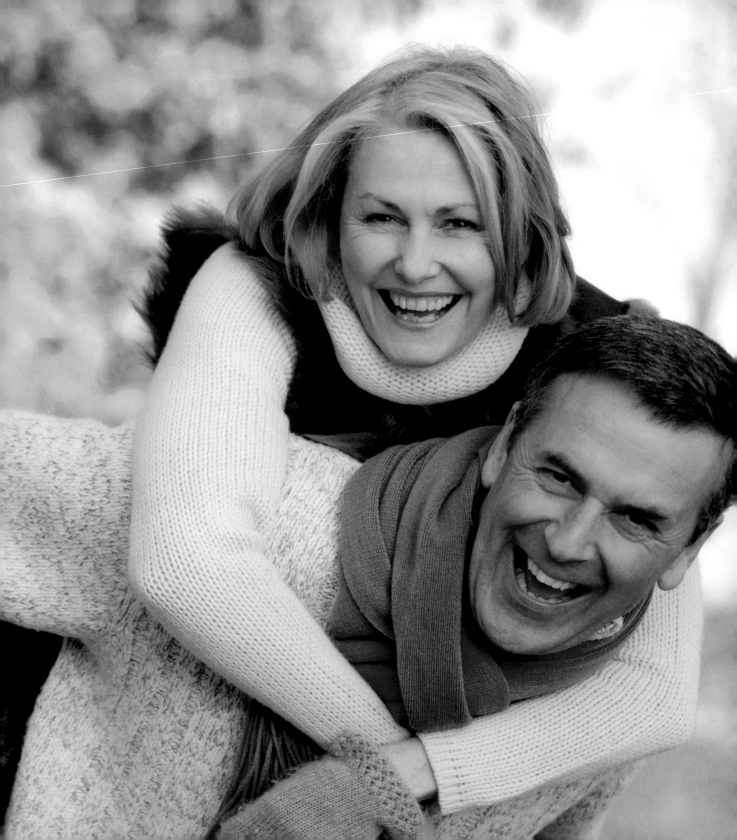

CHAPTER 11

THE ELEMENTS OF AGEING
[INFLAMMATION]

Our bodies have many defence and healing mechanisms. They are designed to quickly turn on when confronted by something harmful, like toxins, trauma or infection. An example of this kind of defence system is inflammation. We all need inflammation at certain times to fight infection or heal wounds. However, left unchecked, inflammation can lead to collateral damage and disease. Ageing is associated with a number of changes in the immune defence system, cumulatively known as 'inflamm-ageing'. More than simply being a marker of harmful processes going on, unfettered inflammation is a significant element of ageing. For example, chronic inflammation can accelerate bone density and cognitive function, as well as destabilise the lining of blood vessels, contributing to heart attacks and strokes. In this chapter, we look at changes in the immune defence system in the ageing body, and some of the ways these pathways can be manipulated to our advantage.

The immune system has many specialised units that work in concert to win our battles. These can be broadly divided into two arms: the innate and adaptive immune systems. The innate system provides an immediate, aggressive but generic response when it recognises anything harmful going on. It is composed of both cells and chemical components, which trigger inflammation. By contrast, the adaptive immune response reacts more slowly, is tailored to specific invaders, and is triggered by specific recognition molecules, the best known being antibodies. This response is utilised in vaccinations, which adapt our immune system to better defend against specific invaders. Both innate and adaptive systems continuously talk to each other to form a defence strategy and ensure a speedy recovery. As we get older, regulation of the innate immune system can become dysfunctional, resulting in chronic low-grade inflammation. At the same time, there is a steady decline in adaptive immunity (known as immuno-senescence). This sees decreased response to vaccines and increased risk from infections, cancer and other diseases.

HOW DOES INFLAMMATION CAUSE DAMAGE?

Although designed to be protective, inflammation in the wrong place and at the wrong time can be destructive to tissues and have a number of adverse effects on human health. A simple example of this is the process of scarring. Scars are the result of inflammatory signals that remodel tissues to wall off damaged areas. While this is helpful to hold our wounds together, scar tissue is not the same as the tissue it replaces and usually results in some compromise of function. For example, excessive scarring in the lungs, blood vessels or heart leaves each of them stiff and dysfunctional.

Inflammation is also a major producer of free radicals (see chapter 8) which are used by the immune system to kill off invading bacteria or get rid of damaged cells. However, free radical damage is rather indiscriminant and results in collateral damage if left firing away. Although the damage may initially be small, if continued it can accumulate and eventually wear us down. For example, cancer is more common in areas of chronic inflammation due to cumulative DNA damage, particularly if the adaptive immunity that keeps cancers in check is also in decline.

Inflammation can also perpetuate disease processes, including heart disease, diabetes, Alzheimer's disease, arthritis, osteoporosis and some cancers, which share a common inflammatory component. For example, in Alzheimer's disease, accumulating brain damage triggers inflammation, which perpetuates further injury. Inflammation is also central to atherosclerosis, the process that ultimately leads to heart attacks and strokes (see chapter 5). Because inflammation is a generic process, anything that enhances it will affect a range of conditions. Essentially, anything that fuels the fire will make the flame burn stronger.

While local inflammation can lead to local problems, its effects can also be widespread, affecting other tissues, even if they are not damaged themselves. This occurs due to the release of inflammatory cytokines, signalling molecules which not only trigger inflammation, but also communicate their effects to all corners of the body. For example, cytokines released by over-stuffed fat cells can render distant cells resistant to the effects of insulin, contributing to impaired glucose tolerance and diabetes (see chapter 6). In the same way, joint inflammation may increase the risk of heart disease and stroke via the cytokines that are released. Depression also appears to be partly triggered by inflammatory cytokines, which is why we feel low when we are sick with the flu. Inflammatory signals can also be directly damaging. For example, some circulating cytokines actually kill the nerve cells of the brain, potentially contributing to the development of cognitive decline with ageing (which is exaggerated in those with chronic inflammation).

BEATING YOURSELF UP (AUTO-IMMUNITY AND AGEING)

We are exposed to a range of foreign substances every day. Some of these are potentially harmful and are therefore rapidly identified and removed by our immune defence systems. At the same time, we don't dispose of our own tissues, which we identify as belonging to us (a good guard dog does not bite its own master, just the burglars). One of the many effects of immuno-senscence and inflamm-ageing is that this system of self-tolerance is slowly eroded. Instead of only reacting against toxic invaders like bacteria, the immune response in ageing individuals sometimes turns on itself, so we essentially beat ourselves up. A number of diseases associated with ageing are examples of this loss of self-tolerance, including rheumatoid arthritis, Sjogren's syndrome, lupus, pulmonary fibrosis, the antiphospholipid syndrome and thyroiditis.

MEASURING INFLAMMATION

There are a number of tests available to identify individuals with chronic inflammation:

We can measure levels of proteins released by the liver into the circulation in response to inflammatory signals (known as acute-phase proteins). The best known of these are C-reactive protein (CRP), fibrinogen, soluble intercellular adhesion molecule-1, soluble CD40 ligand, neopterin and serum amyloid A. In general, high levels of proteins in the bloodstream are associated with the development of disease and disability with age. For example, individuals with CRP concentrations greater than 3.0 mg/L are more likely to go on to have a heart attack or develop dementia or some cancers than those with a level below 1.0 mg/L (low risk).

It is possible to measure circulating levels of cytokines, the chemical messages that trigger inflammation. For example, interleukin-6 (IL-6) and tumour necrosis factor-alpha (TNF-alpha) are elevated in elderly individuals.

During our lives, we are all exposed to viruses that remain dormant within us, held in check by immune defences. Testing the integrity of these defences enables us to tell how well they are doing their job. For example, signs that cytomegalovirus (CMV) is active in our body (as demonstrated by elevated levels of anti-CMV antibodies) is associated with reduced immune function.

Finally, it is possible to measure levels of circulating inflammatory cells. Elevated levels of white cells in circulation indicate increased levels of inflammation and higher levels of risk. Measurement of various white cell populations is also

> DURING OUR LIVES, WE ARE ALL EXPOSED TO VIRUSES THAT REMAIN DORMANT WITHIN US, HELD IN CHECK BY IMMUNE DEFENCES.

possible, which provides more detailed information on specific functions of the immune system.

While high levels of any of these markers have been associated with an increased risk for adverse outcomes in a range of settings, the advantage of one type of measurement over another remains to be established. It is likely that a set of inflammatory bio-markers will provide the best discriminating power, particularly combined with other markers of risk (see chapter 38). However, any value in measuring our inflammation levels comes if we do something when we get the result. If we and our health care provider have no plans, or plan to undertake activities regardless of the result, then spending on expensive tests offers us very little.

TURNING DOWN THE FLAME (TREATING INFLAMMATION)

Elevated markers of inflammation identify an individual at increased risk of disease, disability and premature mortality. Increased levels of inflammatory signals should be considered a warning sign that more work is needed to prevent bad things from happening. Moreover, dealing with all the other risks for ageing is more beneficial in absolute terms in those with high levels of inflammation, as they have the greatest absolute risk. For example, in individuals with high levels of inflammation, lowering LDL (bad) cholesterol or systolic blood pressure may be more beneficial than for those with lower levels, as their absolute risk is greater.

INCREASED LEVELS OF INFLAMMATORY SIGNALS SHOULD BE CONSIDERED A WARNING SIGN THAT MORE WORK IS NEEDED TO PREVENT BAD THINGS FROM HAPPENING.

There is currently little information about the value of directly treating the immune defence system. While decreasing chronic inflammation would seem to be important, there are potential dangers in blocking processes vital for tissue repair and defence against infections. Nonetheless, a number of simple activities have been shown to safely turn down the flame of inflammation. Indeed, all of the very diverse interventions detailed in this book will have some anti-inflammatory effects. This is because the innate immune system is non-specific, responding generically to any hazard. The simplest way to reduce inflammation is not to unnecessarily feed the fire.

OPTIONS TO REDUCE INFLAMMATION

☑ Exercise daily as regular moderate physical activity/fitness is associated with lower levels of inflammatory markers
  - > Join a walking club
  - > Try kayaking or go for a bike ride on the weekend
  - > Walk to the shops instead of driving
  - > Park as far as possible from where you need to go and walk the longer distance

☑ Don't over eat
  - > Read the packet and substitute foods that are less energy-dense, low in fat and rich in water or insoluble fibre
  - > Pay attention to the cues that make you overeat, and reduce your opportunities to lose control
  - > Eat 80% of what you would normally eat. For every four spoonfuls eat three and leave one behind
  - > Avoid eating relating to boredom. If you are bored, don't head to the fridge but go for a walk instead
  - > Avoid snacking when stressed; instead go for a walk or find another diversion apart from food
  - > Avoid overeating at work functions by eating a piece of fruit or a boiled egg before you go
  - > Slow down your eating so you don't eat as much. Also sip water between bites and chew thoroughly before swallowing
  - > Don't eat when watching TV; you'll tend to overeat if you have enough food on your plate. Alternatively only take a small snack to eat when watching TV

☑ Stop smoking
  - > Think about giving up and then put together a plan of attack
  - > Think about the negative effects of smoking – impact on others, yellowing of your teeth and fingers, risk of cancer, high blood pressure, bad breath, gum disease, depression, snoring, early morning cough and diabetes to name a few
  - > See your GP for options to help give up
  - > Call Quitline on 131 848 for assistance

OPTIONS TO REDUCE INFLAMMATION

☑ Substitute fresh and low fat alternatives for pro-inflammatory foods
  > Avoid saturated and trans fats found in fast food and junk food, snack
    foods, high fat animal protein, margarine and dairy spreads, dairy desserts,
    biscuits and pastries
  > Eat grass fed beef and other animal foods. Unlike grain-fed livestock,
    meat that comes from animals fed grass, also contains anti-inflammatory
    omega-3s
  > Avoid simple sugars – minimise lollies, cakes, pastries, sweet biscuits,
    ice-cream and soft drinks
  > Include olive oil in your diet as is a great source of oleic acid, an
    anti-inflammatory oil. Buy extra-virgin olive oil, which has the least amount
    of processing and use it instead of other cooking oils

☑ Eat foods that are naturally high in antioxidants
  > Berries are packed with anti-inflammatory phytonutrients.
  > Choose from blueberries, blackberries, mulberries, raspberries, cherries,
    boysenberries, unsweetened cranberries and strawberries
  > Choose colour on your plate with rainbow fruit and vegetables
  > Add Turmeric for spice to reduce inflammation (¼ teaspoon at least
    3 times a week)
  > Chose low GI whole grain alternatives that are high in antioxidants and fibre
  > Increase your intake of cruciferous vegetables. These include broccoli,
    califlower, Brussels sprouts are also loaded with antioxidants. They offer
    a double whammy in that they provide another important ingredient —
    sulphur — that the body needs to make its own high-powered antioxidants,
    such as one called glutathione
  > Increase your intake of fresh ginger. Brew your own ginger tea - use a peeler
    to remove the skin, then add several thin slices to a cup of hot water and let
    steep for a few minutes
  > Eat garlic every day. Put in salads, soups, steam with veges, mashed
    sweet potato
  > Substitute green tea for other beverages. Make up a thermos and it will last
    for the day

OPTIONS TO REDUCE INFLAMMATION

☑ Increase your intake of omega-3 fats. The suggested dietary targets are 610mg for men and 430mg for women
  > Include deep sea fish as a source of protein
  > Consider a fish oil supplement
  > Increase your intake from vegetarian sources such as flaxseeds (20g contains 4,500mg), nuts, especially walnuts (20g contains 1,800mg), hazelnuts (100g contains 87mg) and brazil nuts, soybeans (100g tofu contains 181mg) and green veggies (50g raw spinach contains 70mg)

☑ Manage your stress
  > Plan your activities – identify at work the what, why, how, when and who will do the jobs at hand. Schedule your obligations and your actions both long-term (weeks or months before) and on a daily basis
  > Organise your time efficiently on a daily basis. Write a to-do list and then prioritise the top 5 things you absolutely have to do that day
  > Try to be flexible in your planning
  > Take regular breaks and break a few minutes in the middle of the day. Relax, and do nothing for a few minutes and do some deep breathing exercises
  > Have a massage at least once a fortnight. Massage is excellent for relaxation and the alleviation of tension. It will improve the quality of your sleep, so contributing to less fatigue during the day
  > Take up a hobby — the best hobbies include social activity as these will take your mind off any issues you have on your mind
  > Give some time to a charitable organisation

☑ Get quality sleep – for a comprehensive list of options go to chapter 26

☑ Go to the doctor and have your hormones checked

☑ Ask your doctor to check your inflammation markers, like hsCRP and fibrinogen, and then do the actions listed to bring them down

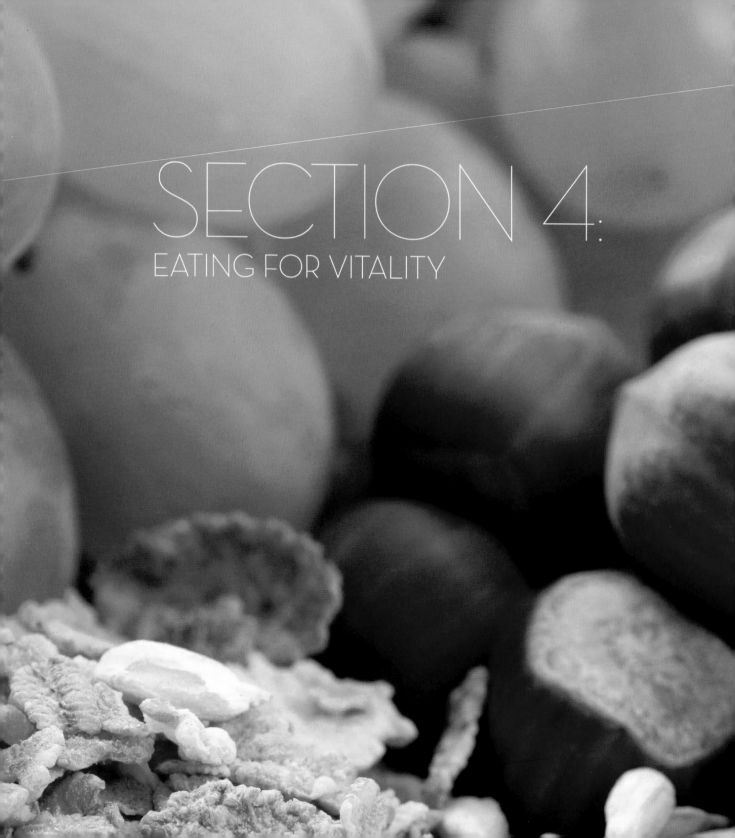

SECTION 4:
EATING FOR VITALITY

All of the changes of ageing are influenced by what we eat. There is a lot to think about! There are the calories and the composition. There are the fats and proteins, sugars and fibre, vitamins and other nutrients. In truth, it's not hard to have a good diet. The biggest challenge is implementing change. This doesn't need to be a drastic, overnight change. Even if you make one tiny change each week, if you can sustain it, over time this will make a considerable difference to your eating habits. For most of us, small steps are all that are necessary. As they become good habits, they lead to better health in our later years. In the following section, we look at simple strategies for achieving a healthy nutrient intake and, with it, slow the ageing process.

KATE'S EXPERIENCE
When I started this process, I was 14 kg overweight and I tried everything from appetite suppressants and fibre tablets to fad diets and hormone modulation to lose weight. I initially focussed on weight until I learnt that the key was to focus on health, then successful weight management would follow. A key health issue for me is that I love sweet food. Sugar also happen to be the 'killer' when it comes to accelerating ageing. There can be no argument about the need to minimise the amount of calories and sugars in your diet.

You need to do whatever it takes to reduce these to a healthy level. Now I have resorted to what some of my friends consider to be excessive means as management tools! I've found that neurofeedback training, hormone modulation and Chinese herbs have been fantastic tools in my arsenal against the war of weight. Having said that, I'm not trying to live longer just so that I have more time to be neurotic about my diet! Another thing to consider is that eating healthy food doesn't mean you have to make sacrifices all the time.

I've found that as my body has 'woken up', it automatically reaches for a healthy choice, rather than processed and unhealthy foods. I also don't need to eat as much food, so I'm more selective. I'm finally in control of what I eat and its consequences, which is a huge relief, given my starting point.

CHAPTER 12

GOOD OILS
BAD FATS

Dietary fat has a bad name and rightly so. It has twice the calories of sugar and protein. Cholesterol clogs our arteries as we get older. Yet fats are more than just the means to a sticky end. In this chapter we look at some of the fats in our body and our diet, and the ways we can maximise their positive effects while minimising their negatives.

THE GOOD OIL

The body is able to synthesise many of the fats it needs for good health. However, some essential fats must be found from our diet (such as Vitamin F). The most well known of these are the omega-3 and omega-6 polyunsaturated fatty acids.

Omega-3 fatty acids are a precursor of many eicosanoids, which control a number of important pathways relevant to ageing, including inflammation, immune function, clotting and cancer growth. There is substantial evidence that a diet high in omega-3 fatty acids can reduce the risk of heart disease and stroke, possibly by lowering blood pressure and cholesterol, stimulating local circulation and preventing clotting. Diets high in omega-3 fats also have beneficial effects on other age-related problems, including cognitive decline, depression, arthritis and varicose veins.

The most nutritionally important omega-3 fatty acids are alpha-linolenic acid and its derivatives: eicosapentaenoic acid (EPA), and docosahexaenoic acid (DHA). It is recommended to eat a gram of EPA and DHA each day from animal fats, or 2-3 g/day of alpha-linolenic acid from plants. This is the equivalent of an oily fish meal two or three times a week. If you can't keep this up, a number of supplements are available which contain large amounts of omega-3, including fish oils and flaxseed (linseed) oil.

Omega-6 fatty acids are essential for making the chemicals that regulate inflammation. However, if our intake of omega-6 fatty acids is too high, this excess leads to increased inflammation, clotting and tissue injury. In a healthy diet, these actions are balanced and negated by omega-3 fats because they compete for the same pathways for their metabolism. However, modern diets typically have too much omega-6 relative to omega-3, often in an excess of 20 to 1. This imbalance has a number of adverse consequences, including depression, heart attack, stroke, arthritis, osteoporosis, inflammation and some forms of cancer.

MONOUNSATURATED FATS

Monounsaturated fats (MUFAs) also have a number of effects on human health, ageing and longevity. A high intake of MUFAs, such as in a Mediterranean diet, can lower blood pressure and cholesterol levels, improve vascular function and reduce our risk of heart disease. The most common MUFA in our diet is oleic acid, found in vegetable and seed oils, nuts, avocado and some meats. Tea oil and olive oil contain more MUFAs than normal canola oils, which in turn have more MUFAs than sunflower, peanut, corn and soybean oils. However, many of these potentially beneficial MUFAs are destroyed by prolonged high temperature cooking or frying. So consider a drizzle on the salad instead.

A DIET RICH IN OMEGA-3'S HAS BENEFICIAL EFFECTS ON THE AGEING PROCESS.

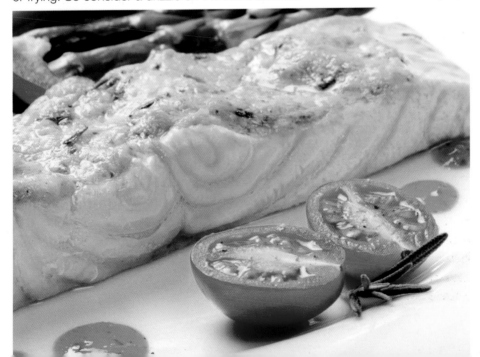

SATURATED (FAT) BOMBING

The intake of saturated fats from our diets can significantly contribute to obesity and heart disease. Saturated fat raises bad (LDL) cholesterol more than dietary cholesterol itself. All natural products have a balance of saturated and unsaturated fats. We should aim to reduce our saturated fat intake to less than 7% of our total calories by limiting our intake of foods high in saturated fat, such as dairy products (especially whole milk, cream cheese and ice cream), palm oils, meat and eggs. We can also choose products with the lowest content of saturated fat. For example, the meat of grass-fed animals and birds contains much lower levels of saturated fat than conventional bulk (grain) fed stocks. Lean cuts should always be preferred.

THE UGLY SISTER (TRANS FATS)

Trans fatty acids are not produced naturally and serve no purpose in human metabolism. Most trans fats are deliberately created during the processing of vegetable oils (by hydrogenation) to make them solid at room temperature, to melt on baking (or eating) or more resistant to going off (rancid) compared to animal fats such as butter. Prolonged deep frying can also generate trans fats, which are then transferred to the food.

Trans fats are toxic to a range of important systems, contributing to heart disease, stroke, diabetes, obesity, insulin resistance, prostate cancer and infertility. In fact, on a pound for pound basis, trans fats increase the risk of heart disease more than any other component in our diet. Even a small intake is sufficient to increase our risk of heart disease. There appears to be no safe limit for trans fats.

The only way is to avoid foods containing them, or choose foods in which the processing has specifically prevented their formation. Although all margarines must now be free of trans fats, many common snack foods, rice cakes, chips and biscuits contain significant amounts of trans fats. Just read the nutritional contents label. For a number or reasons, including trans fats, it is best to avoid deep frying at home, even if we regularly change the oil.

CHOLESTEROL LEVELS INCREASE AS WE GET OLDER, PARTICULARLY AFTER MENOPAUSE IN WOMEN.

BAD AND GOOD CHOLESTEROL

Cholesterol is a lipid found in the membranes of every human cell, where it functions to keep our cell membranes flexible. It also has an important role in the function of bile, which is important for the digestion and absorption of fat, as well as fat-soluble vitamins, such as Vitamins A, D, E and K. Cholesterol is also used in the body to synthesise Vitamin D, as well as a number of hormones important to the ageing process, such as cortisol, estrogens and testosterone.

Each day the body makes about 1 gram of cholesterol and takes in another 20-30% from our diet. Any food that contains animal fat also contains cholesterol, especially egg yolks, beef, poultry and prawns. Even a litre of plant oil contains far less cholesterol than a single egg yolk.

Oil does not dissolve in water, nor does cholesterol, so to transport it around the body it must be packaged in waterproof containers, called lipoproteins. The best known are low density lipoprotein (LDL) and high density lipoprotein (HDL) and there is also very low density lipoprotein (VLDL).

VLDL particles are generally considered the 'bad cholesterol' and carry triglycerides around the body and are implicated in development of hardening of the arteries; they also transform into LDL which can become oxidised. LDL cholesterol levels increase as we get older, particularly after menopause in women. The lower our LDL cholesterol levels, the lower our risk of heart attack, stroke and other diseases of the blood vessels. There is good evidence that lowering LDL cholesterol results in a reduced risk of heart attack and stroke. For every 1.0 mmol/L we lower our LDL cholesterol, our risk of dying from a heart attack reduces by 20%.

Another way to deal with the LDL problem is to offset it with the good cholesterol contained in HDL particles. These remove cholesterol from the walls of blood vessels and transport it back to the liver for excretion or safer storage sites (so-called 'reverse cholesterol transport'). Individuals with high levels of HDL cholesterol have a lower risk of heart disease and stroke and improved longevity. Physical activity is very effective at increasing HDL levels, while smoking and inactivity reduce HDL cholesterol levels and shorten lives.

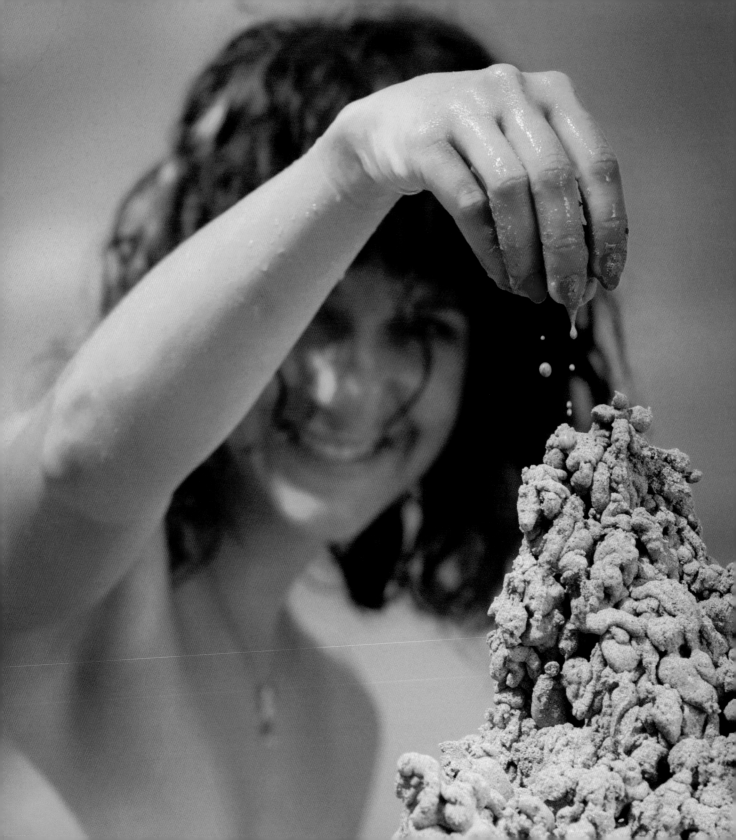

CHAPTER 13
BUILDING YOUR AGEING CASTLE
[PROTEIN & AGEING]

Proteins are the structures that our body builds, from the hair on our head to the nails on our toes. Over half of our body's dry weight is protein. Although there are countless different proteins in every cell of our body, at their core proteins are composed of the same 20 bricks. These bricks are called amino acids. Every protein is made up of chains of amino acids linked together in different amounts and different combinations as determined by our genetic code. The body can also use amino acid building blocks for other purposes, such as the synthesis of hormones and as a fuel source for energy metabolism.

The body can make 11 of the 20 amino acids needed to make a protein. The others must be obtained from food. If any of these nine essential amino acids are lacking in our diet, the body must break down another protein to obtain them. This chapter examines different kinds of dietary protein and its role in slowing ageing.

WHAT PROTEIN SHOULD WE EAT?

When we eat any protein, it is rapidly dismantled by our digestive system. So when we consider the value of any protein in our diet, we are really talking about:

> The other nutrients that are ingested at the same time (such as fats, vitamins and fibre). For example, a steak is packed with animal fats, as well as protein. By comparison, lentils contain less than 5% fat, and have the bonus of fibre, vitamins and minerals.

> Its composition of essential amino acids. For example, most animal sources of protein, such as meat, milk and eggs, have the complete complement of all the essential amino acids. Most plant proteins lack at least one amino acid. However, there is little danger of deficiency in a vegetarian diet, as most involve eating a broad range of plant foods (known as protein combining or complementing). For example, a meal containing rice as well as legumes provides all the essential amino acids found in a typical meat dish. Some special vegetable sources provide a full range of amino acids (so-called 'complete proteins'), including soy products, quinoa, spirulina, buckwheat and amaranth.

> Its biological value. This measures the amount of any dietary protein that ends up being used by the body. Some proteins, like egg white and whey, are almost completely utilised. This is why these are the main ingredients of most protein supplements used by body builders and people with increased protein requirements. Methods of food preparation also impact on the biological value of proteins. For example, prolonged cooking or processing in the presence of fats can destroy some amino acids, reducing their biological value as well as generating toxins and carcinogens.

HOW MUCH PROTEIN SHOULD WE EAT?

Adults need between 45 to 80 grams of protein a day. We regularly consume twice this much. In general, if you are getting enough calories, you are almost always getting enough protein. Most animal products are 20-30% protein. For example, a 100g piece of steak contains about 29g of protein and a 100g piece of fish about 22g. Legumes contain about 15% protein, while soy and nuts contain about 20%.

> ADULTS NEED 45-60 GRAMS OF PROTEIN PER DAY
> WE REGULARLY CONSUME TWICE THIS AMOUNT

Higher protein intakes may be helpful for those undertaking an exercise program, in pregnant women and those with increased protein turnover (eg. recovering from surgery, illness, burns or cancer). In particular, there is some advantage in consuming extra protein around the time of exercise, when muscles are at their most needy.

HIGH-PROTEIN DIETS – BENEFITS AND RISKS

If we eat more protein than our requirements, it cannot be stored as amino acids, but must be added to our fat stockpiles. Although there are less calories in protein than fat, it is still possible to get fat on a high-protein diet if we eat too much. However, as protein makes us feel full faster, we tend to eat less. A number of effective weight loss diets make use of this action, including the Zone diet, Protein Power and the CSIRO diet. These diets do not generally increase the amount of protein in the diet (this would not work on its own), rather they increase the amount of energy coming from protein by reducing carbohydrate intake. In most diets, 10-15% of energy comes from protein, and this is doubled in most of these diets. The other obvious advantage of a high-protein diet is that it usually means eating less carbohydrate and fat.

High-protein diets also have a down-side. Too much animal protein always increases our exposure to animal fat, as well as leading to constipation if fibre intake is not increased at the same time. Vegetable protein doesn't have these same problems. Very high protein diets (> 45% energy as protein) can also cause weakness, nausea and diarrhoea.

AMINO ACID SUPPLEMENTS

A number of dietary supplements contain pre-digested protein (amino acid supplements, elemental diets). While this may be helpful in individuals with a damaged digestive tract, eating high biological value protein achieves the same result as expensive supplements in otherwise healthy individuals. Where possible, amino acids should always be obtained from whole food protein sources. A number of specific amino acid supplements are widely used in clinical nutrition and for health promotion. As few individuals on a conventional diet have inadequate levels of amino acids, these supplements mainly act by stimulating pathways involved in removing the excess load, or by altering the balance of amino acids in the body.

> Arginine is normally obtained from both the diet and cell metabolism. It is used in many proteins, as well as the synthesis of nitric oxide, one of the major regulators of blood flow in the body. Supplements have been used to support immune function, increase growth hormone and reduce erection problems. However, the impact of these effects is probably small when compared to more specific interventions.

> Glutamine is the most abundant amino acid in the body. It is used to make protein, as well as DNA and some brain neurotransmitters. Unlike other amino acids, it can be stored in muscles for later use. Although it can be synthesised in the body under conditions of increased protein turnover (eg. illness, surgery), it becomes essential. In these states, supplements have been shown to be beneficial in aiding recovery. As glutamine readily crosses into the brain, supplements have also been widely used as a memory aid, especially in ageing individuals.

> Tyrosine is a non-essential amino acid that is also used as the starting substrate for many important brain signalling chemicals, including dopamine and noradrenaline. Although supplements have little effect in healthy individuals, in individuals with an activated stress response (eg. sleep deprived, over-worked, emotionally wrought), tyrosine can improve function and mood.

> Tryptophan is an essential amino acid used by the body to make proteins, Vitamin B3 and a number of important brain signaling chemicals. Although present in most protein, it is particularly plentiful in dairy products, meat, eggs, fish, chocolate, oats, bananas, mangoes, nuts and seeds. Tryptophan supplements can aid sleep, possibly by altering levels of the sleep hormones, serotonin and melatonin. It may also be useful in mental diseases associated with low serotonin levels, like depression.

> The branched chain amino acids (leucine, isoleucine and valine) are among the major components of muscle protein. Supplements containing branched chain amino acids, especially leucine, can help build muscle mass.

OPTIONS FOR OPTIMAL PROTEIN INTAKE

☑ Cook plant protein alternatives to meat protein such as legumes, tofu, nuts and seeds, quinoa, amaranth, buckwheat, tofu and tempeh
> Substitute quinoa for rice
> Buy bread which has amaranth as a key ingredient
> Substitute buckwheat pancakes for those made with white flour

☑ Add beans to your diet; you'll also get the added benefit of boosting your soluble fibre intake
> Buy a salad recipe book containing lots of bean dishes
> Make Make your own soup with beans as a key ingredient
> Buy a slow cooker and add beans to casseroles
> Substitute beans for meat in tacos
> Make your own hummus with chickpeas. A great alternative to butter on bread and crackers

☑ Choose seafood instead of meat

☑ Eat soy protein which is found in soy beans, tofu, tempeh, soy flour which is found in soy beans, tofu, tempeh, soy flour and edamame

☑ To ensure you get a full complement of protein from vegetarian sources, combine the following protein sources in at least one meal per day:
> Legumes with grains
> Legumes with nuts
> Grains and nuts

☑ Avoid overcooked and processed protein sources
> Cook fish, chicken or red meat fresh rather than choosing processed, pre-packaged or deli style foods

CHAPTER 14

FINDING YOUR FIBRE
[ROUGHAGE & AGEING]

Some elements in our diet are indigestible. But that does not mean that they are useless. In fact, our bodies make use of most things we eat, even if we don't digest them. One example of this is dietary fibre.

Fibre is only found in plants. It is the indigestible part of plant material (also known as 'roughage'). There are two types of dietary fibre: those that dissolve in water (soluble fibre) and those that do not (insoluble fibre). Most plants contain a mixture of the two (at a ratio of about 3:1 insoluble to soluble) and both forms are vitally important in our diet.

GOOD SOURCES OF FIBRE

Insoluble fibre (such as cellulose and lignin) is found in whole grains, particularly in the outer husk or bran (eg. oat bran, wheat bran, rice bran). Milling or refining removes the bran and therefore much of the fibre. For example, wheat flour made from whole grains contains 10 times the fibre as standard white flour. Lower levels of insoluble fibre are also found in nuts, seeds and refined cereals such as flour. Lignin is also found in the skin of fruit and vegetables, such as strawberries, prunes, tomatoes, potatoes and onions.

Soluble fibre (such as gums, beta-glucans, psyllium, mucilages and pectins) is found in most plant foods, with the highest amounts in oats, bran, barley, legumes, nuts, soy products and some yeasts. Fruit and vegetables also contain significant levels of fibre. Fruits high in fibre include plums, Asian pears, raspberries, blackberries, apples and citrus pulp. Nonlegume vegetables high in fibre include cauliflower, zucchini, broccoli, carrots, Jerusalem artichokes and celery. However, these fibre levels are still lower than in legumes.

Diets that are naturally high in fibre have a number of positive effects on our health to:

> Improve blood sugar levels – soluble fibre slows the absorption of glucose from the foods we eat, which creates a sustained energy release and lowers the strain on insulin production (see chapter 6).

> Reduce bad (LDL) cholesterol levels – about a 10% reduction is seen with psyllium supplements.

> Improve weight management — consuming fibre-rich foods can make us feel satisfied sooner and feel full for longer (and therefore less likely to feel hungry or snack between meals). Soluble fibre can also reduce the absorption of nutrients (including sugars, fats and proteins), meaning their energy is lost to our metabolism (to the gain of our healthy gut bacteria). Even the extra chewing time of high fibre foods helps slow the intake of food and reduce the amount (of calories) we consume.

> Reduce the risk of heart attack — significant cardiovascular benefits are seen in diets rich in insoluble fibre beyond lowering cholesterol. For example, lignins like sesamin and sesamolin from sesame seed have beneficial effects on the immune system and can reduce oxidative stress. The bran and germ of whole grains are also rich in minerals, vitamins, antioxidants and other phytochemicals that have positive effects on heart disease.

> Improves bowel health – insoluble fibre makes the stool more soft and bulky, allowing it to move more easily through the intestine and colon. This is useful for the prevention and management of constipation.

> Helps the work of our gut bacteria – dietary fibre is fermented by the gut bacteria of the large intestine. This process releases gas, as well as a number of beneficial compounds like short-chain fatty acids. These help the absorption of minerals and contribute to lower rates of bowel cancer for those on a high fibre diet.

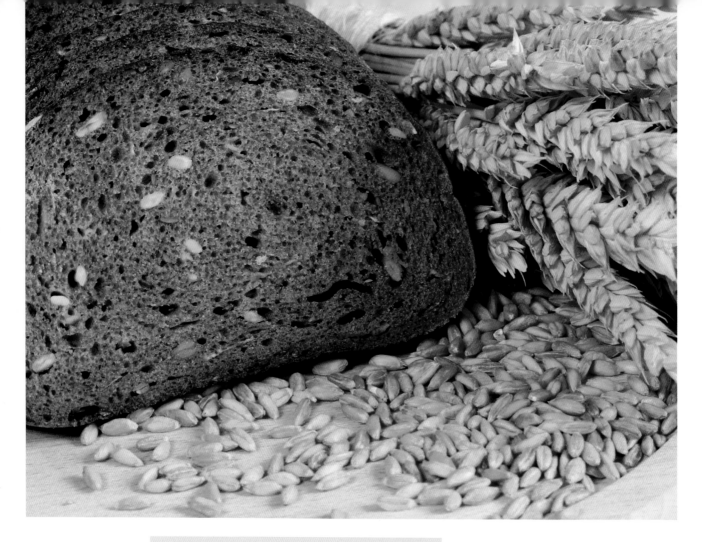

PUTTING THE FIBRE BACK IN OUR LIVES

Current recommendations say we should aim for greater than 30g of fibre each day. The average adult consumes half this amount. One reason is that the most common cereals we eat are heavily refined, meaning that the bran and germ (which contain most of the good bits) have been removed and only the inner starchy part of the grain left behind. Many of our other staples are only rich in starch. Unlike fibre, starch is readily metabolised and used to generate glucose and fat, leading to obesity.

OPTIONS TO INCREASE DIETARY FIBRE

☑ Buy a book with a fibre counter so you'll educate yourself on better fibre choices

☑ Dietary fibre absorbs water so increase your water intake when you increase your fibre intake

☑ Make sure you eat 3 fruits and 5 vegetables per day

☑ Eat brown rice instead of white rice

☑ Eat rolled oats instead of processed, microwave or instant oats

☑ Use oatbran in cooking. Substitute some of the flour in baking for oatbran; add to meat rissoles or meat loaf; use as a coating for crumbed fish or chicken

☑ Eat whole grain bread i.e. whole rye, whole grain spelt, whole grain kamut, whole grain barley, sunflower, linseed (flaxseed) or bulgur

☑ Eat breakfast cereal that says 'whole grain' not just wheat

☑ Use whole grain wheat flour compared to white 'all purpose' flour for baking (it has ten times the fibre content per 100g)

☑ Buy bread from a bakery that uses whole grains or wheat alternatives such as spelt or kamut

☑ Eat brown or wild rice rather than white rice

☑ Include more barley in soups, casseroles, risotto, salads

☑ Eat whole fruit instead of fruit juice

☑ Consider chickpeas, lentils and soybeans instead of steak mince for your next nachos night!

☑ Consider taking fibre supplements. The most commonly used supplement is psyllium made from ispaghula husks – take 2 tsp daily. Fibre supplements containing inulin or fructans can also be used as a sugar substitute

☑ Include dried fruit and nuts as a quick, high fibre snack

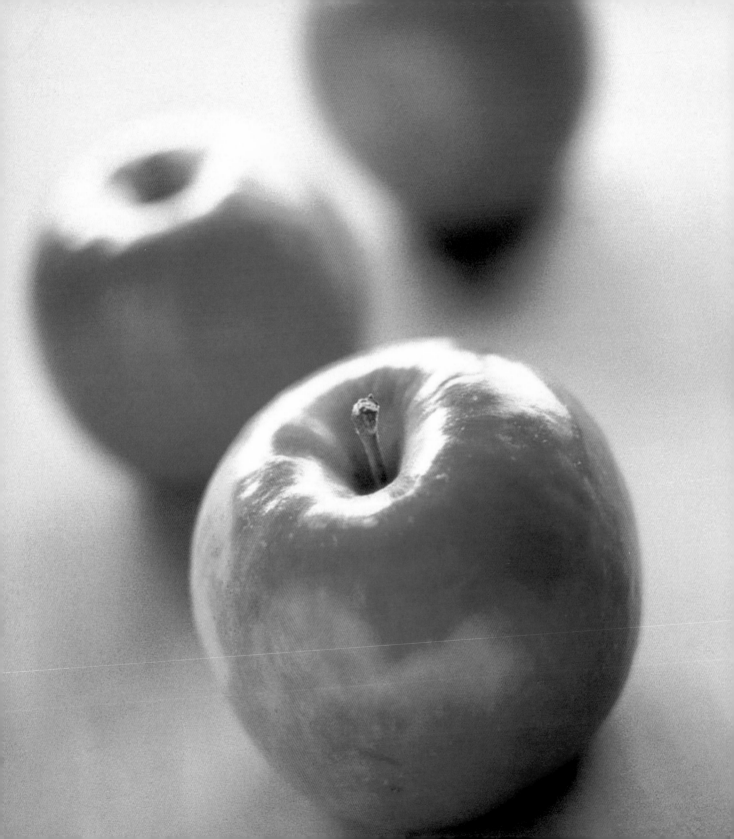

CHAPTER 15

AVOIDING THE POISONS
[TOXINS & AGEING]

We live our lives in a toxic soup - a complex mixture of harmful chemicals and disease causing pathogens. Some of these toxins are of our own making (such as free radicals), while others are acquired from our environment. Fortunately, we have a number of highly developed strategies for intercepting and neutralising toxins before they can damage crucial systems.

Our intestinal barrier prevents most from getting in. This barrier is made up of digestive enzymes, antibodies and large amounts of fluid and mucus to dilute and neutralise noxious substances. A number of different factors influence the functions of the intestinal barrier. For example, a diet high in antioxidants and fibre can improve the functions of the intestinal barrier while stress and alcohol reduce them.

Inside the intestines on any individual, there are more microbes than there have ever been humans walking on the face of the earth - about a hundred trillion, or up to two 2 kilos! For every cell in an adult body, there are about 10 bacteria. These bacteria are not just along for the ride. They pay their way by performing a number of chores, including fermenting any indigestible nutrients that would otherwise be lost in the stool. During this process they release short-chain fatty acids that are an essential tonic for the cells that line the bowel. Fermentation also lowers the pH to prevent growth of harmful bacterial species, allow better absorption of minerals (such as calcium, magnesium and iron) and improve gut motility.

The makeup of bacteria that line our intestines can be significantly modified by what we eat. Nutrients that support or enhance a health gut flora are called prebiotics (as opposed to antibiotics which kill them). Another way to get healthy gut bacteria is to ingest them. This strategy is called probiotic. When probiotics are ingested they quickly establish a healthy, balanced gut flora. At the beginning of the 20th century, it was suggested that disease and ageing could be partly mediated by toxic substances produced by bad bacteria, and that ageing as a result could be slowed by helpful probiotic bacteria by out competing the bad guys for food and space. Although their effect on ageing continues to be debated, supplementing with probiotics may be useful in certain situations, such as after a course of antibiotics. Some probiotics also contain bacteria that can lower our cholesterol levels and managing lactose intolerance. Improving intestinal health can also enhance the immune system, improve resistance to infections and reduce symptoms of allergies, such as eczema.

FIRST PASS

Any toxins absorbed from what we eat and drink, must first pass through the liver, whose job it is to keeping anything harmful from reaching the rest of the body. A number of factors influence the effectiveness of this function. The big ones are drugs, alcohol and calories (leading to diabetes and obesity), which in excess can compromise the integrity of liver detox. Fasting also enhances the liver's ability to clear toxins from the blood stream, which is why it is often part of a detox strategy.

THE BUFFERS (IN THE BLOOD STREAM AND THE FAT)

If any toxins make it past the liver, the blood stream has ways to sideline their effects. For example blood contains proteins whose job it is to bind free toxins and prevent them from interfering with crucial systems. For example, if you take a benzodiazepine (such as Valium), much of it is removed by the liver, but because of its concentrated dose, some reaches the blood. Here over 95% of it is bound by proteins, leaving less than 1% free to interact with receptors in the brain and cause sleepiness. This is just one example of how good a healthy body is at dealing with toxins, even when in highly concentrated form, such as a medicine.

This is also a good example of how our detoxification systems can deteriorate as we get older. When most elderly people take a sleeping pill, their liver is not as effective in removing it at the first pass and the proteins that buffer the toxins in the blood do not work as effiiciently. This means for the same dose there is more free drug available, leading to a stronger effect and longer sedation. This is why our actions to reduce our exposure to harmful toxins are even more important as we get older.

Many toxins are also impounded into our fat, meaning they are not free to interact with more vital systems. Consequently, alongside the liver and kidneys, the highest levels of environmental toxins like dioxin and PCBs, are in fat. This is just one more good reason for a diet low in animal fat.

PASSING INTEREST (URINE AND THE KIDNEYS)

Every five minutes, all the blood in our body is filtered by the kidneys. We even have a spare one to make sure we can deal with any extra demands. In individuals with impaired kidney function, a number of toxins can accumulate (such as AGEs and free radicals). This leads to 'accelerated ageing', and many of the symptoms and diseases of old age occurring in much younger individuals. Keeping our kidneys in peak condition is an important way to age well.

SWEAT IT OUT (PERSPIRATION)

Perspiration is mostly salty water excreted by the skin to keep us cool. It also contains small amounts of minerals, toxins and other chemicals that contribute to body odour. Repeated sauna (60°C for 15 minutes) and other activities to increasing the flow of sweat (eg. exercise) are widely used in detoxification programs, although its impacts are only small. Nonetheless, there can be little doubt about the feelings of wellbeing, relaxation and health that come from sweaty activities.

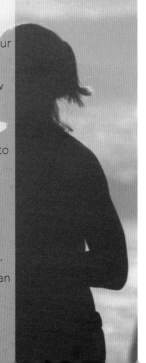

KEEPING YOUR KIDNEYS HEALTHY

PREVENT DIABETES — diabetes is the most common cause of kidney failure and can be prevented by the things you do today, like regular exercise and fighting obesity (see chapter 6).

LOWER YOUR BLOOD PRESSURE — if you can find ways to lower your blood pressure and keep it low, your filters will work better for longer. Regular exercise, staying in a healthy weight range and eating a diet low in salt (<6g/day) and fat can reduce your systolic blood pressure.

DRINK LOTS OF WATER — at least 2 to 3 litres of fluid (about 8-10 glasses) every day. On hot days or if you have exercised you will need to drink more to make up for fluid lost as sweat. You'll know when you've got it right when you are going to the toilet about 3-4 times every day, making a good amount of clear to light yellow urine with little or no odour.

LIMIT ANIMAL PROTEIN — in those with impaired kidney function (eg. half of all individuals over the age of 65), a diet high in animal protein can increase its workload and accelerate the rate of decline in function.

PLASTIC (NOT SO) FANTASTIC

Plastics are chemical polymers that can be moulded into almost any shape for any function. Most plastics contain a range of chemical products, some of which gets into our food and drink, or the environment. Many different toxins have been identified, depending on the type of plastic (which can be identified by the number inside the triangular recycling label). However, in this modern world it is not always easy to spot plastic. Take a look inside a can and you will usually see a solid film of plastic to prevent food from reacting with the metal. This plastic can leach a number of toxins into canned food. The best-known plastic toxins include the phthalates and adipates (contained in type 3 plastics) and polycarbonates (like bisphenol A, in some type 3 and type 7 plastics). The long-term health implications of various chemicals that leach from plastics are poorly understood. We now know that many can disrupt hormonal function. For example, bisphenol A binds and activates oestrogen signalling. Some phthalates may also contribute to the development of allergies and asthma. And while we're making a change, consider the environment and the pollution that these non-degradable plastics can cause. It is not too hard to make a change to limit the plastics that we use (and abuse).

OPTIONS TO REDUCE YOUR EXPOSURE TO TOXINS FROM PLASTICS

☑ Cook and microwave using glass or ceramic containers. If you must use plastic, choose opaque or coloured bottles that are made of safer plastics. Do not heat polycarbonate bottles (#7)

☑ Use microwave-safe plastic wrap (made of polyethylene), or better still, non-bleached paper towels

☑ Limit use of canned food and plastic containers. Use bottles made from glass or stainless steel. Watch out for those large water cooler bottles. Try to avoid #3 and #7 plastics. The safest plastic products are those made of high density polyethylene (HDPE, #2), low density polyethylene (LDPE, #4) or polypropylene (#5, translucent, not transparent)

HEAVY METALS (AND HUMAN HEALTH)

The healthy function of the body requires metals, like iron, zinc and copper. Other metals, such as mercury and arsenic, have no role in human physiology. Although the body tries to put them where metals should go, like a square peg in a round hole they don't fit and get stuck. This can disrupt healthy functions, as well as lead to their progressive accumulation. The ones we should do our best to avoid include:

> Mercury – increased exposure to mercury is associated with hypertension, heart disease and oxidative stress. You should try to limit your intake of long lived predatory fish, such as swordfish, shark, marlin and mackerel, which have mercury levels 10 times higher than most other fish. This doesn't necessarily mean avoiding them altogether, as a single meal is in no way toxic. But you shouldn't make a habit of it. As a source of lean protein and essential fatty acids, fish is too important to keep off the menu, particularly if it is replacing red meat. Just consider the small fry more often.

> Cadmium — chronic exposure has been associated with oxidative stress, high blood pressure, heart disease and some cancers. Increased levels of cadmium are mostly observed in chronic smokers and in those drinking polluted water.

> Arsenic — is the classic poison. In lower doses, it leads to oxidative stress and its consequences including cancer, heart disease, diabetes and accelerated ageing. Outside of industry and polluted water, the main sources of arsenic around the home are fungicides and wood preservatives. Remember not to edge your vegetable patch with treated pine, unless it is arsenic-free! Untreated hardwood is a safer alternative.

> Lead — long-term exposure to lead can cause kidney disease, mental disease, cognitive decline and anaemia. Watch out when stripping old paint by sanding. Some pottery glazes also contain lead which leaches out when exposed to acid liquids, such as soft drinks and fruit juices.

> Aluminium — in individuals with impaired kidney function (and therefore reduced ability to remove aluminium from the body), accumulation of aluminium leads to anaemia, bone thinning and cognitive decline. Any toxicity of aluminium in individuals with healthy detoxification systems remains unproven. There are enough calories in soft drinks to consider avoiding them, without even thinking about the aluminium.

COLLATERAL DAMAGE (PESTICIDE CONTAMINATION)

One of the greatest changes in human agriculture has been the transition from organic practices to farming techniques that involve the use of synthetic herbicides, fungicides, insecticides and other chemicals to increase crop yields or quality. As a result, nearly two out of three products on the supermarket shelf contains pesticide residue. The highest levels are often in foods considered healthy, like fresh fruit and vegetables. Many of these pesticides are carcinogenic or have effects on brain function, hormonal regulation and reproductive health. For the most part, we don't know what the long-term exposure to the low levels of pesticides commonly found in our food will do to our health. However, given the clear association between industrial exposure to pesticides and poor health, it is prudent to try to limit our exposure.

GOING MOULDY (MYCOTOXINS)

One group of naturally occurring environmental toxins are the mycotoxins made by fungi (e.g. moulds, mildew, spores and mushrooms). A number of these chemicals have been shown to impact on human health, including mental disorders, liver and kidney disease and some cancers. The main source of exposure to mycotoxins is your diet. Fresh is always best. Throw away fruit and vegetables that have passed their use by date. Poor quality grain or mouldy vegetable components are sometimes used as animal food. These can accumulate in meat, milk and eggs. Most food safety programs monitor mycotoxin levels in various mass-produced food sources. However, smaller farmers and producers cannot guarantee this kind of quality control. So be careful. Inhaling mycotoxins in a mouldy indoor setting is recognised as a potential source of toxic exposure. Many people have allergies to mould. A simple way to deal with this risk is to check our house and work environment for mould and damp conditions and take the necessary steps to eradicate all traces. Replace old pillows and mattresses if necessary.

TOXINS CAN NEVER BE TOTALLY AVOIDED.

FORMULATING YOUR DETOX PLAN

Slow ageing is about maintaining reserves and limiting damage to secure a healthy future. Toxins can never be totally avoided. Yet, we can take a number of practical actions every day to maximise our detoxification defences and reduce our overall toxic burden. The benefits of one-off detox programs are probably small to insignificant in individuals with a healthy metabolism. However, many people gain substantial stress release from these programs. The mere act of participating in our health also tends to encourage other health seeking behaviours (such as exercise, meditation and more selective dietary choices).

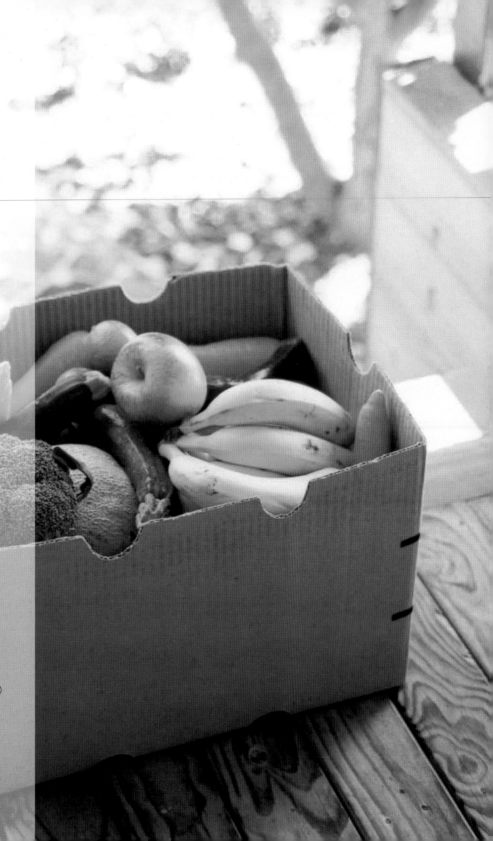

FOODS THAT STIMULATE THE ACTIVITY OF THE LIVER'S DETOXIFICATION ENZYMES INCLUDE:

> DIETARY CRUCIFERS, SUCH AS BROCCOLI, CABBAGE, SPROUTS AND KALE, CONTAIN SULFORAPHANE AND INDOLE-3-CARBINOL.
> EPIGALLOCATECHIN GALLATE CONTAINED IN GREEN TEA.
> CURCUMIN FROM TURMERIC.
> LIMONENE FROM CITRUS PEEL.
> ISOFLAVONES AND LIGNANS FROM SOY FOODS AND FLAX SEED.
> GARLIC, ONION AND LEEK SUPPORT SULPHATION, ONE OF THE 6 PRIMARY PHASES OF LIVER DETOXIFICATION.
> ORAL SUPPLEMENTATION WITH GLYCINE (AN AMINO ACID – SEE CHAPTER 13) HAS ALSO BEEN FOUND TO IMPROVE DETOXIFICATION IN SOME INDIVIDUALS.

OPTIONS TO REDUCE EXPOSURE TO PESTICIDES AND ENVIRONMENTAL TOXINS

☑ Choose organic produce (grown without pesticides). If you cannot change to organic foods completely, go organic with the foods you eat most often. Additional nutritional benefits, environmental considerations and support of sustainable farming practices are also valuable considerations
  > Try an online organic food supply service
  > Do your weekly shopping at an organic food market
  > Grow herbs in pots on your balcony
  > Find organic foods at www.organicfooddirectory.com.au

☑ Wash your fruit and vegetables with a fragrance-free olive oil soap or specific fruit and vegetable wash

☑ Eat low fat and vegetarian protein sources such as tofu, tempeh, legumes, quinoa, nuts and seed to reduce your exposure to chemical residues in animal fat (as well as animal fat itself)

☑ Consume a wide variety of foods to lessen your potential exposure to pesticides loaded on any one food
  > Try a new fruit or vegetable each week. Be creative with your cooking
  > Include grains such as quinoa, amaranth, spelt and kamut as replacements for wheat

☑ Start a garden and grow your own crops, particularly those with a high risk of pesticide residue, such as green leafy vegetables, spinach, strawberries and broccoli

☑ Wear appropriate protective gear to avoid pesticide exposure at home, at work or in the garden

☑ Use 'old-fashioned' cleaning, pesticide and gardening remedies, such as bicarbonate and vinegar

OPTIONS TO REDUCE EXPOSURE TO PESTICIDES AND ENVIRONMENTAL TOXINS

☑ Dust and vacuum weekly. Toxins like polybrominated diphenylethers (PBDEs) are found in fire retardants in carpet underlay, bedding and polyurethane foams in furniture. These can settle into the dust in your house. This is especially important if you are pregnant, have a young child or a pet, which can transfer the dust through its movements

☑ Don't use stain-protection treatment (the 'extra' they try to sell you when you buy a new pair of shoes or furniture). These treatments usually contain perfluorinated chemicals (PFOAs) which incidentally are also widely used in everyday items such as food packaging, pesticides, clothing, upholstery, carpets and personal care products

☑ Avoid using pots and pans that have a non-stick coating. PFOAs are also often used in the production of the non-stick surfaces and when the pan gets scratched or worn, the chemicals can be released into the air

☑ Check the ingredients before buying personal grooming products. Shampoos, lotions and makeup can contain a number of toxins like parabens and phthalates, which have been identified as hormone disruptors and may be linked to certain cancers
   > Read the label. Avoid anything with paraben (often used as a suffix, as in methylparaben) or phthalate (listed as dibutyl and diethylhexyl or just 'fragrance')
   > Check out www.cosmeticsdatabase.com for a list of toxic ingredients in thousands of personal-care products

CHAPTER 16

DRINK TO YOUR HEALTH
[DRINKS & AGEING]

Throughout the ages, our imagination has been captured by stories of the 'fountain of youth' - bestowing health and vitality on those who drink from it. Equally, poisons that take life away are always depicted in liquid form. In considering our own ageing, we must also consider the potential benefits and hazards of what we drink.

FLUID FIXATIONS

Water is both the source of life and medium for its flow. Over 70% of our body is water. It helps us feel at home, even if we are no longer aquatic. The human body is very good at keeping the inner sea inside us in balance. If we start becoming dry, we feel 'thirsty', and our urine becomes dark and our stools hard. If fluid is drunk in excess, increased losses via more urine restores the balance.

Not drinking enough fluid increases our risk of kidney stones, constipation and piles. The resulting bowel sluggishness may also contribute to an increased risk for colon cancer. Skin and mucous membranes also become dry if we don't drink enough, which can lead to flaking, cracking and reduced density. Inadequate fluid intake can also lead to a drop in mental and physical performance, impairing our co-ordination, concentration, and slowing our thinking. There is also some evidence suggesting thirst can sometimes be mistaken for hunger, so under-drinking may contribute to overeating in some people.

Most adults should drink at least 2 to 3 litres (8 to 10 glasses) of fluid every day. On hot days, or if we have exercised, we need to drink more to make up for fluid lost as sweat. We know we've got it right when we make a good amount of clear to light yellow urine with little or no odour.

DRINKING WATER

Water is an ideal drink that is cheap, readily available and contains no calories. There are now many water products on the market that compete with the taps in our homes, on the basis that they 'taste' better, lack contamination or have additional 'health benefits' such as minerals and trace elements. There are also a range of purification technologies which have their own positives and negatives.

Certainly high quality filtered water has many merits (like less chlorine and fluoride) that make it more enjoyable to drink and use in cooking. However, tap water quality in most Western countries is excellent, highly regulated and monitored. At the same time, plastic bottles may leach small amounts of toxins (such as phthalates and Bisphenol A – see chapter 15) and have an environmental impact as pollution. In the end, the choice of water is largely pragmatic. Choose the one where we will actually drink 8 -10 glasses a day. This is more important than the source. But you will be amazed at how much more water we drink when it tastes better.

THE DREADED BOOZE

Alcohol can be both good and bad, often at the same time. Quite apart from the psychosocial and relaxant effects, alcohol has a number of positive effects on health and wellbeing. However, binge drinking and excessive chronic intake are a leading cause of preventable death, particularly in young adults and men, but also increasingly, in women. Its individual and social costs are even more significant. Overall, excess alcohol contributes to the global burden of disease to a greater extent than smoking.

Alcohol affects the mind and the body in a number of ways:

> Alcohol inhibits the functions of the brain, especially at the front end whose job it is to think through what we are doing. When this area is boozed we lose some of your inhibitions. This is why alcohol seems relaxing and takes away (thoughts of) your worries. This disinhibition can also lead to bad choices, such as dancing on tables or driver error. More alcohol and other areas of the brain are also affected, leading to disturbed balance, slurred speech, blurred vision and other symptoms recognizable as being drunk.

> Long term alcohol use can lead to dependency. Going without a drink can trigger symptoms including nausea, fatigue, shakes, or even hallucinations.

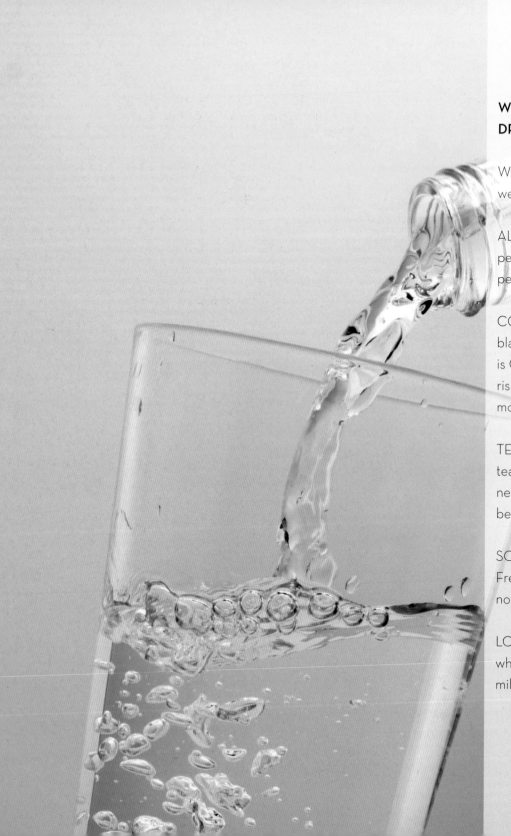

WHAT SHOULD WE BE DRINKING

WATER: When we can, however we can.

ALCOHOL: Fewer than 4 drinks per day in a man and fewer than 2 per day in a woman is optimal.

COFFEE: Up to 2 to 3 cups of black coffee (not lattes) every day is OK. More than this increases risks, dependence and makes us more dehydrated.

TEA: 2-3 cups a day is fine. Green tea if we like it (if we don't we'll never do it regularly or get the benefits).

SOFT DRINKS: Never ever. Fresh fruit juices from whole fruit, not the processed stuff.

LOW-FAT MILK: to wet wholegrain cereal and if you add milk to your tea and coffee.

> Alcohol affects our sleep. While we may feel groggy, deep sleep and dream sleep are suppressed. This, along with the hangover, can make us grumpy and tired the next day.

> Alcohol blocks pathways normally used to retain water, so we pee more. For every standard drink, beyond normal losses, we lose about 150 mls of urine. Have at least one glass of water for every glass of alcohol. This is why most good restaurants have two glasses. It's not an either or thing, so use them both.

> Most alcohol is removed by the liver's detoxification systems, which use up B group vitamins in the process. Chronic drinking can therefore deplete our stores of essential nutrients like retinol, Vitamin C, and BETA-carotene.

> Alcohol is rich in calories. Drinking it adds to our calorie burden, manifested most graphically in the 'beer belly'.

There is no doubt that drinking too much is bad for us. Heavy drinkers have more heart disease, hypertension, dementia and some cancers (especially breast and colon cancer), quiet apart from its individual and social costs. Yet there are some drinking habits that are associated with improved health and longevity.

A moderate habit is associated with improved survival and a lower risk of heart attacks, strokes, heart failure, diabetes, and some cancers when compared to those who don't drink at all or drink only occasionally. This means less than four drinks per day for men and less than two per day for women, as women achieve higher concentrations of alcohol in the blood and become more impaired than men after drinking equivalent amounts of alcohol. The best outcomes are seen with a regular intake of half to one drink per day in both men and women.

Daily alcohol intake provides superior benefits, especially in men, compared with less frequent consumption, possibly because the effects of alcohol on metabolism are short-lived. Irregular heavy drinking bouts, even if accompanied by usual moderation can undo any benefits. Everyone should still have one or two alcohol-free days every week.

Alcohol is probably most beneficial (and less intoxicating) when consumed with a meal, away from sleep. This kind of drinking pattern can also be easier to regulate and the right bottle can also add significantly to the experience and flavour of a meal.

WHAT CONSTITUTES A STANDARD DRINK:
> WINE – 100MLS OR ABOUT 2/3RD OF A GLASS (12.5% ALCOHOL)
> SPIRITS – 30MLS OR ONE SHOT (40% ALCOHOL)
> BEER – ONE CAN OF MID STRENGTH BEER (3.5% ALCOHOL)

The benefits of a moderate alcohol intake are seen regardless of the beverage. However, red wine has some advantages over beer or spirits. One reason may be that lifestyle factors that permit a regular limited intake are more common with wine drinkers. In addition, red wine contains a number of antioxidants including resveratrol (see chapter 8). However, beer also contains antioxidants (eg. isohumulones from hops) some of which may better absorbed than those in wine. Light beers may have a number of advantages, as the potential for intoxication and abuse is reduced along with the alcohol content. Many also contain reduced calories, while retaining both flavor and flavanoids. By contrast, most spirits are largely devoid of phytonutrients, and are more readily abused. There is not enough evidence to suggest that non-drinkers should start drinking and there are many effective ways to get antioxidants into our diet, other than red wine and beer (see chapter 8).

COFFEE, COFFEE, COFFEE... (THE HEALTH BUZZ)

Coffee is the most widely-consumed stimulant in the world. Coffee was, and largely still is, viewed as a tonic with revitalising properties for the sick and the weary. However, coffee is not a health drink. It is clearly addictive and there are many better sources of phytonutrients. But what effects is the coffee fix having on our health?

In fact, the effects of coffee are mixed, probably because coffee is a complex mixture of different compounds from the bean as well as generated or excluded in the processes of fermentation, roasting and preparation. Some of these may be beneficial for human health, like vitamins, antioxidants and minerals. Others, like acrylamide and diterpene are noxious chemicals. Coffee beans grown using sustainable organic practices and in the absence of synthetic pesticides herbicides and fertilizers also have number of positives for the coffee drinker.

The most well known component is caffeine, the main stimulant in coffee. It acts by blocking receptors in the brain whose job it is to dull brain activity. So by preventing dulling, it stimulates. This may seem useful on Monday mornings or when we'd rather be in bed. But it also increases our blood pressure and metabolism, stiffens our arteries and makes us pee more. If we drink caffeine regularly, even as little as a cup a day, we can suffer withdrawal symptoms if we stop. The more coffee we drink, the more likely we will experience the need for a cup! Some of the feeling we get from our morning 'fix' of coffee is relief of this withdrawal.

Overall, a regular moderate intake of coffee (2-3 cups a day) does not appear to be harmful to health. Black coffee (not lattes) may slightly reduce the risk of heart disease, diabetes, Parkinson's disease, Alzheimer's disease, hip fracture and liver disease. For heart disease and diabetes, at least, this is not the caffeine, as the same benefits are also seen in those who drink decaffeinated coffee, especially when prepared in the absence of chemical solvents (e.g. the Swiss Water method). It could be that there is something about coffee drinkers that protects them (e.g. they have less stress in the mornings, the social ritual, or even the stress of daily withdrawal).

A NICE CUP OF TEA IN THE MORNING

Tea is second only to water in its global consumption. In western countries, the most widely drunk tea is black tea, prepared from leaves that have been fermented and oxidised. About half of the adult population drinks 2 to 3 cups a day. By contrast, oolong tea is partially oxidised and green tea is minimally processed before drying. This creates a range of different flavours, astringencies and caffeine content (which is generally greater the less processing). In each case, the tea leaf is then steeped in hot or boiling water to release the complex mixture of chemicals contained within.

The health properties of tea are readily confused with the stimulant effects of its caffeine content. Black teas contain about half the caffeine of most coffees, while many green teas contain more caffeine than coffee. Contained within the tea leaf are also a number of beneficial compounds including flavonoid antioxidants (catechins or tannins, vitamins and minerals. Some, but not all, of these are lost or transformed during prolonged drying and oxidization required to make to make the tea leaves black. Adding milk to black tea may also reduce the availability of antioxidants. Nonetheless, health benefits have been described in adults drinking 2-3 cups of black tea a day. For example, a regular cup of tea is associated with a small reduction in the risk of heart attacks and strokes. Tea drinking may also improve bone density and reduce the risk of fractures in women.

SOFT DRINKS HAVE NO PART IN A RATIONAL PLAN FOR SLOW AGEING.

Green teas have a greater antioxidant potential, and with it, potentially greater benefits for human health. A number of studies have shown that the intake of green tea is associated with reduced rates of some cancers, heart disease and cognitive decline with advancing age. It should be remembered to never brew green tea with boiling water, as this can damage some of its antioxidants, as well as increase the release of caffeine and other bitter tasting compounds. Because not everyone likes the taste or has time to drink three cups a day, extracts are available that can be taken in pill form, standardised to contain 80% total polyphenols and 55% epigallocatechin gallate (see chapter 8).

LIQUID CALORIES (SOFT DRINKS)

Soft drinks are a major source of excess calories, largely derived from high-fructose corn syrup. By displacing water that has no calories, soft drinks have significantly contributed to weight gain, obesity and diabetes. Unlike food calories, our body is not programmed to know when it has had enough energy from a drink. Drinking is driven by thirst not hunger. Soft drinks have no part in a rational plan for slow ageing.

Because of the well-known hazards of soft drink calories, many health conscious drinkers have embraced diet versions, which contain less or none of the calories contained in their fully sugared parents. In most cases, sugars are replaced with sweeteners such as aspartame or saccharin, which have no nutritional value. However, artificial sweeteners trigger responses that make us eat more. Most diet drinks are also acidic and will promote tooth decay. In addition most contain significant amounts of caffeine that increases blood pressure, stiffens our arteries, make us pee more and leads to dependency.

JUICES AND MILK

Juices carry some of the benefits of the fruits from which they are extracted, as well as all their potential hazards (like pesticides). A freshly prepared juice offers an excellent source of antioxidants, vitamins and minerals. A puree of whole fruit contains more essential nutrients and fibre than a squeeze of the same fruit. The benefits of juice appear to be greatest when taken with a meal, like breakfast, as the dietary fibre slows the absorption of fruit sugars and allows the antioxidants to peak at the right time, with a burst in metabolic activity that follows eating.

Most off-the-shelf fruit drinks have undergone a degree of processing that significantly diminishes their nutritional value. Though marketed as '100% juice' and a 'healthier alternative to soft drinks', these typically contain as many or more calories as soft drinks. In fact the sugars used in most soft drinks are the same as those in concentrated apple juice used in the bulk of fruit drinks. The regular consumption of high-calorie high-GI fruit drinks probably contributes to increased rate of diabetes and obesity both in adults and children.

Milk is a complex food designed for baby cows. It contains a range of essential nutrients (depending on the cow's diet or breed) which may have positive effects for human health. However, milk and cream also contain accumulated pesticides and saturated fat which adds to our cholesterol levels and our waistlines. Casein (dairy protein) intolerance can be the trigger for many atopic health conditions such as colic, eczema, asthma, chronic tonsillitis and dermatitis and if you suffer from any of these chronically see your nutritional doctor for more information. Many diet conscious individuals have embraced low fat milk. Diets that include low-fat milk have a slightly reduced risk of high blood pressure, heart disease, cancer, fracture risk and obesity. Avoiding milk altogether doesn't seem necessary. Those unable to drink milk because of lactose intolerance do not have better health or live longer.

OPTIONS TO OPTIMISE YOUR FLUID INTAKE

☑ Drink 500ml of water first thing in the morning to flush your digestive tract and rehydrate your system from the overnight dry

☑ Drink water at regular intervals throughout the day
> Set objectives such as drinking before you leave the house, and first thing upon your return, or before you start work
> Set your alarm so you have a drink every hour
> Have a glass of water each time you need a break from work

☑ Drink before meals (15 to 20 minutes before) or 1 to 3 hours after meals

☑ Drink when you are more active - whether that be mental or physical activity

☑ For clear thinking or more energy, take a sip of water

☑ Keep a bottle on the desk or carry one (preferably made of glass, stainless steel, HDPE or LDPE plastic)

☑ Add fresh squeezed juice to your water. You may see water as boring but drinking like ageing, must be a positive experience, not a chore!

GETTING THE ESSENTIALS
[VITAMINS & MINERALS]

Every cell in our body requires an optimal level of nutrition in order to function normally. Most people eat far too much. Yet even if we overeat, we can still fail to get enough of the important micronutrients that are essential to function and age normally. This is because many of the excess calories in our diets are empty calories, instead of being packed with the essential micronutrients (vitamins, minerals and other biochemicals) needed for optimal health and wellbeing. Even minor deficiencies can increase risk factors for major chronic diseases, such as heart disease, diabetes, cancer and osteoporosis.

The best way to make sure we get what we need is to consume the kind of balanced and varied diet described elsewhere in this book. People whose diets include highly processed foods with little fresh fruit and vegetables are likely to have an inadequate intake of many micronutrients.

RECOMMENDED DIETARY INTAKE

The Recommended Dietary Intake (RDI) is one way to check whether we are getting enough nutrients (see table at end of the chapter). RDIs are available on the nutritional content of most food labels. The RDI is the average daily dietary intake level that is sufficient to meet the nutrient requirements of 98% of healthy individuals. However, they are not the same as our individual requirements for health. The amount we need to minimise DNA damage or to be truly vibrant and healthy is sometimes much more than the RDI. RDIs also don't take into account conditions in which requirements may be higher. For example, higher nutrient intake is required by stress, living in polluted environments, active lifestyles, certain polymorphisms in genes or even when we have a cold, when our body cannot get or cannot efficiently use all the nutrients it needs.

Given these demands this is when we may benefit from nutritional supplements. Of course supplements, particularly multivitamins, are also widely used by people hoping to offset a poor diet. For an increasing number of people, multivitamins now constitute a substantial proportion of their total vitamin and mineral intake. However, regardless of any hype, a tablet can never provide the full complement of nutrients and phytochemicals of a varied diet. A poor diet should never be used as an excuse for supplementation.

THE ESSENTIAL VITAMINS

Vitamins are chemicals that are essential for good health. They cannot be generated in sufficient quantities by our body, so we must rely on our diet (or supplements) to get what we need. Vitamins act in all parts of the body with diverse functions, including antioxidant effects, regulation of growth and metabolism. Vitamins are broadly classified by their biological activities, so any one vitamin may refer to a family of different natural chemicals. Some of the most important vitamins are discussed below:

VITAMIN A

Vitamin A (retinol) is a family of natural antioxidants found in both plant and animal products. In plants, it is present in yellow, orange and red carotenoids, such as beta-carotene, which can be converted into Vitamin A during digestion. Vitamin A is high in liver, eggs and dairy, as well a range of dark green and orange-yellow fruit and vegetables, including carrots, broccoli leaves, kale, sweet potato, spinach, romaine lettuce, apricots and capsicum. Increased consumption of fruit and vegetables rich in Vitamin A is associated with lower oxidative damage. Fresh is always best, as Vitamin A is light and heat sensitive can be depleted from food during preparation, cooking or storage.

Vitamin A and beta-carotene are important natural antioxidants. Vitamin A maintains production of cells that divide and regenerate repeatedly, such as those in the skin, as well as the immune system. Vitamin A is also important for vision, particularly at night. Consuming less than the RDI can lead to dry eyes, poor night vision and increased susceptibility to some diseases. Too much Vitamin A (more than 3 mg) can lead to yellowing of the skin, damage to the liver or vision, and may increase the risk of hip fractures. It may also damage unborn babies and should not be used by pregnant women.

The most common Vitamin A supplement is beta-carotene. There are two kinds of beta-carotene supplements - those made from natural sources eg. palm oil,

VITAMIN A MAINTAINS
PRODUCTION OF
CELLS THAT DIVIDE
AND REGENERATE
REPEATEDLY, SUCH AS
THOSE IN THE SKIN.

algae and D. salina, and those manufactured synthetically (all trans beta-carotene). The naturally-sourced carotenes appear to have better antioxidant activity and less side-effects.

When used on its own in people with a normal diet, Vitamin A or betacarotene alone has not significantly improved survival rates or shown benefits for other age-related complications such as age-related blindness or cancer. In fact, some studies suggest that betacarotene when taken in excess may act to promote cancer formation and liver damage in some circumstances, such as for smokers, alcoholics and genetically predisposed individuals.

VITAMIN E

Vitamin E (α,β,γ and δ tocopherol) is a natural antioxidant found in leafy green vegetables, nuts and seeds, whole grains, fortified cereals and some vegetable oils. Many of the vegetable oils sold in supermarkets have had the Vitamin E removed during processing. As an antioxidant, it is particularly effective at scavenging free radicals, thereby preventing damage to lipids of our cell membranes and circulating fats. It also has significant effects on inflammation, immune function and fertility.

The standard daily Western diet contains 3 or 4 mg of Vitamin E, less than half the RDI. Vitamin E is available in supplement form from both synthetic and natural sources. The natural form is more potent and better absorbed and should be preferred over synthetic Vitamin E. Natural Vitamin E may be sold as alpha(α), beta(β), gamma(γ) and delta(δ) tocopherol. Although   is most abundant in food, supplements that contain 'mixed tocopherols' are emerging as the preferred form of Vitamin E supplements. When used on its own in clinical trials, alpha tocopherol has shown no beneficial effects in terms of heart attack, stroke, cataracts, cancer or longevity. Most clinical studies have used high dose supplements (50-500 mg per day). Such doses (>300mg) may also lead to headaches, fatigue and gastrointestinal upset.

VITAMIN C

Vitamin C (ascorbate) is a natural antioxidant found in fruit (such as citrus, currants, strawberries and tomatoes) and vegetables (such as Brassica and peppers). It is also found in high levels in liver, brain and oysters. Significant amounts of vitamin C are lost during storage and cooking of food, so fresh sources are best. Ascorbate is widely used as a food preservative, especially in processed juices.

Vitamin C is a non-specific antioxidant, with additional actions on a range of other systems, including hormone synthesis, wound healing and iron absorption.

Most healthy diets would include 3 or 4 times the RDI. Large doses of Vitamin C (up to 2 g) are generally well tolerated, although in some people doses above this range may result in nausea or diarrhoea. This can be lessened by using a buffered form of Vitamin C, such as calcium or other mineral ascorbates (which also hang around for longer in the blood than garden variety vitamin C) or a Vitamin C 'mix' that combines Vitamin C with chlorophyll, hesparin, rutin and other bioflavonoids.

Diets naturally rich in ascorbate are associated with reduced illness and longevity. Short-term supplementation with Vitamin C has been shown to have a number of health-giving effects, including beneficial actions on vascular and immune function. High-dose Vitamin C supplementation can also reduce the severity and duration of symptoms of cold and flu. At this time, trials with Vitamin C supplements have shown no long-term benefits on longevity, cancer risk, heart disease or other age-related complications.

VITAMIN B12

Vitamin B12 (cyanocobalamin) only comes from animal products, such as meat, poultry, fish, eggs and milk. Because plants cannot make B12, strict vegetarians must take supplements or fortified foods to stay healthy (or alternatively soften their stance and include dairy products in their diet). The absorption and processing of B12 in the human body is complex, involving the combined functions of healthy saliva, stomach and intestinal functions, and subsequent storage in a healthy liver. Consequently, the absorption of Vitamin B12 is precarious and often impaired, as we get older.

Vitamin B12 is important for healthy functioning and ageing. It has a key role in the synthesis of DNA and fat, which it shares with folate. In fact, many of the functions of Vitamin B12 can still be performed if sufficient folate is present. However, even when folate levels are adequate, reduced B12 levels can lead to fatigue, depression, cognitive decline and possibly cancer. And if folate levels are low (usually because the diet is low in fruit, leafy vegetables or legumes), the effects of even minor reductions in Vitamin B12 levels are magnified.

Vitamin B12 levels are easy to measure in the blood. Concentrations under 160 pmol/L are thought to indicate deficiency. Borderline-low levels may also be significant if folate levels are also low, or in the presence of high blood levels of methylmalonic acid or homocysteine, both of which are normally metabolised by B12 dependent enzymes. Using this criteria, 5% to 20% of all adults will develop B12 deficiency during their lifetime. However, waiting for this deficiency to occur is not an option. If more than a year of low levels has passed, any damage is generally permanent, although further decline may be slowed. Preventative supplementation is a much better alternative.

A number of supplements are available, including oral crystalline B12 and injectable forms. There are no side-effects with increased intake of B12, so some ageing specialists recommend taking an oral B12 supplement (2.4 µg/d) every day from age 50. This amount can be found in most B-group supplements, or in fortified foods such as cereals. A regular intake of low fat grass fed meat, like kangaroo, also does the trick. Bigger doses are needed to correct an established B12 deficiency. Taking folate at the same time may also be useful, so take your 'roo with a salad.

FOLATE

Folate (folic acid, Vitamin B9) is an important regulator of metabolism. As the name suggests, it is highest in the foliage of leafy vegetables, such as spinach and lettuce. It is also found in legumes, whole grain cereals, seeds, many fruits and 'Vegemite'. Many baking products and breakfast cereals have also been fortified with folate. As a result, most diets contain the recommended RDI of 400 µg per day. Higher levels may be required in some circumstances, such as pregnant women or alcoholics.

Folate supplements (up to 1mg per day) have useful effects in the ageing body. Folate supplements have positive actions on short-term memory and mental agility. Increasing our intake of folate, Vitamin B12 or Vitamin B6 will lower our levels of homocysteine, a risk marker for heart disease. While there is no evidence that this translates to fewer heart attacks, some improvements have been observed in people taking folate supplements, including lower blood pressure. While diets naturally high in folate are associated with a lower risk of some cancers, these benefits have not been seen in people taking folate supplements. We should never take folate supplements if our B12 levels are low, as this can exacerbate the problem.

VITAMIN B6

Vitamin B6 (pyridoxine) is an essential regulator of metabolism, nerve function and gene expression, acting as a cofactor for many of the key enzymes in the body.

Vitamin B6 is found in many foods, including meat, poultry, fish, whole grain products, vegetables, beans and nuts. Cooking, storage and processing results in significant loss of Vitamin B6, so fresh is always best. Too much alcohol or coffee may deplete our Vitamin B6 stores (but supplements are not the answer to this problem). However, a standard diet usually contains three to four times the RDI, so deficiency is almost never seen.

Vitamin B6 supplements (up to 50mg per day) have been popular for the treatment of a diverse range of conditions, including heart disease, cognitive decline, hangovers and PMS. There is no evidence that it significantly benefits any of these conditions. However, for people with a certain genetic pattern, B6 supplements may reduce the risk of some cancers.

TOO MUCH ALCOHOL OR COFFEE MAY DEPLETE OUR VITAMIN B6 STORES.

VITAMIN K

Vitamin K is essential for the normal clotting of blood, as well as bone and joint metabolism. Most comes from our gut bacteria in the form of Vitamin K2. Keeping our intestines healthy with a diet rich in fibre and low in overcooked animal protein and fat is the best way to keep up our Vitamin K supplies. People who have problems with their intestines may become more dependent on their diet for Vitamin K.

Because our gut bacteria do such a good job, the RDI for Vitamin K is small, equivalent to a daily teaspoon of fresh parsley. Other good dietary sources of Vitamin K1 include leafy green vegetables, Brassica, avocado and kiwi fruit. Vitamin K2 is found in meat, eggs and dairy products, so vegetarians must rely on their gut or supplements.

Even in otherwise healthy individuals, a good dietary intake of Vitamin K is associated with a lower risk of bone fractures and some cancers, especially in postmenopausal women. Some studies have suggested supplements containing Vitamin K2 (but not K1) may also have beneficial effects on bone and other health parameters.

VITAMIN D

Vitamin D is not a true vitamin as we can make all we need by getting adequate sun exposure. However, if we are not getting regular sun exposure, we depend on our diet (or supplements) to maintain our levels. Oily fish, such as herring, are naturally rich in Vitamin D. Vitamin D is also widely available in fortified products such as cereals, bread and milk. However, we don't have to consume any Vitamin D in our diet. Even 10 minutes of sunshine twice a week provides more Vitamin D than eating fish every day.

Even in sunny states, over half of all retirees have suboptimal levels of Vitamin D due to a combination of reduced exposure to sunlight and declining metabolic function of the skin, liver and kidneys. This accelerates bone thinning and loss of muscle strength, and contributes to aches and pains. Vitamin D deficiency may also exacerbate several age-related diseases, including diabetes cardiovascular disease and some cancers.

A simple blood test can measure our stores of Vitamin D. In those not exposed to sunlight or eating fortified foods, a regular dose of Vitamin D3 (10µg) is usually sufficient to maintain healthy levels. A number of supplements contain an inactive form of Vitamin D, which can be activated by the body when needed. These include Vitamin D2 (from plants or yeast), which is less potent than Vitamin D3 (from animal sources), so it needs to be given in three times higher doses to achieve the same effect. Eg 10µg of Vitamin D3 is equivalent to 30µg of Vitamin D2. Vitamin D should always be taken in combination with calcium supplements for increased calcium intake.

VITAMIN B1

Vitamin B1 (thiamine) is a family of chemicals that plays an essential role in metabolism and heart and brain function. Most thiamine in our diets comes from cereal grains. However, processing and refining, which removes the germ, reduces the thiamine content of cereal tenfold.

Thiamine deficiency can be seen in those with a poor diet or chronic disease such as alcoholism or diabetes, which increases the body's demand for thiamine. In these cases, supplements may have useful effects to maintain heart and cognitive functions.

In otherwise healthy individuals, thiamine supplements have not been shown to have any reproducible effects. This is possible because excess thiamine is lost rapidly into the urine. For the same reason an upper limit of safety has not been possible to define. Benfotiamine, a form of thiamine that accumulates better, may prove more useful and has been shown to reduce AGE levels (see chapter 10).

VITAMIN B2

Vitamin B2 (riboflavin) is another B-group vitamin that is essential for growth and metabolism. It is orange-yellow in colour and is the main reason why our urine turns bright yellow after taking multivitamins. It is highest in green leafy vegetables, legumes, bananas, eggs, dairy products, meat and Vegemite. However, it is destroyed by exposure to light, so the shorter it has been left on the shelf, the higher its levels. Riboflavin is widely used to fortify foods such as cereals, fruit and energy drinks.

Because any excess is lost in urine, rather than stored, we must replenish it every day. Consequently, it is easy to become deficient in riboflavin with poor dietary choices. Typically this results in cracked lips, a red and painful tongue, or dry skin and eyes. In men, B2 deficiency is one reason for an itchy scrotum. The long-term implications of deficiency in adults are unclear. Supplements also have an important role in women by improving the response to iron supplements and in helping prevent cataracts.

VITAMIN B3

Vitamin B3 (niacin) is a family of compounds essential to the body for energy metabolism, DNA repair and mental function. Niacin is widely found in a normal diet, including meat, grains, dairy, fruit and vegetables. In Western society, deficiency is only seen in those who, for whatever reason, eat little or nothing.

Niacin supplements are able to lower bad (LDL) cholesterol and increase good (HDL) cholesterol. However, in some people, these high doses (1 - 6g/day) can cause flushing, skin problems and gastrointestinal upset. Taking an aspirin half an hour before, or using a sustained release preparation can lessen this.

VITAMIN B5

Vitamin B5 (panthothenate) is another B-group vitamin that is essential to metabolise carbohydrates, proteins and fats for their energy. B5 is found in almost every food, with the highest amounts in whole grain/bran, legumes, eggs and meat. Because it is so prevalent and healthy gut bacteria can also make some for us, deficiency is rare. Many multivitamins contain B5 in doses up to 2g per day, which is many times the RDI. Again most is lost into the urine. However, in these high doses, B5 has been reported to lower cholesterol levels and reduce stress and joint stiffness. None of these claims have been validated.

A number of minerals (or trace elements) are also essential requirements for well-being. Only very small quantities of minerals are needed (generally less than 100 ug/day), but any deficiency can have a profound effect on health.

IRON

Iron is essential for good health. It is a key component of haemoglobin, the molecule that delivers oxygen around our body and provides the energy we need to function. It is so important that our body has ways of storing iron so it doesn't suddenly run out. Nevertheless, a shortage of iron is the most common mineral deficiency, affecting nearly a third of adult Australians, especially women. By reducing our energy levels, low iron levels impact on all aspects of performance and quality of life, from exercise and thinking, to sleep.

It is recommended that men take more than 8 mg of iron per day, and menstruating women take more than twice this amount (18mg). However, partly due to our intake of empty calories, at least a third of adults do not consume anywhere near enough. Yet iron is found in many foods. It is highest in liver, red meat, fish and poultry, as well as legumes and green leafy vegetables such as spinach (hence the energy of Popeye).

Absorption of iron from our diet is inefficient, especially from plant sources, and less than a quarter is absorbed. This means that vegetarians need almost twice as much dietary iron per day than meat-eaters. Combining foods rich in Vitamin C with foods rich in iron can boost iron absorption e.g. squeezing some lemon juice over beans or salad. A number of foods, especially cereals, are also fortified with iron.

Iron supplements are widely taken by women, often as part of a women's multivitamin. Supplemental iron is generally available as ferrous and ferric salts, with ferrous being the best absorbed (especially ferrous fumarate). Commencing iron supplementation can sometimes cause gastrointestinal upset, which may be off-putting. This can be minimised by taking iron chelates, dividing the dose, taking it with food or starting with a small dose and gradually building up. This requirement for individual flexibility is the major limitation of most generic multivitamin products.

CALCIUM

Calcium is a key regulator of many of the body's functions. Brain, muscle and nerve activity all depend on calcium levels remaining constant, so blood concentrations are kept under tight control throughout our lives. Whether we drink milk or not, our levels hardly budge. This is achieved by having an enormous store that can release or absorb large amounts of calcium according to our body's needs. This store is bone. If calcium in our diet is insufficient to offset normal losses in urine, bone is broken down to retrieve its calcium. Conversely, if calcium intake is increased, bone manufacture occurs and more calcium is deposited as insurance against hard times.

It is recommended that we all consume more than 1g of calcium per day. Most of us consume far less. Calcium can be obtained from dairy products, as well as seaweed, nuts, seeds, legumes and green leafy vegetables. Many products are also fortified with calcium, including orange juice and soy milk.

The ability to get the most out of the calcium in our diet is critically dependent on our levels of Vitamin D, so most people who take supplements use these in combination. Alternatively, we can grow our greens in the sunshine of our own garden to get both for free. Other simple things we can do to keep calcium in our bones includes reducing excessive intake of salt, caffeine and alcohol, thus reducing the loss of calcium into urine. Soluble fibre in our diet can also improve calcium absorption.

THE ABILITY TO GET THE MOST OUT OF CALCIUM IN OUR DIET IS CRITICALLY DEPENDENT ON OUR LEVELS OF VITAMIN D, SO MOST PEOPLE WHO TAKE SUPPLEMENTS USE THESE IN COMBINATION.

Inadequate calcium intake is associated with an increased risk of osteoporosis, hypertension and some cancers in later life. For those not getting enough calcium in their diet, a range of supplements is available. These are best taken with food and spread throughout the day, rather than all at once, to get the best absorption. The various supplements contain different amounts of elemental calcium, so we need to be careful to read the label and adjust the dose to achieve 1- 2g per day.

Some supplements can cause constipation or bloating, particularly those predominantly comprised of calcium carbonate. As a cheap alternative to supplements, a pinch of finely ground eggshell into meals will also do the trick. Hydroxyapatite is widely marketed as a 'bone-building' supplement. It is essentially ground bone. Hydroxyapatite is an excellent source of calcium and a good way to maintain bone mass. It may also contain other chemical elements and toxins that can accumulate in bone, so choose a product that has been fully tested and certified, or is definitively toxin-free.

ZINC

Zinc is essential for growth, metabolism, detoxification and healing. Yet 75% of Australians don't receive their RDI of zinc. This is more of a problem because, unlike iron, we do not store zinc in our bodies, so we need a daily fix to maintain our levels.

The best sources are seafood (oysters, crab, lobster), meat and poultry. Many cereals and other products are fortified with zinc. Although whole grains, legumes and nuts contain lesser amounts of zinc, fibre in plants may partially inhibit zinc absorption, so strict vegetarians need to take twice as much zinc in a vegetarian diet. Other groups at high risk of low zinc levels include alcoholics and those with digestive diseases.

Low levels of zinc can lead to lethargy, delayed healing of wounds and increased susceptibility to infection. Zinc concentrations are correlated with sperm-count, with the lowest zinc concentrations found in infertile men. When zinc levels are low, our sense of taste and smell may also be impaired. This principle is utilised in the simple zinc taste test in which a dilute solution of zinc sulphate is used to test our sense of taste. If an immediate, strong and unpleasant taste is experienced, then our levels are OK. But if the response is not immediate or we don't taste anything it could indicate low zinc levels.

Zinc is widely used in multivitamins, as well as over-the-counter preparations that reduce the duration and severity of cold symptoms. These are fine to maintain our levels. However, correcting deficiency may take a higher dose than can be provided by ordinary supplements, due to zinc blockade (where low zinc levels impairs the absorption of all minerals).

The effect of zinc supplements on ageing is unclear, although some studies suggest that supplements may reduce the risk of oesophageal cancer and age-related damage to the retina.

MAGNESIUM

Magnesium is a key regulator of the body, supporting the function of muscles, bones, the immune system, brain and heart. Like calcium, the body tries to keep magnesium levels constant, storing any excess in the bone, from where it can be released if dietary intake is inadequate. And this is often the case. Two out of every three adults do not reach the RDI, through diets low in the best sources of magnesium including green leafy vegetables, legumes, nuts and whole grains.

Low levels of magnesium can lead to weakness and lethargy, cramps and low mood. There is some suggestion that magnesium supplements can reduce the risk of diabetes, hypertension, heart disease and osteoporosis in those at increased risk of these conditions. Magnesium can also be a potent laxative (e.g. milk of magnesia). Good supplements containing chelates won't have this effect.

SELENIUM

Selenium is a natural component of many of the body's enzymes, including the antioxidant defence enzymes. High levels of selenium are found in meat, tuna and eggs. Plants grown in selenium-rich soil (some regions in some countries) contain increased levels of selenium, especially wheat germ, nuts (particularly Brazil nuts), turnips, garlic and oranges.

Although most adults have sufficient selenium for their metabolic functions, supplementation (even in non-deficient people) has been shown to increase natural antioxidant activity and boost immunity and thyroid function. In clinical studies, selenium supplements have been shown to reduce the risk of some cancers and improve overall survival.

IODINE

Iodine is an essential trace mineral that is important for the function of the thyroid gland, which regulates the body's metabolic rate. Most of the iodine we get from our diet comes from the sea (fish or seaweed) or iodised table salt. If we don't eat any seafood or salt, it is easy to fall below the RDI. Too little iodine can lead to fatigue, cognitive decline, depression, weight gain or increased size of the thyroid as it tries to compensate. Iodine deficiency may also contribute to an increased risk of breast cancer. Most multivitamins contain at least 200ug of iodine.

CHROMIUM

Chromium is an important factor in the regulation of sugar and fat metabolism. Levels are highest in meat, whole grain products, fruit and vegetables, especially brassica such as broccoli. As with iron, absorption of chromium is assisted by Vitamin C. Deficiency is rare since most adults get their RDI from a normal diet. However, high sugar levels, regular exercise, stress and ageing can all increase chromium losses, which need to be offset by increased chromium intake.

The impact of deficiency on health and ageing is controversial. It has been suggested that chromium supplements may promote weight loss, enhance energy and lower lipid and sugar levels in the blood, although none of these claims are proven.

SHOULD WE BE TAKING MULTIVITAMINS?

It is possible to get all the vitamins and minerals we need by replacing energy dense, nutrient-poor foods and drinks with a fresh and balanced diet, not to mention innumerable other positive effects on health and well-being that cannot be provided by supplements. People who eat very few fruits and vegetables should not see supplements as a solution. Nor should taking supplements mean we don't need to take care of our diet.

Far from being a panacea, multivitamins are best used as an adjunct to a good diet. Multivitamins are easiest and most widely available source of all the vitamins and minerals required for health. There a number of different formulations and most contain the RDI for Vitamin A, B1, B2, B3, B5, B6, B9, C, D3, E and K1, as well as a range of different minerals, with or without iron. This means there is less to think about, allowing us to focus on our food choices (especially lessening our calories) without being tied up in recommended intakes. Not all micronutrients can be found in fruit and vegetables, while meat and dairy is not an option for many. A regular multivitamin takes up the slack.

If it is not possible to eat a variety of healthy foods (e.g. special diets, food intolerance/allergies) or if we have restricted our calorie intake to the point where our nutrient intake falls, then dietary supplements can be an important way to maintain optimal levels.

Many essential nutrients are not stored in the human body and must be replenished every day. While establishing and maintaining a healthy diet solves this issue, sometimes we need a little help. Let's be realistic, multivitamins are the most practical way to cover all our bases today and offer increased freedom for making eating choices, without having to chase the RDI every day.

Multivitamins also provide cover for times of extra need. For example, multivitamins are widely used the day-after a night of excess, when our B vitamins are depleted while metabolising alcohol and passing more urine. The same can be said about the ageing body, which needs more help to get the job done. Equally increased levels of activity also have additional nutritional requirements for its benefits to be fully realised.

Some argue that only people with an established deficiency should take supplements. However, waiting for this deficiency to occur is like waiting to become unwell before doing something about it. In some cases, like that of low B12 levels, by the time we realise we are deficient; the adverse effects may be permanent.

Preventative approaches are a much better alternative than simply reactive ones. And again regular multivitamins are the most straightforward means for prevention.

The current evidence suggests that regular supplementation with one or a range of different vitamins and minerals in motivated individuals without deficiency has no overall benefits in preventing cancer, heart disease or other age-related phenomena. But this does not mean multivitamins can't work to maintain quality of life, health and well-being. Every woman knows how lethargic she feels when her iron stores are low. No trial has shown that iron supplements make women live longer or prevent cancer, but that doesn't mean they don't work. The same may be said for multivitamin supplements. Even though nutritional supplements have not been proven to slow the aging process or extend life, there is enough scientific evidence to support that they might have this ability, particular when are diets provide inadequate supplies. Who has the time to wait and see whether generational studies will show what we have been missing?

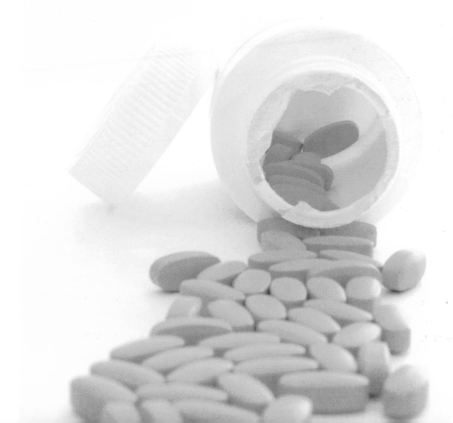

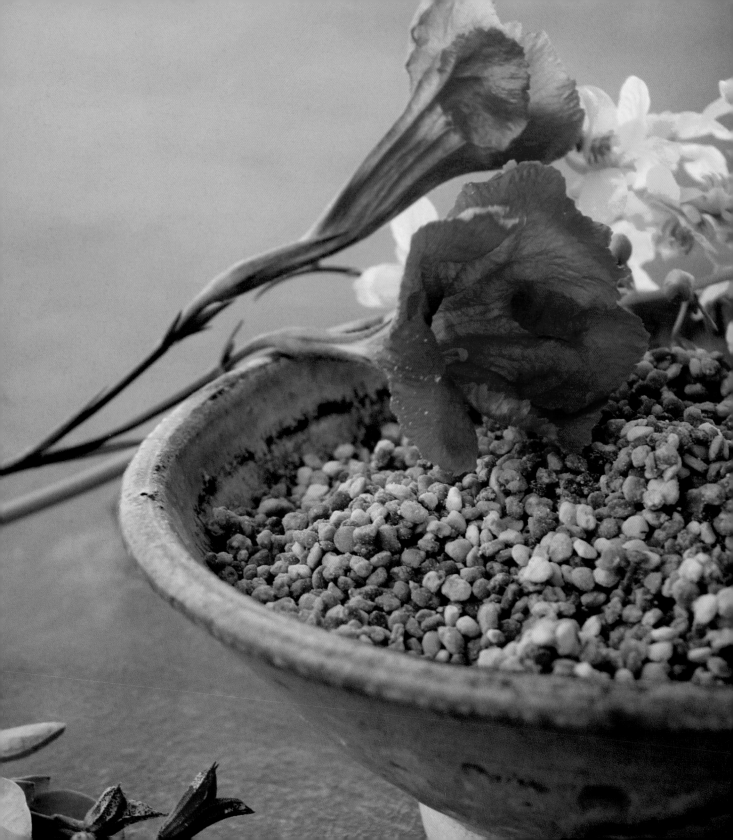

SUGGESTED INTAKE OF KEY ESSENTIAL NUTRIENTS FOR ADULTS

Vitamin	RDI (Men)	Dietary Target	RDI (Women)	Dietary Target	Upper Limit
Vitamin A	900µg	1,500µg	700µg	1,220µg	3,000mg
Vitamin B1 (thiamine)	1.2mg	2.5-5mg	1.1mg	2.5-5mg	not defined
Vitamin B2 (riboflavin)	1.3mg	5-10mg	1.1mg	5-10mg	not defined
Vitamin B3 (niacin)	16mg	16mg	14mg	14mg	35mg
Vitamin B5 (panthothenate)	6mg	10-100mg	4mg	10-100mg	not defined
Vitamin B6 (pyridoxine)	1.7mg	10-20mg	1.3mg	10-20mg	50mg
Vitamin B12 (cyanocobalamin)	2.4µg	5-10µg	2.4µg	5-10µg	not defined
Folic Acid	400µg	600µg	400µg	600µg	1,000µg
Vitamin C	45mg	220mg	45mg	190mg	not defined
Vitamin D (cholecalciferol)	10µg	sun dependent	10µg	sun dependent	80µg
Vitamin E (d-alpha-tocopherol)	10mg	20mg	7mg	14mg	300mg
Vitamin K	70µg	120µg	60µg	90µg	not defined
Mineral	RDI (Men)	Dietary Target	RDI (Women)	Dietary Target	Upper Limit
Iron	8mg	15mg	18mg	30mg	45mg
Calcium	1,000mg	1,200mg	1,000mg	1,200mg	3,500mg
Zinc	14mg	20mg	8mg	20mg	40mg
Magnesium	420mg	420mg	320mg	320mg	350mg
Chromium	35µg	50-100µg	25µg	50-100µg	not defined
Iodine	150µg	200µg	150µg	200µg	1,100µg
Selenium	70µg	100-200µg	60µg	100-200µg	200µg

*Intake above these levels will be required to correct deficiency or deal with additional specific needs.

Regular intake above this level may place you at risk of side-effects. This threshold will be lower in some individuals, depending on their tolerance, metabolism and other factors.

8 SIMPLE STRATEGIES TO MAKE IT HAPPEN
[A SLOW AGEING DIET]

Do we eat on the run? Or only when we have moment to spare? Do we eat when stressed, tired or grumpy. Did we actually notice what we were eating or did we eat whatever is on hand? Do we eat in a disruptive environment or while doing other things (e.g. watching TV, working, studying etc).

This is what is really meant by fast food. It's opposite is SLOW, and is what this book is all about - taking the time to become engaged with our diet and our choices as though they matter. In any diet there is a lot to think about! There are the calories and the composition. There are the fats and proteins, sugars and fibre. There are the vitamins and other nutrients. So how do we arrive at slow and healthy diet?

STRATEGY 1: FRESH IS BEST (UNPROCESSED IS BETTER)

A healthy diet is generally one that results in us eating more fresh food. If we follow it, and stick to it, a diet high in fresh produce is always associated with a healthier and longer life.

But there is fresh, and then there is really fresh. The nutrients in fresh food convey their health-giving properties. Consequently, the greatest benefits can be achieved when those nutrients are at their highest. The more transportation, handling, storage and processing is involved, the lower the nutrient levels of food. Nutrient losses occur with every freeze and thaw cycle (transported in the back of your car, leaving the packet out, etc) and even more nutrients are lost during cooking.

> The best way to buy and store fruit and vegetables is whole. Buying freshly-cut fruit and vegetables may seem an attractive option, but only if you're ready to eat them. Cutting them up and exposing their contents to light results in the loss of nutritional properties. The less processed a food is, the higher the nutritional value.

> Only buy fresh what you can eat within the next five days. When you run out, walk to the shop and buy some more. Exercise and nutrition at the same time!

> Eat as soon as possible after purchase. The longer we leave it, the more likely it will lose nutrients. Putting it in the fridge slows this process, but does not stop it.

> Choose your fruit and vegetables carefully. We normally have a wide range, so be picky. Choose the freshest of the fresh. Any outward sign that it is past its prime usually means that its nutrients are also past their prime! Buy early in the day from a local farmers market that brings in fresh produce. Arriving early means we get the pick of the bunch and cooler temperatures means the food stays fresher for longer. If we have a long drive home, keep an esky in our car for storage and grab an ice pack before we leave home. In our hot climate, the car trip home can wilt many vegies and damage their nutrients.

> Fruit and vegies should be stored in different drawers because ripe fruit releases chemicals that cause some vegies to lose their nutrients quicker.

> Frozen foods are not devoid of benefits. Frozen vegetables are often nutritionally better than so called 'fresh' produce imported out-of-season from distant climates. In fact, carotenes, which are sensitive to light, are preserved better in the dark of a freezer than exposed to light on a pantry shelf. This is why frozen peas may have more carotene than fresh peas from the shelf. Overall, the level of nutrients is about the same for both frozen and off-the-shelf vegetables, although both have lost more nutrients than truly fresh produce. But any vegetables are better than no vegetables. Having fruit and vegetables ready to eat in your refrigerator, rather than ice cream, may make it easier for us to make healthy choices.

A simple way to make the most of any produce is to remember the SLOW foods acronym:

"Slow foods ® are those that are Seasonal, Local, Organic and Whole."

Foods that are in season are more likely to be fresh and thus richer in nutrients. Where possible, buy local produce, which has normally been subject to less storage and handling. Imported food may look peachy, but it has probably been on the road a lot longer.

Modern farming techniques involve the use of synthetic herbicides, fungicides, insecticides and other chemicals to increase crop yields or quality. Nearly two out of every three products on the supermarket shelf contains pesticide residue. The highest levels are often seen in foods that are considered healthy, such as juices and fresh fruit and vegetables, especially strawberries, stone-fruit, tomatoes, lettuce and capsicum. Organic food (grown without hazardous chemicals) often has 20% to 40% greater nutrient content than non-organic products (and are usually grown locally with minimal processing and handling). The greater concentrations of phytochemicals in organic food not only contribute to wellbeing, they also often improve the flavour. In addition, organic farming is better for the environment and involves more sustainable farming practices.

Simple tips for switching to organic produce include:

> Substitute those foods that often have the highest chemical residue. The ones to think about are strawberries, capsicums, stone-fruit such as apricots, cherries and peaches, spinach and lettuce, grapes, carrots, apples and pears, celery and green beans.

> Substitute those foods that we eat the most often e.g. dairy products, eggs, meat, poultry.

> Substitute those packaged goods in your pantry e.g. cereals, rice, pasta, canned legumes.

STRATEGY 2: ENERGY-DENSE FOODS MAY SINK US FASTER

In the human body, excess calories are converted into fat. Limiting our energy intake has a range of effects that help slow ageing, not least of which is avoiding becoming overweight. In any successful diet, there must be a way to control calories, while maintaining a nutritionally-rich intake of vitamins, minerals, antioxidants and other valuable elements.

SLOW FOODS® ARE THOSE FOODS THAT ARE SEASONAL LOCAL ORGANIC AND WHOLE.

One trick is to try to exchange your intake of foods that are essentially concentrated calories (so-called 'energy-dense' foods) for foods that have fewer calories, yet just as many nutrients. The goal is to make excess calories harder to obtain, so every mouthful contains less energy. Typical energy-dense foods are often dry (e.g. chips, biscuits, confectionary, cereals), although soft drinks and fruit drinks are notable exceptions to this rule. Fat is also twice as energy-dense as sugar or protein, so the same amount of fat counts twice as much towards weight gain. Even a small quantity of food rich in fat, like a piece of cheese has a higher energy content when compared to the same size of grapes.

We can reduce our calorie intake simply by substituting foods that are less energy-dense. It is possible to eat the same volume of food and yet consume significantly less calories. Less energy-dense foods are generally low-fat and rich in fibre and water, such as fresh fruit and non-starchy vegetables or soups. Many of these foods can be served in portion sizes that still make us feel full, while adding less to energy accrual. We might think that eating low-energy foods would just make us hungrier, but this is not true. If we reduce the energy density of your food by 25%, we reduce our energy intake by a similar amount. As a result, adults who regularly eat fruit, vegetables and other foods with reduced energy density have a lower risk of weight gain as they age.

Another trick is to limit access. Sometimes we eat simply because food is there! This does not mean having a house devoid of food, it means ensuring it is easier to access fruit and harder to get to the ice cream, sweets, biscuits and chips. Plan our environment and make it easier for us and our familes to get into good habits.

Another way to get the most out of low-energy food is to eat a portion of soup or salad as a first course to enhance satisfaction and reduce overeating during the rest of the meal. But a word of caution - the ingredients matter. Once calories start being added (some cheese, bread and egg, etc), the energy content of a first course can quickly climb.

Nowadays most food labels list energy density (measured as kJ/g), along with other nutrient contents. For example, the energy in a packet of nacho chips is around 2,000 kj/100g (almost the same as butter – and we'd never eat 100g of butter in one sitting!), while most fruit and vegetables are less that 400 kj/100g. When we're starting out, don't radically change our diet. Just take the time to read the labels and choose ones that have low density.

STRATEGY 3: (S)LOW AND STEADY WINS THE RACE

Slow works for ageing. It also works for digestion and metabolism. Fast food generally means fast calories and a fast track to energy excess and weight gain. Fast foods are over-processed, overcooked and poor in nutrients and fibre. One way to a slow diet is to avoid fast food.

 But there is even more we can do. When we eat any food, it must be digested and absorbed. If this can be slowed, it takes a load off our system and reduces the chances of burnout with age, e.g. diabetes. One way to slow is to spread our meals out, allowing our body to deal with the calories in its own time. Although this works for most people, if some people suddenly start eating multiple courses (particularly if they are also high in calories), they can quickly start to put on weight. An alternative approach for these people is to eat foods that deliver their nutrients at a slow pace.

This can be better appreciated by considering how quickly a food causes a rise in our blood sugar or Glycemic index (GI). Low-GI foods (< 55) are slow foods.

They deliver their sugar load more slowly, so our sugar levels remain steadier. These foods are less likely to contribute to production of fat. High-GI foods (> 70) are fast foods that break down their sugars quickly during digestion. Refined sugars need very little digestion, resulting in a rapid rise in our blood sugar level, and the foods that contain them (soft drink, icing, etc) have a high-GI. The GI of our diet is strongly associated with our risk of heart disease, diabetes and obesity, so reducing our load by switching to low-GI foods is a simple way to reduce these risks. Low-GI foods also make us feel full and keep us satisfied and sustained for longer. Many foods now carry the GI symbol. An improved version of the glycemic index incorporates both the GI level and the sugar quantity or Glycemic load (GL). The GL of our meal or daily diet correlates with the effort required to keep our metabolism in check, so if we keep our GL low, we also keep the work of our metabolism at manageable levels and better preserve it for the long-term.

Another simple way to slow digestion and absorption is to include more fibre in our diet. Fibre transforms the contents of our intestines into a gel that releases its nutrients gradually and completely. Most diets contain too little fibre because we don't eat enough fruit and vegetables and the cereals and grains we consume are often heavily refined. Just by replacing refined products with wholegrain equivalents, without even changing our diet, we can more than double our intake of total and soluble fibre. By mixing wholegrain products with our meal (eg. bran with cornflakes), we can feel full sooner (thereby eating less corn flakes) and reduce our GI to more manageable levels.

STRATEGY 4: MAKING THE MOST OF EVERY MOUTHFUL

We have to eat. So when we are eating, why not make the most of a great opportunity? Many foods contain what are known as 'empty calories'. These are calories that give us energy, but few other nutrients. Soft drinks, sweets and snacks rich in processed fats and carbohydrate (ie. high-energy foods) are classic examples.

On the other hand, some foods are 'nutrient-dense' and deliver a complete nutritional package. If we want to stick to our plan of limiting calorie intake while maintaining a balanced diet, we need to reconnect nutrients with calories and substitute empty-calorie foods with nutrient-dense foods.

Fruit and vegetables, whole grains, nuts and seeds all provide substantial amounts of nutrients (known as phytonutrients) and generally fewer calories. But it is not just plants that have nutrients. Lean meat is more nutrientdense than mince. Low-fat yoghurt is more nutrient-dense than full-cream milk. These foods give us more return for every calorie, so are worth the investment. When we choose foods based on nutrient-density, we will find it's much easier to achieve a better diet.

Actions to slow your mealtime down:

> Plan your meals in advance so that they aren't last minute
> Turn off the TV
> Take the time to cook and savour a meal
> Take 10 minutes out before you eat to relax and prepare your body for receiving nourishment – practice breathing, do a mini meditation or just involve yourself in the cooking process
> Sit down at the table and eat with your family
> Remember to chew and taste your food (and complement the chef)

STRATEGY 5: PHYTOCHEMICALS FOLLOW THE RAINBOW

All plant products - fruit, vegetables, nuts, grains, legumes and seeds - contain a number of chemicals (phytochemicals), some of which have been shown to have beneficial properties for health and ageing.

However, plants are more than the sum of their known phytonutrients. Individually, none of these components can wholly explain the benefits acquired from eating at least five serves of fruit and vegetables per day. This is why a good diet beats a handful of tablets every time – the combination of different elements in food; the attention and commitment to a dietaryregimen; and certainly more tasty and probably cheaper too. And most of all, because it works, and has done for centuries.

Rather than only looking for lycopenes or favouring flavonoids, a simple way to make sure we access all the phytochemicals we need is to follow the rainbow. Look to fill your diet with every bright colour of the rainbow every day.

> Red - lycopenes and ellagic acid.
> Orange and deep yellow - high in beta-carotene. (The darker the colour, the more beta-carotene).
> Dark green - vegetables that contain lutein and zeaxanthin.
> Blue, purple and dark red - flavonoids, including berries.
> Green, white and purple - cruciferous vegetables are high in sulphurous phytochemicals. The same colours in legumes indicate lignins.

INCREASE THE VARIETY OF FOODS WE EAT

Many of us get into the habit of eating the same foods - day in, day out. If we routinely find ourselves eating iceberg lettuce, try some new varieties, such as rocket or baby spinach. Instead of potato, try a different colour – maybe sweet potato or pumpkin.

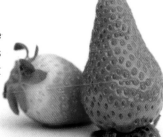

Which phytochemical?	What are they good for?	Where from?	How much? How to prepare?
Flavonoid: Anthrocyanidins, especially Cyanidin	Very strong antioxidants, improve insulin sensitivity, anti-inflammatory in arthritis, protect against skin cancer from UV radiation	The skins of red-coloured berries, apples, pears, peaches, plums, dark chocolate	1 serve of 1 of these fruits daily. 30gm of good quality dark chocolate regularly
Yellow flavonoid: Luteolin (a flavone)	Anti-inflammatory, anti-cancer, anti-allergenic, helps promote healthy glucose levels, reduces risk of cataracts and colon cancer	Celery, green peppers, parsley, artichoke leaves, olive oil, rosemary, lemons, sage, peppermint, thyme	Mix all these greens in a salad and eat most days. Cook artichokes in water for 30 mins, cool, then mix lemon vinaigrette. Pull off oll the leaves, dip and eat
Flavonoid: Catechins	Anti-ageing, anti-inflammatory, protects against cancer, skin cancer and atherosclerosis	Tea (particularly green and white), chocolate, grapes, berries, apples	Drink green tea daily. 1 30gm of good quality dark chocolate regularly
Flavonoid: Quercetin	Anti-allergy, anti-inflammatory, protects against cancer, prostatitis, asthma and bronchitis	Yellow onions, scallions, kale, broccoli, apples, berries, tea	Red apples eaten with the skin are best - 'an apple a day
Tetraterpene: Lycopene (a red carotenoid)	Anti-inflammatory, acts against cell damage	Tomato (raw, paste, sauce, puree, soup), watermelon, pink grapefruit, baked beans	Tomatoes cooked with skins and some fat 3 times per week. ½ cup of these fruits 3 times per week
Isoflavones: Daidzein and Genistein	Relieves menopausal symptoms, inhibits arteriosclerosis, protects prostate from cancer and enlargement, prevents osteoporosis	Soy - beans, tempeh, miso, tofu, soy milk, soy yoghurt	Soy copes with processing so get your ½ cup from cooked, tinned or packaged soy products 3 times per week
Isothiocyanate precursors: Glucosinolates	Anti-tumour, anti-cancer, supports liver detoxification pathways	Bok choy, broccoli, brussels sprouts, cabbage, cauliflower, horseradish, kale, kohlrabi, mustard, radish, rutabaga, turnip, watercress	2 serves per day from this list. Cook but only ever so lightly - steam or a quick stir-fry
Stilbene: Resveratrol	Anti-inflammatory, antiarteriosclerotic, anti-cancer and anti-ageing actions. (These findings not in humans, but the research is promising)	Grapes, wine, grape juice, peanuts, berries of Vaccinum species, including blueberries, bilberries, cranberries	Red wine/grape juice - 4 glasses a week. 1 serve per day of any of the berries. 20 peanuts 3 times per week

Which phytochemical?	What are they good for?	Where from?	How much? How to prepare?
Tetraterpenes: Beta-carotene (orange carotenoid) pawpaw	Protects against cancer, antioxidant, anti-ageing, prevents Vitamin A deficiency	Pumpkin, carrot, sweet potato, spinach, kale, red pepper,	1 cup of root vegetables - cut, stir fried and cooked with oil. Fruit is always best raw every day
Lignans: Enterdiol	Protects against breast cancer, promotes ovulation, reduces pre/peri-menopausal symptoms, decreases insulin resistance, lowers cholesterol	Linseeds (flax) and sesame seeds 1 tablespoon of flax oil per day, or add ground flax to any meal.	Sprinkle sesame seeds or spoon tahini on salads

NUTRIGENOMICS IS ONE WAY TO GET MORE SELECTIVE IN OUR DIET

What is nutrigenomics? Different foods interact with specific genes to increase the risk of diseases. Across the population, these genes can subtly differ. These differences can partly explain why our own response to the diet may be different from another person. Some genes, good and bad, just need the right environment to make themselves felt, and finding the right diet is one way to get the balance right. For example, fat in the diet is especially bad for those whose genes mean they can't handle bad (LDL) cholesterol, but it is less of a problem in those with a strong cholesterol removal pathway.

How does it work? A simple mouth swab or blood tests is all we need. A number of commercial agencies offer this kind of DNA testing and then it depends on the ability of the practitioner to interpret the results. The costs are coming down but still cost hundreds of dollars for an analysis of a specific set of variations believed to influence disease risk and to be diet responsive.

Does it tell us what best to do? Although nutrigenomics is supposed to provide and individualised diet, for the most part, any dietary recommendations that result from such tests are probably not too different from those suggested in this book. At the moment, the cost of these tests may be greater than their advertised benefits. But this area is constantly evolving. WATCH THIS SPACE.

Not all fats are bad. Neither are they all good. The same can be said for carbohydrate and protein. Just as important as diet composition is the need to choose the right stuff. Getting carried away with 'I need 30% protein' is less valuable than finding the right source of dietary protein for your needs.

All natural products have a balance of saturated and unsaturated fats. It is the saturated fat - packed in tight - that we should try to limit in our diet. Foods containing a higher proportion of saturated fat include butter, coconut, dairy products (especially cream cheese and milk chocolate), meat and eggs. In each case, there are low-fat alternatives. So read the label, compare and choose the one that has the least saturated fat. Keep in mind that low fat sometimes means high carbs.

Some fats are essential for good health, including the omega-3 polyunsaturated fatty acids. Good sources of omega-3 include cold-water oily fish, meat from animals that eat grass, organic eggs, flax seed (linseed), kiwifruit, black raspberries and walnuts.

When we feel we have to use some oil on a salad or in a meal, choose the good oil:

> For high temperature cooking try grape-seed, rice bran, peanut, macadamia oils as these are more stable. However, prolonged or very high temperatures (e.g. deep frying) will destroy many of the antioxidants and phytochemicals contained in the oil. Prolonged deep frying can also generate trans fats. Even if we use trans fat free oil we need to change it regularly.

> Consider a drizzle on the salad, like the Greeks do, not spa bath for potatoes (as the French would fry). For dressings and flavour, try sesame, olive, or walnut oils. Try some fresh 'hand-picked' oils from local producers. They taste much better.

> Choose organic or virgin (not refined) oils where we can, as these contain more polyphenols. 'First cold press' means that it came from the first press and generally contains the most phytonutrients. '100% Pure Olive Oil' is often the lowest quality available. Good quality extra virgin olive oil should have a distinct green colour, and be stored in the dark. If your oil is light or yellow, its polyphenol content is probably also low.

> Use canola oil sparingly as well as butter as oil surrogates in your cooking.

GO FOR VARIETY AND TRY SOMETHING NEW	
Vegetable oil/canola oil for cooking	Peanut oil (organic), rice bran oil and macadamia oil (good for high temperature cooking)
Margarine	Organic butter, non-organic butter, olive oil and butter blend, hummus, drizzled olive oil, avocado

THE RIGHT PROTEIN

All protein is digested into amino acids, whether the protein comes from an animal or a plant, so when considering our protein, we are really considering its complement of amino acids, as well other nutrients and toxins that are ingested at the same time. These should be our main concern when looking for protein. 'Does it come with fat or calories?' - so we choose the leanest meat. "Can I get it with added vitamin and fibre?" - so substitute plant proteins, or perhaps fish, for your omega-3 dose.

Plant proteins – eat a broad range of plant foods ad libitum

> A mixed vegetable meal can provide all the protein of a steak, with far less fat, and provide the bonus of fibre, vitamins and minerals.

> Complete protein requirements are found in soy products, quinoa, spirulina, buckwheat and amaranth. Try substituting rice with quinoa as it is a high protein grain with a nutty flavour similar to rice.

> Tofu and soy are good vegetarian protein sources with the added benefits of isoflavones. Use tofu in stir fries, curries and casseroles as an animal protein substitute.

> While canned foods are not the first choice with most foods, canned legumes retain their nutritional value and are quicker and more convenient than preparing beans at home. Choose from lentils, kidney beans, chick peas, broad beans, baked beans (drain off the sauce), mixed bean varieties and use them in salads, Mexican style dishes, soups and stews.

Red meat – eat it no more than twice a week (one serve = 100g or a piece the size of the palm of your hand)

> Chose lean cuts and lean meats (such as kangaroo).

> We can get the added bonus of essential fatty acids by choosing meat from grass fed rather than grain fed herds.

> Don't overcook your beef for flavour. Find another way.

> Avoid cured, smoked and processed meats.

Chicken - eat it no more than twice a week (one serve = 100g, one drumstick or half a small chicken breast)

> Discard the skin and chose lean cuts.

> We are after protein not pesticides or antibiotics, so choose organic.

> We can get the added bonus of essential fatty acids by choosing free range chickens rather than factory fed ones (modern farming methods have led to the development of chicken feed that produces an imbalance of omega-6: omega-3 (the ratio needs to be less than 4:1). Chickens that eat vegetable matter high in omega-3 fatty acids, along with insects and fresh green grass, supplemented with fresh fruit and small amounts of corn produce eggs that have a ratio of 1.5:1, whereas grain-fed chicken eggs have a ratio of 20:1.

> Don't overcook your chicken.

Eggs - eat no more than 7 eggs a week

> We can get the added bonus of essential fatty acids by choosing free range eggs rather than factory fed hens.

> Keep a few chickens in your own backyard. They are great consumers of kitchen scraps!

Milk - no more than 1 cup per day (so minimise your milk consumption)

> Grass fed cows have much higher levels of essential fatty acids.

> We are after calcium, but calcium can be found elsewhere (see chapter 34).

> Saturated fat is our enemy. Low fat milk has less fat but also less fat-soluble vitamins (e.g. vitamin A, D, E and K) and less available calcium. Fortified products can make up for these changes (e.g. choose fortified low fat milk).

> Choose probiotic dairy products such as yoghurt to get calcium and the added bonus of intestinal health. But watch out, low fat generally means high sugar and high GI, so it's best mixed with fibre (e.g. bran for breakfast).

GO FOR VARIETY AND TRY SOMETHING NEW	
Milk	Rice milk, soy milk, almond milk, goat's milk
Cow's milk yoghurt	Keffir, sheep's milk yoghurt, soy milk yoghurt
Ice cream	Frozen fruit smoothie or sorbet
Cream	Coconut cream
Cow's milk cheese	Sheep or goat's milk cheese. In general hard cheeses are a better alternative if we can tolerate cow's milk e.g. parmesan. Avoid soft cheeses

Fish – up to 7 serves per week (1 serve = 100-150g of fish or the size of your palm)

> All fish are an excellent source of lean protein.

> Cold water oily fish (such as salmon, herring, mackerel, anchovies, sardines and to a lesser extent tuna) have the added bonus of essential fatty acids.

> If the fish is farmed then it is generally higher in omega-6 and lower in omega-3.

> Long-living predatory fish, like swordfish and shark, may accumulate toxins such as heavy metals PCBs, furans and dioxins.

> Canned tuna has less chemical residues than fresh tuna because the smaller fish are used in the canning process.

> As omega-3's are generally unstable in heat, any health benefits may be lost, along with the omega-3 by frying or overcooking fish.

THE RIGHT CARBOHYDRATE

We run on sugars for energy, but we need not be run down by them. It's not hard to keep track of our sugar load by looking at the glycemic index and the carbohydrate content of our food. Replacing refined sugars and the foods that contain them with fruit products is one simple, yet valuable, change.

To provide sustained energy and greater nutritional value, we need to change our focus from simple sugars to complex-carbohydrate containing foods. Finding low GI substitutes will also help. Just by replacing refined products with wholegrain equivalents, without ever changing our diet, we can more than double our intake of total and soluble fibre. This also gives us the added bonus of phytonutrients contained in the germ.

Whole grains

> 3-5 serves per day (1 serve = 1 slice of bread, 1/2 a cup of rice, cereal or pasta)

Rice

> Use brown rice that keeps the germ instead of white varieties.

> Try Basmati or wild rice as they have a lower GI than Jasmine or short grain rice.

> Soak washed brown rice for 20 minutes in warm water prior to cooking it. This process stimulates germination, and releases more of its nutrients.

> Avoid 'easy-cook' or 'one minute rice', as its nutrient value has usually been depleted and generally has a higher GI.

Bread/crackers/baking

> Switch to whole grain bread, or bread that is high in whole rye, whole grain barley, sunflower, linseed (flaxseed) or bulgur. Keep in mind that multigrain breads are white bread with seeds. While the seeds have nutritional value, the best choice is a wholegrain seeded bread. White flour has had the nutritious 'germ' removed and with it much of the nutritional value.

> Use whole grain wheat flour compared to white 'all purpose' flour for baking (it has ten times the fibre content).

> Buy from the bakery that uses whole grains (if they don't know, find a shop that knows what they are putting into their food!).

> Avoid crispy snacks such as chips, rice crackers and white crackers. Substitute with vegetable sticks and humus, avocado dips or use wholegrain alternatives based on rye, whole wheat or other grains.

> Experiment with wheat flour substitutes such as spelt, amaranth or kamut flour. Try spelt and kamut bread or rye crackers instead of wheat based breads.

> Try sprouted breads for their added nutritional value.

Pasta

> Substitute brown pasta for normal yellow varieties.

> Avoid rice and corn pastas unless we are on a gluten free diet as they have a high GI.

> Swap pasta for vegetables (grated cauliflower as a pasta substitute).

Breakfast cereals

> Try a breakfast cereal that says 'whole grain' not just wheat.

> Consider oat bran rather than just oats, as brans are more concentrated and therefore we need to eat less to carry the same benefit.

> Avoid highly processed cereals, especially those with a high GI. Avoid microwave and instant or quick cook oats. The more processed (literally chopped up into finer pieces) the higher GI our cereal becomes. Instead choose unprocessed cereals such as untoasted muesli, Bircher muesli and porridge. Choose rolled oats as they are a low GI sustained source of energy.

> Mix with products that slow the absorption of sugar (e.g. have strawberries or fruit with your cereal).

Sugar

> Substituting refined sugars and the foods that contain them (soft drinks, icing, etc) with fruit products is one simple, yet valuable, change.

> Substitute highly processed (white) sugar with unrefined Rapadura. This is different from raw, brown or black sugar, Demerara or sucanat. Rapadura contains vitamins, minerals and other trace elements as well as the sweet taste that we all love. You'll also be helping the planet as Rapadura comes from organically grown sugar cane from Colombia and Brazil through fair trade programs.

GO FOR VARIETY AND TRY SOMETHING NEW

White bread	Sourdough wholegrain, brown wholegrain bread
Wheat bread	Spelt bread, kamut bread, rice bread, white wheat pasta
White wheat pasta	Wholemeal pasta
Wheat pasta	Kamut, Spelt or wholegrain rice pasta. White corn and rice pasta have a very high GI so if we can find them go for the wholegrain varieties
White rice	Brown long or short grain rice (long grain has a lower GI than short grain brown rice), basmati rice
White biscuits/crackers	Wholemeal biscuits, brown rice cakes
Wheat biscuits	Brown rice cakes, rye crackers
Rice and pasta alternatives	Quinoa, Amaranth, Buckwheat, grated cauliflower, potato, pumpkin, sweet potato
Rolled oats	Brown rice flakes, Spelt flakes
Packaged cereals	Rolled oats raw in muesli or as porridge, brown rice flakes, Spelt flakes, cooked brown rice

STRATEGY 7: BE PREPARED

Some foods need to be cooked, such as meat, potatoes and red beans. Depending on the way that food is cooked, there may be considerable loss of nutrients. The longer and the hotter we cook food, by any method, the greater the nutrient loss. Overcooking also swells starches and softens food, which speeds up digestion and absorption, increasing the GI. Simple tips to reduce nutrient loss include:

> Serve fresh and unprocessed (raw) fruit and vegetables when possible.

> Cut and cook vegetables in large pieces (to minimise surface area for loss).

> Prepare vegetables as close to cooking time as possible.

> Cook vegetables until just tender to retain nutrients, vibrant colours and texture. For most vegetables, changes in colour provide clues about nutrient loss. They are usually done when at their brightest.

> Use the minimum amount of water to keep food moist, but don't cook without it, even in a frying pan.

> Avoid long exposure to heat or high heat. For example, frying at high temperatures destroys most heatsensitive vitamins.

> Cook what we need to eat, then eat it. The longer we leave it around, the less nutrients it will have.

> Rinsing rice and pasta is unnecessary and results in the loss of some nutrients. Similarly, browning your risotto rice before adding water can reduce its nutritional value.

> Avoid microwaving vegetables as research shows important phytochemicals are lost in the process. Instead, lightly stir-fry or steam your vegetables.

Cooking is not all about losses. It is also about many gains. The cooking process generates new chemicals that we perceive as flavour, aroma and texture. These add to the experience of eating, but may also generate a range of toxic compounds. The most well known of these include the cancer-causing polycyclic aromatic hydrocarbons generated in cooked meat, acrylamide in baked products and AGEs, which form when sugars and fats in food chemically react with protein to result in browning. Another important group of toxins generated in cooking are the trans fats. For example, prolonged deep frying can transform oils into trans fats, which are then transferred to the food. Examples include snack foods (eg. rice cakes, chips, biscuits), fried foods and baked goods. The best way to avoid trans fats is to read the label and avoid foods containing them, or choose foods in which the processing has specifically prevented their formation. For example, all margarines in Australia are now free of trans fats, as are most global fast foods (mostly because of the threat of litigation). It is best to avoid deep frying at home, even if we use oil free of trans fats and change it regularly.

Natural sources of flavour add their own unique benefits. For example, spices have a range of healthy influences. Rosemary, oregano, turmeric and curcumin have strong antioxidant contents. Chilli and black pepper boosts circulation. Fennel is a digestive aid, while cinnamon improves sugar metabolism. So why not put some spice back into your life and cook your meal a little less tonight?

STRATEGY 8: HARNESS THE SUPERFOODS

Most foods contain useful nutrients that we use to build and renew. Yet all foods were not created equally. Some are in a class of their own when it comes to positive effects on health and ageing. They may sometimes look a bit ordinary, but inside they are power-packed with antioxidants, vitamins, minerals, fibre and other phytonutrients to maintain and enhance function. These are often called superfoods. They often form part of traditional cures or folklore. To make the most of each mouthful in our slow ageing diet, we should eat them whenever we can. At least half of our diet should preferably comprise superfoods.

Some of the most common superfoods include:
> Berries (of all sorts)
> The Allium family (onions, shallots, leeks, garlic, chives, etc)
> The Crucifers (spinach, broccoli, bok choy, rocket cabbage, kale, greens, etc)
> Legumes (beans, lentils, peas, sprouts, peanuts, etc)
> Whole nuts and seeds
> Probiotic yoghurt
> All fruits
> Dark chocolate
> Green tea

SLOW AGEING FOOD PRINCIPLES

1. Awareness is the first rule of SLOW ageing. Some advocate starting with a clean slate. Clear out your pantry and fridge of all the unnecessary, out of date, energy-dense and otherwise unhealthy foods. For most of us, a healthy change does not need to be this drastic. The most important part is to actually notice what's on our plate and think about the impact it may be having on our health.

2. The second step is planning and setting goals. Start with the low hanging fruit. For example, stop buying that packet of chips or eat a small amount with really healthy dips and vegetable sticks as your dinner (rather than a snack).

3. The third step is to make our diet a positive experience, not a punishment. Get excited about the diet we plan to implement. Enjoy the experience of new foods and new recipes. Relish the new connections we can make through our food choices (maybe the grower, the seller or the environment).

4. The choices we make must be ones that are sustainable for the long-term. Otherwise they are simply a fad.

5. Don't be exclusive. A diet won't be effective if it isn't part of an overall plan with a range of different strategies. There are so many theories on nutrition management that it is difficult at times to put them into any practical context. Many diets have been popularised on the back of only one or two of these useful concepts. The challenge is to understand where all these approaches fit when trying to work out a long-term program for ourselves. No matter what the advertising says, there is no one diet that will work for everybody. Any diet also needs to be part of an overall plan with a range of different strategies. For example, a diet may have benefits for weight control, but for those to be sustained they are best combined with other techniques, like exercise and stress management. A diet won't be effective if it isn't part of an overall plan. Don't be exclusive. In fact it may even be counterproductive.

6. When we plan to make a change it is easier if we have some help. There are many dieticians, nutritionists and other specialists out there who can offer advice and support.

7. Finally, for our diet to work, like Goldilocks, we have to be selective. We have to try a few different products to find the one that is best suited to our needs. The bulk of nutritional information is written as universal recommendations, a 'one size fits all' approach, without recognising that people and our nutritional needs are different. It is important to personalise nutrition recommendations when putting them into practice. A number of differences also exist between one individual and the next in our absorption, distribution, metabolism, and excretion of dietary nutrients. So one way of getting our diet 'just right' is to better understand our particular requirements.

Now we have the principles, the next step is their application. The next chapter shows what to do on a daily basis so we achieve optimal health through selection of food.

CHAPTER 19

THE SLOW AGEING EATING PLAN

In the last chapter, we covered many different elements of good nutrition. How do we make all of these different goals happen in one shopping trip? How does anyone ever keep score and come out on top? We could give control over to some else, to tell you what to eat and when to eat. Many pre-made meals and diets are now available, as though we were flying on a plane. This can work for a short journey, but when we're in it for the long haul, this kind of strategy doesn't teach self-reliance.

EATING TO SLOW AGEING

In truth, it's not really that hard to have a good diet. For most of us, very small changes are all that are necessary, which by becoming good habits and being magnified by decades of use become real effectors of health in our later years. For example, the average weight gain each year as we get older is equivalent to two extra spoonfuls a day. We can really get all the nutrients we really need from food by making informed dietary choices. It doesn't mean spending lots of money or conforming to radical or restrictive formulas. It doesn't even mean being vegetarian. It simply means making the right choices for you. A SLOW diet is ours for the making, and most importantly, something we can really do today and keep doing it.

☑ Eat these foods every day :
> Fresh fruit – choose 3 serves per day (one serve = one piece of fruit or half a cup)
> Legumes – choose 1-3 servings per day (1 serve = half a cup)
> Fresh vegetables – 5-7 servings per day (1 serve = half a cup)
> Fresh herbs and spices – as an alternative to over cooking for flavor
> Nuts and seeds – 1 serve daily (1 serve = 7-10 nuts)
> Whole grains – 3-5 serves per day (1 serve = 1 slice of whole grain bread, a cup of brown rice, unprocessed cereal or whole grain pasta)
> Water – 2-3 litres per day (one glass = 300mls)
> Green or black tea – 1-2 cups per day

☑ Eat these a few times a week :
> Fresh fish – up to 7 serves per week (one serve = 100-150g or the size of your palm)
> Eggs – up to 7 eggs per week
> Milk and cheese – optional up to 7 serves per week (one serve = one cup of milk or 30g of cheese)
> Yoghurt – optional up to 7 serves per week
> Dark chocolate - optional up to 5 serves per week (one serve = two squares of chocolate)
> Low fat red meat – a maximum of 2 serves per week (one serve = 100g or the size of your palm)
> Chicken – a maximum of 2 serves per week (one serve = 100g, one drumstick or a small breast of chicken)

☑ Avoid (fast foods) where possible :
> Ice-cream
> Highly processed foods e.g. toasted cereals
> Bakery goods, pastries, biscuits
> Lollies and candy
> Crisps
> Fried food
> Processed and deli meats
> Soft drink
> Food with preservatives

Breakfast options:

> Natural, live low fat yoghurt with freshly chopped fruits and a teaspoon of LSA (linseed, sunflower and almond meal)
> Muesli made from oats, fresh sunflower, pumpkin and sesame seeds and raisins with natural low fat yoghurt and some apple juice, rice milk or low fat milk
> Spelt toast with a poached egg
> Rolled oat porridge with live yoghurt, LSA, stewed apple and honey

Mid morning and afternoon options:

> Fresh fruit, raw nuts and seeds such as almonds, hazelnuts, Brazils, pumpkin and sunflower seeds
> Raw vegetables such as carrots, broccoli, celery with dips such as hummus, yoghurt and garlic or salsa (as long as they are fresh or at least contain no preservatives)
> Wholegrain biscuits or half a slice of wholegrain toast with avocado

Lunch options:

> Serve of wholemeal pasta with tuna fish, tomato, celery and spring onion, with olive oil and lemon juice
> Rice salad with many types of fresh vegetables, cottage cheese, pumpkin seeds, olive oil, lemon juice and freshly ground pepper
> Homemade chicken and vegetable soup including celery, potato, zucchini and mung bean lentils
> Wholegrain sandwich or wrap with salad avocado and Greek feta cheese

Dinner options:

> Hot meal of grilled fresh fish, chicken or lean red meat or a vegetarian alternative made from beans, lentils or soya
> Serve with a large helping of freshly steamed or lightly stir-fried vegetables 'Steam-fry' vegetables by using just the tiniest drop of oil and adding a couple of tablespoons of water to, in effect, steam them. Add a serve of rice, pasta, quinoa or other wholegrain
> Instead of steamed vegetables, we could have a large fresh salad using a lemon and olive oil dressing. In the salad include different green leaves (rocket,

marionette, cos, romaine), tomato or cherry tomato, cucumber, grated carrot
and fresh beetroot, mung bean sprouts, capsicum, shallots chopped finely,
fresh asparagus….and any of the other fresh vegetables

Drink options :

> At least six glasses of water, fresh fruit and vegetable juices, occasional
  'smoothies' - freshly made with fruits/fruit juices and yoghurt, herbal and fruit
  teas (beware of artificially flavoured or sweetened ones)

THE SLOW AGEING FOOD BASKET – A SNAPSHOT

FOOD	DAILY	WEEKLY	SERVE SIZE	SERVES	CATEGORY
Fish		√	140g	4-7	Protein, essential fats
Red meat, chicken		√	100g (Lean)	2	Protein
Tofu		√	100g	3	Protein
Avocado, olive oil	√		15g (1tbspoon)	2-3	Fat
Berries	√		1/3 cup	1	Complex carbohydrates, micro nutrients
Fruit	√		1 medium piece	2	Complex carbohydrates, nutrients
Vegetables	√		75g (½ cup)	5-7	Complex carbohydrates, nutrients
Legumes	√		75g (½ cup)	1	Fibre, nutrients
Nuts and seeds	√		¼ cup	1	Sterols, fats protein, micro nutrients
Wholegrains	√		½ -1 slice bread	3-5	Complex carbohydrates
Yoghurt, cheese, milk	√		Yoghurt - 200g, Milk - 250ml Cheese–30g	1	Protein, probiotics

HOW NOT TO SABOTAGE YOUR PLANS:

Here are some suggestions for various common scenarios that mean we can still enjoy life without sabotaging our new health habits.

The coffee shop - one of the largest fat traps out there. We are lured in with a promise of escape from our worldly worries, a chance to have a good catch up with friends and a way of forming new friends and business relationships. Pretty much everything on the menu falls into the treat zone and self control is required. Safest bets are a cup of exotic green, black or herbal tea, black coffee, a fresh squeezed juice or a fruit smoothie. A larger drink may allow for us to bypass the baked sweet treats. Next best alternative is to stick to skim milk cappuccino (skinny cappuccino) which at least provides some low fat protein and fills our tummy a bit. Sometimes it comes with a wee biscuit that can satisfy that little indulgent inner self. Get into the habit of always ordering with water, or even a sparkling water with a squeeze of lemon, so you don't end up dry from the caffeine.

Celebrations and family get-togethers - there are three rules of engagement for the continuing round of birthdays, anniversaries, weddings, sporting events and the lazy Sunday afternoon get-togethers:

☑ If we are asked to bring a dish then bring one that is in line with our own goals. Spend a little time thinking what might be popular and dress it up well. People will be impressed, conversation will get started and we will be surprised how many people say that they have been meaning to eat healthier but did not know it could taste this good.

☑ Feed our body first, then treat it second. With a whole smorgasbord of food awaiting us at these events it can be hard not to throw all caution to the wind and pig out! The best strategy is to fill our plates with the most beneficial foods possible, thus feeding our body properly. Fill up with some more of these foods if you feel the need. Once we are satiated, we might then carefully contemplate which of the desserts will tingle our tastebuds. We'll find that just a few mouthfuls will be enough and there will be little or no guilt attached.

☑ Speaking of guilt beware of family induced emotional eating as in "Oh, I made this especially for you" while someone is passing you a 3 kg slice of triple layer chocolate cake. There are as many different variations as there are families, so be on the lookout. Be polite by declaring your state of blissful fullness and have a bite or two, or ask to take it home to enjoy later (and do with it what you will... single male neighbours and university students always seem to be willing recipients).

After work -do what you can to keep control. If you can't then don't even start!

Binge drinking is a leading cause of preventable death, particularly in young adults and men, but also increasingly, in women. When drinking socially, most people don't even notice when we switch to lemon lime and bitters after our second drink. Get into the habit of ordering more water, more sparkling water or more soda lime and bitters after the first or second 'toast'. Our body, brain liver and skin will thank us for it....the next morning and for the next decade.

At play - daytime activities can also have their own challenges. Think of what activities you do regularly, what kind of refreshments are served and what you may be 'mindlessly' indulging in. Always order the healthiest item, or choose the path of least damage, no matter what. Healthy living comes from healthy regular habits, getting together with friends is good for us, we can make it even better. Choose water, tea, fruit, veggie sticks and salads where possible.

WHAT'S ON THE MENU TONIGHT?

Eating is one of life's great pleasures and it still can be, if we know where to look. There are so many interesting tasty and healthy foods out there. Because we are looking after our health or our waists, doesn't mean that we have to eat cardboard. For any diet to be successful it cannot be a punishment, the medicine we had to take to get and maintain our health. Become connected with our dietary choices is also not about becoming a fussy eater or being neurotic. It can be as much fun, even more than ever, before. The moment when we realise "Hey, this food is actually interesting... I wonder what this tastes like?... What nutrients does it have? Where does it come from?" is the moment that slow begins, and a whole world of choices opens up.

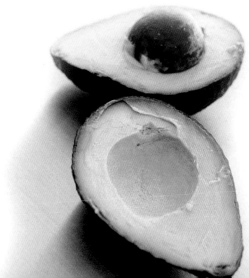

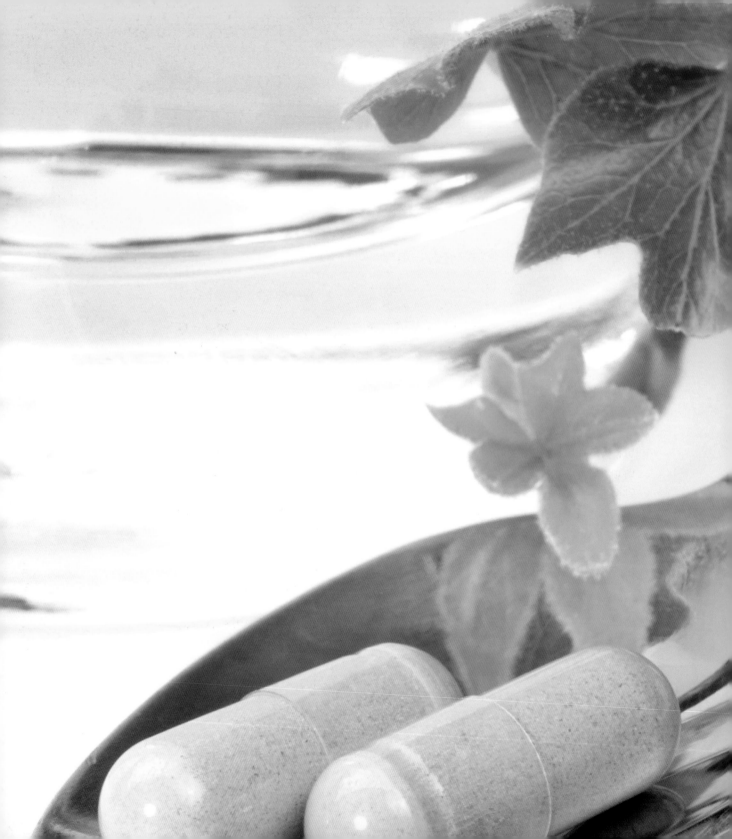

CHAPTER 20
CHOOSING THE
RIGHT SUPPLEMENTS
[THE SLOW AGEING SHOPPING LIST]

Every cell in our body requires an optimal level of nutrition in order to function normally. In the real world, the everyday demands on our nutritional status and reserves are surprisingly common and given these demands, we may not be able to meet the nutritional needs of our cells by diet alone. A state of inadequate supply or excessive demand can quickly lead to nutritional imbalances. While in the short term our ability to compensate may be enough to overcome any imbalance, the cascade effect from inadequate supply or excessive demand in the medium or long term may manifest as a disease and hasten ageing.

Higher nutrient levels are necessitated by stress, living in polluted environments, illness, active lifestyles and poor dietary habits. Additionally, optimal health is more than simply the absence of scurvy or rickets. Many modern illnesses like heart disease and diabetes, which affect our ageing process, can result from consumption of nutrients at levels higher than the RDI but less than the optimal. The amount of any given nutrient we need each day to be truly vibrant and well is often much more than the RDI.

Although there is substantial overlap, supplements can be divided roughly into three groups:

The first and largest of these are the dietary supplements that are intended to provide nutrients that may be inadequate in our diet, such as fatty acids (see chapter 12), fibre (see chapter 14), vitamins and minerals (see chapter 17). There is a growing body of evidence to show that some illnesses and the things we perceive as ageing are partly determined by what we don't eat enough of. Few if any supplements have been proven to be beneficial in the form that they are marketed. However, there is indirect evidence that some of the constituents of a fabulous diet have protective effects to support specific bodily reserves, and help modify the threshold for disease. Their best sources of nutrients are whole foods and a balanced and varied diet such as that detailed in the previous chapter. While a multivitamin can never substitute for daily servings of fresh fruits and vegetables, not all nutrients are contained in fruits and vegetables.

The second group are preparations that use specific natural ingredients with known health actions to convey health benefits, rather than simply adding to dietary intake. Many reflect their use in traditional medicines or 'natural remedies'. The most commonly used are herbal supplements (aka botanicals), which harness the medicinal properties of phytochemicals. One example is green tea or epigallocatechin gallate (EGCG), the antioxidant contained within it. Others include non-plant products such as those derived from fungi (e.g. mushrooms), insects (e.g. bee pollen), fish or animal products. Unlike dietary supplements there is no RDI, so it is less easy to know how much to take to mimic a state of optimal health. Many preparations also contain mixtures of multiple components in varying proportions. If using herbal supplements, it is far better to start with a single-herb product unless it has been prescribed by a health care professional. If we know what we are getting and how much, we can control its use and any interactions much better.

The third and final group of supplements broadly attempts to replace actual components of our body, either by stimulating pathways or directly giving us what we are missing. These things cannot be found in a healthy diet or fully delivered from the medicinal properties of plants or other natural products. This is the most rapidly growing area of supplement use. The most common of these are hormonal supplements like melatonin and DHEA. Others include bacteria (e.g. probiotics - see chapter 15), and the building blocks for healthy connective tissue, hydroxyapetite and glucosamine.

But which of these supplements should be in our shopping trolley? When we try to keep up with all the research on promising supplements, we end up consuming about 40 plus pills per day. Is there a SLOW solution for this problem too? In fact the slow principles enunciated in this book provide a useful framework to look at some of reasons why we take or should take supplements, and how to make the most of our many, many options.

STEP 1: ENGAGEMENT AND AWARENESS (WHAT)

While manufacturers rely on expansive claims to sell their product, you should be less enthusiastic about such claims.

It is very important to see beyond the hype of a 'breakthrough' or 'magic' product, in the same way we are skeptical of a 'miracle cure'. Be openminded, but trust our instincts! Many products are sold by buzz words claiming that they detoxify, purify and/or energise. Also be aware of concepts that are vague and impossible to measure. Some others claim to be more potent, contain MEGA doses or provide a cheap alternative. Even the term 'natural' is often used to advertise rather than inform. Do not be swayed by advertising. What we choose are the ingredients not the wrapper. Try making a shopping list. If we can't write what we want, we really shouldn't be shopping for supplements. It begins by understanding what we want to try, learning about it and getting advice. When we go to the pharmacy or the health food store, we should ask questions. If they don't know how something is or what's in it, we need to find answers elsewhere. One way is to read up on the options available to us.

Important steps to evaluate each product include:

> Read labels carefully and research products where possible. Product labels tell us which nutrients are included and the amount contained in each dose.
> Critically evaluate claims of treatment success. Look at the 'trackrecord' of the compound; what is the exact impact the compound has on the body in clinical trials. Gather information from a variety of sources and evaluate the information carefully. It is often useful to get help (we have tried to help in this book but there are many professionals out there who can tell you a lot more). Even though supplements have not been proven to slow the ageing process or extend life, there is enough promising scientific evidence (in animals and other life forms) to support that they might have this ability and who has the time to wait and see whether generational studies will show conclusively that they do the same thing in humans as they do in animals? Somewhere along the line we have to take an educated guess. The trick is the educated part, not the guess work.
> Look at the cost. The most expensive is the one we put in the cupboard and never use. But the super cheap ones in the dump bins may not give us what we bargained for. Some of the best selling products are best selling only because they are cheap, not because they contain quality ingredients or actually work. Cut price products should be questioned why they are produced or sold so cheaply.
> Look at our budget. Taking a range of supplements can be a major spend over a long period of time so it is best to plan well. Look at our budget for supplementation. No point in being ad hoc. Put our list together, know exactly why we've selected these (remind ourselves every now and again) and budget for these.
> Look at the dose we are taking. For nutritional supplements there is an RDI, which gives us an idea of how much we need on average to prevent deficiency.

This is not the same as the amount you personally require to maintain, and stay in peak condition (which can be much higher). As a starting point to maintain good health, choose to take a dose that falls within the lower end of the therapeutic range (see table in chapter 17). To correct a deficiency we will need to take a bigger dose, in the middle to upper dosing range. Once our levels have optimised, we can maintain them with foods rich in the specific nutrient and/or a maintenance dose.

> Try to avoid the hype of 'megadoses' that provide vast excesses on our recommended daily intake. This also lulls us into a false sense of security when missing doses or taking supplements intermittently. This is different for stored (fat soluble) vitamins like vitamin D, where large doses such as supplied by a good dose of sunlight can get us though the darkest winter. However most advertised 'megadoses' are usually selling water-soluble vitamins and the greater part of these tablets rapidly ends up in the toilet.

> Look at how they are stored. Just as in food, many supplements lose their value the longer they are stored, especially in hot and humid places, such as in the bathroom. Throw out the old and expired supplements in our cupboard.

STEP 2: THE GOALS OF SUPPLEMENT TAKING (WHY)

Before embarking on a course of supplements, we should assess our needs and motivation. Why do we really want to take all these? Are we fearful of becoming ill, of being diseased, of losing control? Fear is neither a good place nor a good reason to start. There are many more positive targets and more practical ones than simply allaying our fears.

> When choosing supplements it is important to have a simple goal in mind. Write down your motivations for taking supplements.

> Use the results of your testing to establish personal areas of focus and a nutrient plan which will meet that need.

> Identify whether you can achieve the same health benefits by eating or avoiding certain foods rather than taking a supplement.

> Determine the difference between what you need to take and any additional supplements you would like to take.

> Pinpoint the specific biochemical issues or system you want to address.

Possible aims of a supplement strategy
> Reduce oxidative stress
> Reduce advanced glycation
> Reduce excessive inflammation
> Improved intestinal health
> Assist in the elimination of waste products.
> Optimise nutritional status / correct deficiencies
> Stress adaptation/relaxation
> Replace depleted hormone levels
> Improve sleep, sex, or cognitive function
> Supporting ageing of a specific body system e.g.bone, skin, joints, etc

STEP 3: SUPPLEMENTING FOR LONG-TERM HEALTH (HOW)

Slow solutions are those that can be incorporated into our daily routine. Supplements are no exception. They are not for whenever we remember to take them, or for lining our bathroom cupboard. They are not for taking in one fad of enthusiasm and then stopping when the fashion changes. This may do more harm than good. For example, antioxidants also stimulate pro-oxidant pathways to balance our systems. This isn't a problem while the antioxidant remains around, but may be an issue if they are stopped. This may be one reason why the best successes are achieved by a diet high in antioxidants, as we are less likely to forget to eat than to take a pill. Sustainability must be a key goal when choosing supplements especially when compared to dietary changes. One way to get the most of our supplement plan is to establish a routine.

STEP 4: SUPPLEMENTING IS A POSITIVE EXPERIENCE

Supplements are not the bitter pill we had to swallow in order to ensure good health, or a punishment for the nutritionally wicked. We will never stay this kind of course. If we are going to embrace supplements, like any relationship, it helps to like what we are hugging.
> Information is important. We need to know as much as we can about our supplement.
> Nothing is without side effects in some individuals. This is especially the case if it actually works. Find out what they are. While we need to be conscious of unwanted effects, we also need to actively take steps to minimise them. This can be as simple as timing and optimising the dosage, or shopping around for a formulation that sits right with you.

> Introduce supplements one at a time and note any positive or negative changes over a week or two. Pay attention and keep a record. If you feel neutral or good, then introduce a new supplement until you are taking all of the supplements in your plan. If you don't care how you feel, you have to ask why you are taking the supplements in the first place!

> Track the benefits. Make note of any improvements or changes in your health when taking supplements. While this is a subjective measure, it is also one of the best measures of personal health. If the supplement we are taking is for prevention, then we may not notice an obvious change in our own health outcomes. However, there may be changes in our biochemical tests. Ask your health care provider to go over these with you at appropriate intervals.

STEP 5: DON'T BE EXCLUSIVE

The best option is never contained in a single pill. Although supplements are often regarded as 'alternative medicines', they cannot be regarded as an alternative to a good diet, exercise, lifestyle or other healthy practices mentioned in this book. This includes cancer screening and lowering of blood pressure and cholesterol levels. In fact these activities are even more important to live long enough to make the most of our supplements. For this reason, it is better to consider supplements as synergistic or complementary therapies used in addition to, and to the advantage of other interventions.

For example, starting any dietary supplements should also be accompanied by a review of our diet plan. We might find that substituting fresh broccoli for pasta is a cheaper and more tasty alternative. Or we might identify that there is not enough B12 or iron in our current vegetarian diet that may be more readily corrected with supplements, so dietary changes can proceed at a slower pace or with a different focus (such as weight control).

Supplements can also help us get through periods when our health focus is elsewhere, like work/relationship stress, weight gain or disease. Rather than dropping one ball while trying to pick up another, supplements can give us the time and resilience for more holistic interventions.

STEP 6: DON'T GO IT ALONE

There are almost too many options available; certainly too many to be covered in this book. One place to start is to ask for a little help. There are many professionals out there to offer advice and make practical suggestions. A growing number of doctors and health care professionals are able to offer useful advice about the role supplements can have in our aims for ageing well.

If one doctor doesn't understand, find one that does or consider a provider who is knowledgeable in this area. Look to find someone who will be a guide or a coach, rather than one who says you must only do something their way. Shop around. Assess their credentials. Gather information from a variety of sources and evaluate the information carefully. If you know someone who's gone there, ask them about their experiences. Call the provider to request an interview.

STEP 7: IT'S ABOUT YOU, GOLDILOCKS

No matter what we read on the Internet, everybody is different. So find out about yourself, and listen to the feedback. Follow progress as we go and set new goals as we are doing it. It is important to follow our successes and failures. Keep a log or a journal to follow how we are performing. Use testing to establish your areas of focus and choose supplements at the right dose that will meet that need. Not everything will work. Some of us will not tolerate some of the very concentrated products on the market. Some will not work at the doses we can get in some supplements. Others will fit like a glove. Following Goldilocks, and test what best works for you.

SOME SLOW AGEING SUPPLEMENTS

Following is a list of supplements mentioned in this book. You will not, of course, choose to use every one. Based on what our testing tells us about where we are at with our ageing process, we will choose supplements that target our specific areas of need. A word of caution, don't try to do too much at once. Supplementation isn't a case of taking the kitchen sink – in fact quite the opposite. If you feel you need to be taking every single nutrient or new ageing discovery, think again. This is about slow ageing and sometimes, the slow and steady path is the best one.

AVOIDING HEARTACHE (CHAPTER 5)

Aspirin - As prescribed by your doctor

Vitamin K2 - As prescribed by your doctor

Omega 3 Fatty Acids - Dose 3-5g of fish oil per day

TOPIC OF CANCER (CHAPTER 7)

See specific doses in antioxidant section

ANTIOXIDANTS (CHAPTER 8)

Vitamin A (retinol) - Antioxidant, vision, immune function. RDI 1.5 mg/day

Vitamin E (tocopherol) - Antioxidant, inflammation, immune function, fertility. RDI 20mg/day

Vitamin C (ascorbate) - Antioxidant, hormone synthesis, wound healing, iron absorption. RDI 35mg/day.

Selenium - Antioxidant, anti-cancer, immune support, thyroid support. RDI 77mcg/day

Coenzyme Q10 - Antioxidant, boosts mitochondrial function and energy production. Dose 30-150mg/day

Alpha-lipoic acid - Universal antioxidant, anti-atherogenic, metal chelator, anti-inflammatory, anti-diabetic, neuroprotective. Dose 50 to 150mg/day

Carnosine - Antioxidant (brain & eyes), reduces AGE production. Dose 100-200mg/day

Lycopenes - Antioxidant, 6.5mg/day or a tablespoon of tomato paste everyday in your cooking

Lutein - Antioxidant (eyes). Dose 6-10mg/day

Soy isoflavones - Dose 40mg/day

Hesperidin and Rutin - Maintains capillary integrity, anti-inflammatory. Dose 500-1000mg daily

Grape seed extract - Antioxidant, maintains capillary integrity, anti-inflammatory, anticancer, neuroprotective. Dose up to 12g of dried herb daily

Resveratrol - Anti-ageing, anticancer, anti-inflammatory, anti-diabetic, antioxidant, anti-atherogenic. A 240ml glass of red wine provides approximately 640-720 mcg of resveratrol, while a handful of peanuts provides about 73 mcg of resveratrol. For slow ageing take up to 20mg in supplement form daily

Green tea - Antioxidant, cholesterol lowering, anti-cancer, UV protective. Dose 3-8 cups per day

Quercetin - Strengthening capillaries and other connective tissue, anti-inflammatory. Dose 50 to 1000mg/day

Indole-3-carbinol (I-3-C) - Anti-cancer (breast, cervical), oestrogen detoxifying. Dose 300-400mg/day

Ginkgo - Antioxidant, circulation stimulant, increases memory & concentration, blood thinning, slow ageing (brain). Dose from 120 to 240mg of extract/day. Products should be standardised to 24% 'ginkgo flavonglycosides' as this is the form used in clinical trials

ADVANCED GLYCATION INHIBITORS (CHAPTER 10)

Benfotiamine - Reduces AGEs, stimulates metabolism, restores thiamine. Dose 100-200mg/day

Pyridoxamine - Reduces AGEs, prevents lipid damage. Dose 25-50mg/day

Carnosine - Reduces AGEs, prevents lipid damage. Dose 100mg to 200mg/day

Alpha-lipoic acid (lipoate) - Reduces AGEs, antioxidant, anti-inflammatory. Dose 50-150mg/day

GOOD FATS (CHAPTER 12)

Omega 3 fatty acids - Anti inflammatory, (2700mg of EPA + DHA), neuro-protective (1000mg of DHA + EPA per day)

FINDING YOUR FIBRE (CHAPTER 14)

Psyllium husks (dose 5-15g per day with at least 300mg of water)

Bran fibre (dose 5-10g per day with food or water)

AVOIDING THE POISONS (CHAPTER 15)

Curcumin – Dose 1/3 teaspoon of Turmeric 3 time a week up to as much as you like or 3.5-8g/day

Green Tea (ECGC) – Dose 3-8 cups per day

Soy Isoflavones – Dose 40mg/day

VITAMINS AND MINERAL SUPPLEMENTS (CHAPTER 17)

Vitamin A (retinol) 2500iu

Betacarotene 15 milligrams (mg)

Vitamin B1 (Thiamine) 2.5-5mg

Vitamin B2 (Riboflavin) 5-10mg

Vitamin B3 (Niacin) 16mg

Vitamin B5 (Panthothenate) 10-100mg

Vitamin B6 (Pyridoxine 10-20mg

Vitamin B12 (cyanocobalamin) 5-10mcg

Folic Acid 400mcg

Vitamin C 220mg

Vitamin D (cholecalciferol) 200 to 400iu

Vitamin E (d-alpha-tocopherol) 500iu

Vitamin K 120mcg

Calcium 1200mg

Chromium 50 to 200mcg

Iodine 200mcg

Iron 15-30mg (gender dependent)

Magnesium 320-420mg

Manganese 2 to 5mg

Selenium 100-200mcg

Zinc 20mg

Please note: the doses listed are the suggested intake of key essential nutrients for adults. Higher doses may be required for optimal nutrition or to manage a deficiency state.

THE AGEING BRAIN (CHAPTER 23)

DMAE – Dose up to 1600mg (starting with low doses)

BUILDING STRESS RESILIENCE (CHAPTER 25)

St John's Wort - Dose up to 1800 mg of dried herb three times daily (standardised for 0.3% hypericin)

SEX (CHAPTER 27)

Nettle Root - Dose 600-1200mg of dried herb/day

Panax Ginseng - Dose 900mg/day

Ginkgo - Dose 120-240mg of extract/day

Horny Goat Weed - Dose 6-12 000mg of dried herb/day

Withania - Dose 3g/day

Tribulus Terrestris - Dose 6-12 g of dried herb/day (standardised to 40% furostanol saponin)

Arginine - 1000-2000mg/day

Zinc - Dose 30mg of elemental zinc/day

FEMALE HORMONES (CHAPTER 28)

HRT - Dose as directed by your prescribing doctor

Bioidentical hormones - Dose as directed by your prescribing doctor

Phyto-oestrogens - 40mg of soy isoflavones

TESTOSTERONE (CHAPTER 29)

Testosterone

Androstenedione

Androstenediol

Dehydroepiandrosterone (DHEA)

All supplements in this section are as prescribed by your doctor for your individual needs.

DHEA (CHAPTER 30)

DHEA (Dose as directed by your prescribing doctor)

GROWTH HORMONE (CHAPTER 31)

Growth hormone (Dose as directed by your prescribing doctor)

MELATONIN (CHAPTER 32)

Melatonin

Tryptophan

Supplements in this chapter are as prescribed by your doctor or health care professional for your individual needs.

SKIN & AGEING (CHAPTER 33)

Antioxidants - vitamin C, E, lipoic acid, lycopene, lutein – see Antioxidant section
Soy Isoflavones - 40mg/day
Glucosamine - Dose 500 - 1500mg/day
GAGs - Dose 380mg/day
Grapeseed - Dose 6-12g of dried herb/day

BONES & JOINTS (CHAPTER 34)

Calcium Citrate - Dose 1500mg/day
Hydroxyapitate - Dose 1500mg/day
Vitamin D - RDI 200 to 400iu
Vitamin K - RDI 80 mcg
Magnesium - Dose 250-750mg/day at bedtime
Glucosamine - Dose 500-1500mg/day
Chondroitin - Dose 400-1200mg/day
Glucosamine - Dose 500mg three times per day
Chondroitin sulphate - Dose 400mg three times per day

THE PELVIC FLOOR (CHAPTER 35)

Glucosamine - Dose 500mg three times per day
Chondroitin sulphate - Dose 400mg three times per day

THE PROSTATE (CHAPTER 35)

Lycopene - 6.5mg/day or a tablespoon of tomato paste everyday in your cooking
Zinc - Dose 30mg of elemental zinc/day
Saw Palmetto - Dose 320mg of extract/day (standardised to 85-95% fatty acids)

EYES (CHAPTER 36)

Vitamin A (retinol) - RDI 1.5 mg/day
Leutin - Dose 10mg/day
Zinc - Dose 30mg of elemental zinc/day

SECTION 5:
SURVIVAL OF THE FITTEST

CHAPTER 21: WHY YOU SHOULD MOVE...NOW!
CHAPTER 22: THE SLOW AGEING EXERCISE PLAN

Most adults don't engage in regular physical activity and their lives are poorer and shorter for it. Exercise can slow down, halt and possibly even reverse many of the trends associated with ageing. Exercise can fight weight gain, increase strength and stress resilience, prevent the diseases of ageing such as cardiovascular disease, and of course help you look and feel fantastic. In this section, we look at how exercise works and help you find ways to make it work for you.

KATE'S EXPERIENCE
Since getting serious about exercise, I have never felt stronger, more energised and confident in my life. I'm attracting men who are gorgeous, young and vital, who never looked my way before. I have never enjoyed this level of attention before.

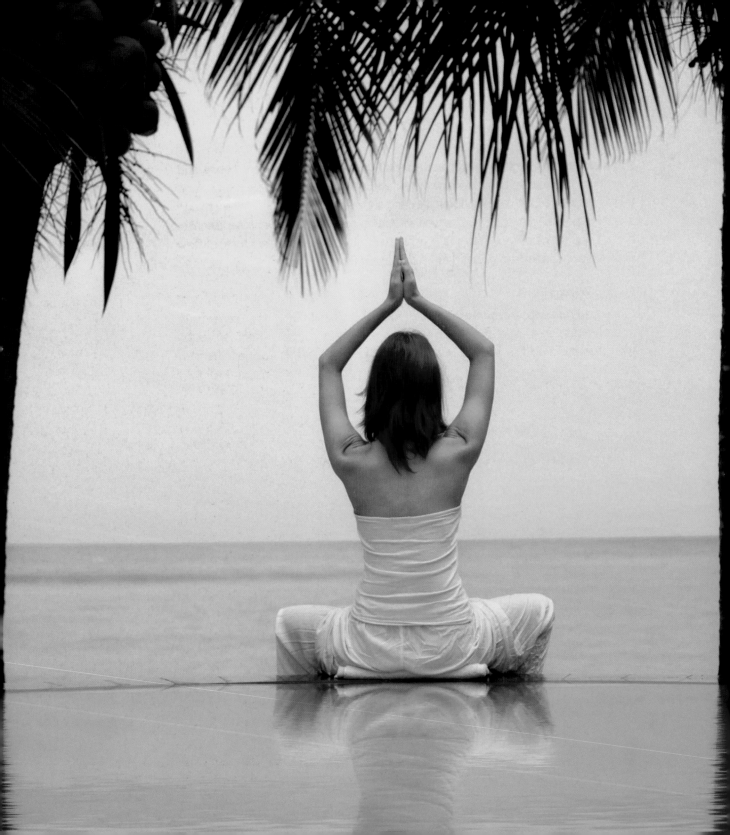

CHAPTER 21
WHY YOU SHOULD MOVE...NOW!

The majority of adults do not get enough physical activity to optimise health and improve their quality life. If we are sedentary, the risk of premature death and disease increases to the same extent as being a smoker. By contrast, regular activity not only increases level of fitness and health, but also has been shown to increase our lifespan by approximately 3 to 5 years. Equally, we can have the best diet, eat handfuls of supplements and have a positive attitude, but if we are sedentary many of these benefits may be lost. But how does exercise work for us?

Firstly, exercise burns calories that would otherwise be deposited as fat around our abdominal area. Consequently, regular exercise is an important means to reduce our abdominal fat levels and assist with weight control but it also improves the proportion of muscle tissue to body fat - a change that reverses the effect of ageing. However, the value of regular exercise is not just about reducing body fat; the effects are wide ranging, slowing down the normal ageing process in many body systems.

Secondly, physical activity modifies many of the factors that contribute to ageing and disease, including heart disease, diabetes, dementia, depression, osteoporosis and cancer. For example, exercise reduces the effects of free radicals, inflammation, AGEs, stress and assists in the reduction of high cholesterol, glucose and blood pressure levels. Exercise is also able to modify hormones that impact the ageing process, including reducing blood insulin levels (and insulin resistance), and increasing the anti-aging hormones, growth hormone, testosterone and DHEA (see section 7).

Thirdly, regular and progressively increasing levels of different types of exercise or 'physical training', stimulates specific body systems which results in adaptations to its natural defence pathways. These adaptations we call 'getting fit'. For example, if the heart and circulatory system is overloaded by a regular walking program, the capacity of this system also increases, so we can do more with less effort and fatigue. Regular exercise will also improve the body's repair and regeneration mechanisms that protect against future damage during exercise.

Fourthly, if muscles are progressively overloaded during resistance training will adapt to become bigger and stronger. Stronger muscles will preserve capacity to

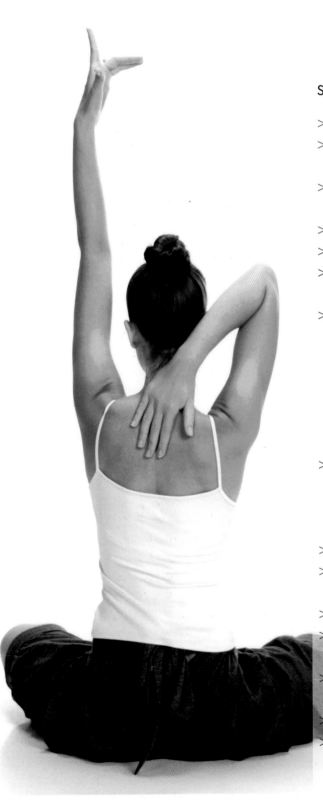

SOME OF THE MANY BENEFITS OF EXERCISE

> Enhanced quality and quantity of life
> Improved physical capacity so we can carry out daily tasks with less effort and fatigue
> Improved appearance (body composition, muscle tone, body shape)
> Improved stress resilience
> Improved weight and appetite control
> Improved sugar control and a reduced risk of diabetes
> Improved cardiovascular function and reduced risk factors for heart disease and stroke, including lower (bad) LDL cholesterol, increased blood vessel elasticity, reduced abdominal fat, lower blood pressure, reduced oxidative stress, improved sugar control and reduced AGEs
> Improved bone density and reduce risk of falls and fracture (especially high-impact and weight-bearing activities such as jogging or skipping or strength training)
> Improved balance, coordination and posture
> Improved regulation of insulin, growth hormone, testosterone and DHEA
> Strengthened adaptive immunity
> Improved cognitive functions and reduced risk of dementia
> Reduced risk of some cancers, especially colon, breast and prostate cancer
> Improved mood and feelings of well-being
> Improved sleep patterns

carry out daily tasks and maintain our quality of life when we are older. Strength training also increases the bone strength, thus reducing our risk of a fracture during a fall. Increased levels of endurance, strength and balance increase the threshold for disability and dependence as we age. Increases in physical activity and functional capacity are increasingly useful as we get older.

Other protective mechanisms also improve. Although exercise releases free radicals, the higher antioxidant levels that result from becoming fit, means that oxidative stress is also lower in the long-term. Being fit also makes us think better. Exercise stimulates the growth and development of brain cells, increasing their capacity for learning and memory and slowing the loss in mental performance and diseases associated with the ageing process.

HOW MUCH EXERCISE SHOULD WE DO?

For most of us, it is more exercise than we are doing right now. The minimum activity level is walking (or other similar activity) at a moderate pace for 30 minutes on most days or 150 minutes/week. This will result in significant health benefits when compared to being sedentary. However, doing even more than this minimum level of exercise, and incorporating other forms of activity, such as strength training, will result in additional health benefits. People who have the highest levels of physical activity and fitness invariably have the lowest risk of premature death and disease.

HOW OFTEN SHOULD WE EXERCISE?

We should undertake at least 30 minutes of moderate-intensity exercise, on at least every second day, otherwise the health benefit will be lost. Even better health outcomes are seen with longer and more frequent workouts. But like any slow solution, it is best to take the time to progressively increase our level of activity and with it our fitness and health. When starting a program after a period of inactivity, exercising 3-4 times/week on alternate days is recommended, allowing a day of recovery between each session to assist recovery and adaptation to occur. The recovery days should be used to engage in lower intensity or a different type of exercise, such as resistance training, so the exercise stress is rotated.

HOW HARD SHOULD WE GO?

To maximise the fitness and health benefits as we get fitter, we need to increase the exercise intensity from moderate to higher intensity. Rather than working at an intensity that would be perceived as 'easy', we need to exercise level which we would rate as 'somewhat hard' to 'hard'. However, you should exercise at a level that still enables you to conduct a conversation, which is often referred to as 'talking pace'. If you cannot talk while you are exercising, you are working too hard.

When undertaking aerobic exercise, such as walking or cycling, another simple way to determine if we are working at an appropriate exercise intensity is to monitor our heart rate during exercise. This can either be done by periodically taking the pulse over a 30-second period during aerobic training, or by using a heart rate monitor. Research has shown that to achieve an optimum aerobic training effect, you need to work at above a minimum threshold heart rate. This threshold heart rate is based on a percentage of your maximal heart rate.

As a guide to establishing your aerobic threshold and your training 'zone', you must first estimate your maximal heart rate. This is calculated as:

Maximum Heart Rate = 220 – age
e.g. for a healthy 50-year-old the max heart rate is 220 – 50 = 170 bpm

Sedentary individuals just starting an exercise program should initially aim to do sufficient work to get their hearts beating between 65-75% of their maximal rate (ie. 110-128 beats per minute in a healthy 50-year-old). For individuals who are currently active, they should aim to work at 75-85% of their maximal capacity (ie. 129-145 beats per minute in a healthy 50-year-old). This will ensure you are obtaining the maximum benefit from your training, without overstressing your heart and circulatory system. By self programming your heart rate monitor, the monitor will determine the optimal heart rate zone for you based on your age and heart rate. Many treadmills and bikes will have heart rate measuring hand pads on them as well.

It must be emphasised that this calculation applies only to healthy individuals. Those with chronic diseases or on medication will need individualised advice as to their appropriate and safe training zones. These individuals must seek advice from a doctor, an accredited exercise physiologist and/or a suitably qualified allied health professional to determine their heart rate training zones. Only healthy athletes would be recommended to exceed these levels for specific performance benefits. Short, repeated bursts of more vigorous exercise (such as performed in interval training) may have some additional health benefits. However, high intensity resistance or strength training has been shown to provide specific benefits when training individuals to increase their bone or muscle mass, and those with a chronic depressive illness.

WHAT FORM OF EXERCISE SHOULD WE DO ?

Similar health benefits of physical activity can be achieved whether performed as a structured daily session (exercise) or as unstructured activity spread over the course of a day. Often it is easier to 'accumulate' moderate-intensity physical activity as part of a busy lifestyle, by walking around the workplace, taking the stairs rather than the lift, walking to the bus stop, or parking a little further away from the office and walking into work. Taking all the little opportunities to exercise when we can, can be as beneficial as a session in the gym and may be more convenient. The most important aspect is to ensure that your physical activity is incorporated into your day, rather than being sedentary.

There are many different kinds of exercise, from sports to more formal programs. Each has its own benefits and limitations. The best results are achieved in 'slow' programs, which balance these different types and target our individual requirements.

AEROBIC EXERCISE

Aerobic exercise is performed when the exercise is continuous and prolonged for more that three minutes. Aerobic exercise requires oxygen to be supplied to the muscles to keep them contracting. Aerobic activities include walking or jogging, cycling, swimming, aerobics, circuit weight training and sports, such as soccer, squash and tennis, where there are repeated bursts of high intensity activity over the course of a game.

Regular aerobic exercise improves the functional capacity of the heart, lungs and blood vessels to deliver oxygen to our body and increases our aerobic fitness. This can be measured as the VO^2max (also known as aerobic capacity, endurance exercise potential). It is assessed by measuring an individual's oxygen consumption as the exercise intensity is progressively increased each minute, until physical exhaustion is achieved. The test may be performed on a treadmill, bike or rowing machine (often referred to an ergometer). The oxygen consumption is calculated by measuring the volume and composition of expired air, with the maximum value achieved near the end of the test, being the VO^2max.

Although aerobic fitness is strongly associated with improved health and wellbeing, it must not be viewed in isolation. In general, most forms of aerobic training does not increase muscle strength or bone mass, which buffer the impacts of ageing.

Although aerobic fitness relies on continuous activities, additional improvements can be achieved in active individuals, by alternating short bursts of near-maximal exertion with intervals of lower intensity activity. This form of training is known as 'interval training'. This may involve short periods of jogging as part of a basic walking program and progress to including multiple sprints of 100 - 200m with alternate periods of walking or jogging. Swimmers may include a couple of faster laps followed by slower laps. The higher-intensity phase should be sufficiently long and strenuous enough that you are out of breath. Recovery periods should be only long enough to result in a partial recovery before the next exercise interval begins. The total of burst-recovery repeats should initially total some 15-20 minutes and be preceded by 10-15 mins of warming up and concluded by 10-15 mins of cooling down and stretching.

Interval training is generally more strenuous than continuous aerobic training, and generally requires increased levels of motivation. It can be included in your basic aerobic exercise program on 1-2 occasions/week. It should only be completed by healthy individuals and those with no history of muscle or joint injury. If interval running forms part of a program, then it is best to run on a soft surface to reduce the stress on muscle and joints (to avoid the risk of developing a chronic injury).

ANAEROBIC EXERCISE

Anaerobic exercise means undertaking short bursts of intense exertion performed at close to, or above 100% effort, like fast running or lifting heavy weights. Because the energy required for this kind of activity is at or above the maximal ability to supply oxygen to fuel the muscles (i.e. above the VO^2 max), anaerobic exercise must use stored energy in the muscles. However, this store is limited and maximal exertion cannot be sustained for more than 2-3 minutes. While anaerobic exercise will burn more energy in a period of time, when compared to aerobic exercise, the body will be unable to sustain this level of exercise for more than a few minutes without a period of recovery.

STRENGTH TRAINING

Strength training involves the repeated generation of a muscle force against a resistance. This form of training increases muscle strength, endurance and over time results in an increase in muscle size, called hypertrophy. This may involve working against gravity (e.g. weights, squatting exercises) or elastic/hydraulic resistance. To achieve improvements, our muscles must to be progressively 'overloaded', as the muscles become stronger. The process of overload, then stimulates adaptive processes that increases strength of the muscles, bones, ligaments, tendons, and cartilage that slow down the ageing process. Strength training is primarily anaerobic activity, however by undertaking a series of resistance training activities with only short periods of rest between them, so the exercise heart rate is kept high, may also result in increased aerobic fitness. This is called circuit weight training.

Strength training programs are designed to apply resistance to specific muscles using an exercise that is continued until muscle fatigue ensues. When starting a strength training program, resistance applied is varied so that the exercise can only be repeated 6 to 12 times. This corresponds to at 65-85% of maximal capacity (often referred to as the one repetition maximum or 1RM). This is called a 'set' of repetitions. Generally, three sets of each exercise, with a 60 to 90 second recovery period between each set, are required to provide the best stimulus to increase muscle strength. A strength program would generally consist of 8 -10 exercises, that stress the major muscles of the legs, upper back, chest, shoulders and arms and importantly the trunk or core muscles of the abdominal wall. As the body adapts to its training load, training is progressively increased by increasing the applied resistance or load, the number of sets, by reducing the time between sets or changing the sequence of exercises, so the muscle is blitzed by exercises that apply similar stresses.

Strength training should be conducted at least 2-3 times/week, on alternate days so the muscles have a chance to regenerate and become stronger as a result of repeated sessions. If strength training is to be conducted every day, it is advisable to split the program into two segments (i.e. upper and lower body), so each muscle has 48 hours to recover between each session.

COMMON MISCONCEPTIONS ABOUT STRENGTH TRAINING

Weight training causes women to bulk up and look masculine. As women have only one tenth the level of testosterone like men, women undertaking weight training do not 'bulk up' like men and look masculine. However, women undertaking weight training can obtain significant strength gains and improve their overall body shape - all very desirable benefits.

Weight training will make you gain weight. As muscle is more dense than fat, increasing your muscle mass may make you weigh more (according to the scales). But it is more common to lose weight as abdominal fat stores decline and body composition and shape changes. Skinfold callipers can easily assess if change in body weight is due to a change in muscle or fat mass.

Weight training will convert fat into muscle. The energy requirements of resistance exercise will burn fat stores, and reduce body fat stores. Muscle mass will increase as a result of strength training but fat is not 'converted' into muscle.

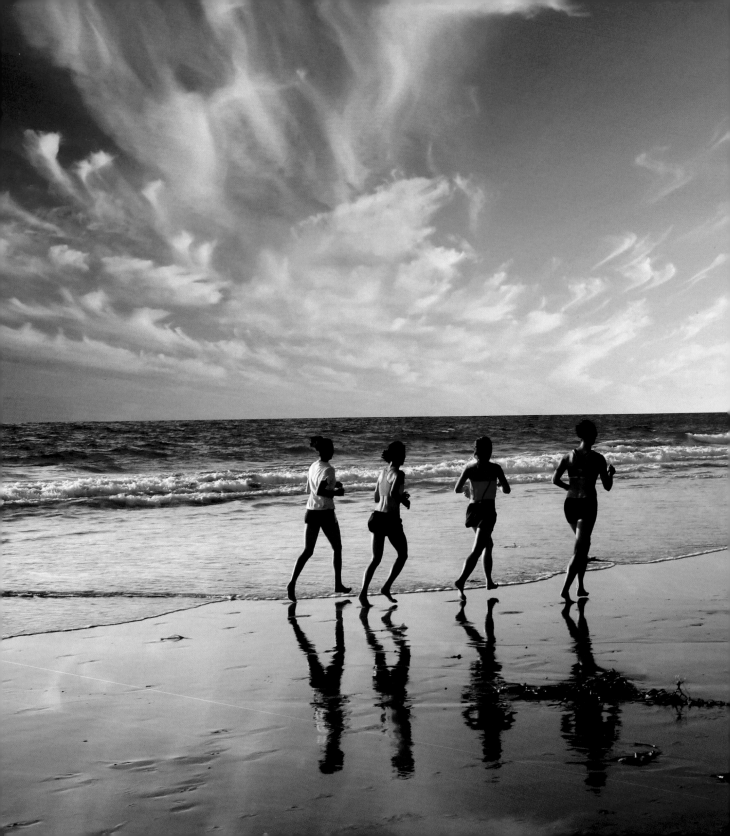

CHAPTER 22

THE SLOW AGEING EXERCISE PLAN

To ensure we achieve the benefits of a regular physical activity program we must make our exercise session a not-negotiable priority each day. 'Slow exercise' is about being open to the many opportunities we have, every day, to accumulate a range of physical activities that will make a real difference to our health. The average yearly weight gain for adults is equivalent to walking an extra half a km every day or 4 km/week. It doesn't seem much, but it all adds up over a lifetime to better health. The most exciting thing is that there are a multitude of activity options to try. The only barrier to our success is the willingness to take responsibility for our activity levels.

1. AWARENESS AND UNDERSTANDING EXERCISE

The first step of slow exercise is awareness and understanding. In the previous chapter, we explored how exercise works to improve health and the basic principles behind different types of exercise. It is also important that we determine any barriers to us undertaking a regular exercise program. Based on your health needs, examine the type and amount of physical activity you need and consider the strategies that will ensure your regular participation. Lack of time, energy, or motivation are the most common barriers to regular participation in an exercise program, but as we age, chronic injury, joint pain and poor health may also be important. All of these barriers can be overcome by clearly identifying your exercise and health priorities, and by seeking professional advice as required.

For those with health problems and those over 45, it is wise to obtain a 'medical clearance' before undertaking any exercise program. This usually involves a comprehensive medical history and health screen. This appointment can also help to can also target the right exercise for your particular requirements and mindful of your particular limitations. A health and musculoskeletal assessment by an accredited exercise physiologist or health professional can ensure that the optimal benefits are achieved for each individual with a minimum risk of injury or other adverse consequences. Individuals with chronic disease may also be eligible for an Enhanced Primary Care (EPC) Plan, which provides a referral to a relevant allied health professional, who can assist with specific health goals. The EPC Plan, which is drawn up by a GP enables you to access a Medicare Rebate for up to five appointments per year for services such as exercise physiology, physiotherapy, dietetics, osteopathy and chiropractic.

2. STRATEGIC PLANNING AND TARGETING OF APPROPRIATE GOALS FOR EXERCISE

Slow is about setting achievable goals and setting up short term steps to obtain these goals. Establishing a clear goal keeps us on track and give us purpose, but there must also be accompanied by a daily plan of how to put these into action.

People exercise for different reasons at different times of their lives. To get the most from your exercise, it helps to know what you want to achieve and how you are going to achieve it. Setting specific and measurable short-term and long-term targets provide the incentive to drive you to action.

Before starting a successful exercise program, it is also useful to undergo some assessment of your current level of fitness, including specific tests of strength, endurance, flexibility, balance and posture. Many of these tests can be conducted by an accredited exercise physiologist, physiotherapist, or qualified personal trainer. These practitioners can also help to make sure these objectives are realistic or we can set ourselves up for failure. Setting behavioural goals each day such as walking 10,000 steps or completing our strength program every second day, rather than specific weight loss targets, are more sensible and readily within our control.

Achieving our goals in small increments each week, will ultimately produce the results we desire. It is important to allocate time for exercise in your diary and set weekly and monthly objectives. Start slowly with small, easily achievable amounts of exercise that you can build upon gradually. If you want to loose 20kgs (which may take 6-12 months) you need to set more short-term weekly targets, to maintain steady and consistent progress. Slow progress will be more sustainable in the long term!

3. ACCENT THE POSITIVE OF EXERCISE, AVOID THE NEGATIVE

Exercise must be an enjoyable positive experience and something you look forward to each day. An exercise session can also become an enjoyable social occasion

AN EXERCISE SESSION CAN ALSO BECOME AN ENJOYABLE SOCIAL OCCASION WITH FRIENDS AND FAMILY.

with friends and family. Also if you choose an activity you enjoy, chances are you will do it more often. Choose an activity you have enjoyed in the past and have the skills and knowledge required to ensure regular participation. Involve a reliable exercise partner, friend or if required, a trainer to share the experience and to assist with motivation and compliance.

If one exercise doesn't work for you, then find an alternative. Find ways to make working out a joy. Maybe put on enjoyable music to support the activity you are doing, listen to interesting books or podcasts. When you start to get positive reinforcement by people around you, it will become easier and even more enjoyable.

If you find you are fatigued or your muscles are sore after your first session, then understand these feelings will be short lived. This is precisely what it takes to make our muscles adapt and get stronger. If you find your muscles are sore for more than 48 hours after your exercise session, you may need to reduce the amount, or the intensity of your program, and reduce your expectations, until your body is more able to cope with the program.

4. MAKING CHOICES THAT ARE SUSTAINABLE FOR THE LONG-TERM

Exercise is a good habit we need to establish for our lifetime. It takes a few months to develop habits. But with persistence, we can make exercise something we do routinely, and something we 'miss', when we don't get enough. Exercise itself can become addictive!

There are so many options. Structured exercise programs are widely available, but we can also structure exercise into our regular daily commitments, such as to walk or cycle to work, or to take the kids to school and then jog back. It all adds up in the long term. Small incremental steps are much easier to sustain. Avoid making multiple lifestyle changes all at once, as this may lead to increased levels of stress, frustration and failure. As your fitness improves begin introducing different types of exercise in a series of stages. For example, this may mean getting a walking program well underway, before starting strength training.

5. ENJOY VARIETY

Exercise programs should not be exclusive and one program does not suit everyone. A balanced multi-component exercise program works best.

Slow exercise is not exclusive. There is no one magic exercise program or exercise machine that is the answer or 'works in only three weeks'. Different forms of exercise training produce specific fitness and health outcomes. The best results come from a balanced exercise program, that incorporates a mix of resistance, aerobic and

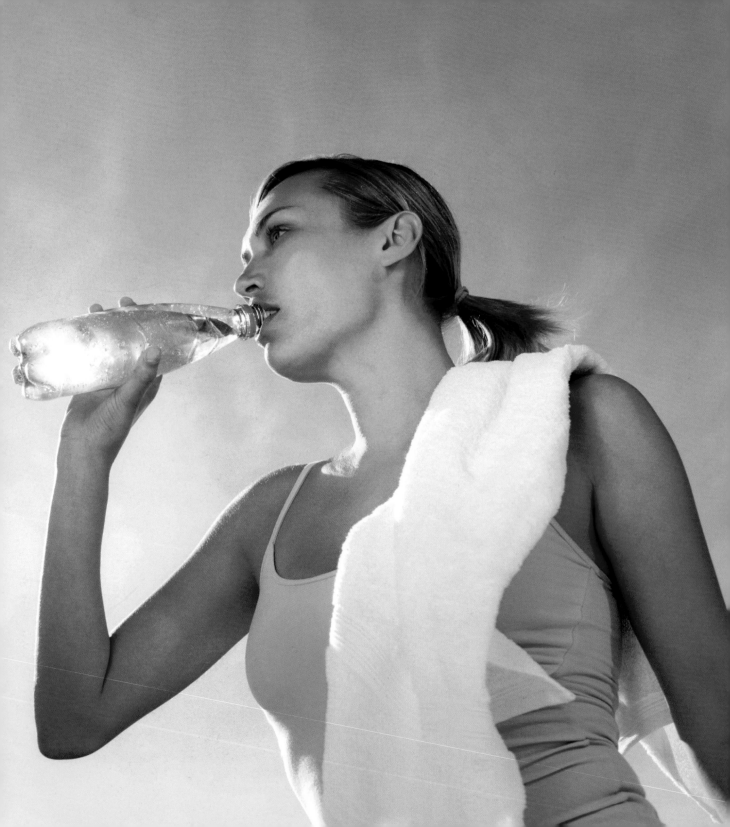

stretching programs to ensure that you gain the many available benefits. For example, aerobic exercise will adapt the cardiorespiratory system, while resistance training will increase muscle strength.

6. SUPPORT IS OUT THERE, GET HELP

Exercise is not about just having weights, a bicycle or a rowing machine. It is about using them regularly and effectively to improve your physical fitness. It is no good purchasing a set of weights or a treadmill that ends up in the back of the garage gathering dust. There are many allied health professionals and personal trainers that can be consulted to assist in achieving your specific health and fitness outcomes. These individuals can define your goals based on our health needs, as well as providing the motivation and support to keep you on the right track.

7. BE SELECTIVE AND MONITOR YOUR PROGRESS

Slow ageing exercise is about doing the right exercise, in the right doses and at the right pace to achieve your individual goals and needs. There is no one solution to achieving the best results for you. The rate of progress will differ for different individuals, so do not compare your rate of progress or measure yourself against others.

It is also important to monitor your progress and achievements, in order to stay on track. Chart the average distances and times of a walking/jogging program and see how you have improved. Keep a record in a diary. Document how weights increase as you undertake your strength program. Watch how your waistline decreases using a tape measure or the changes in you belt size. Monitor your resting heart rate each morning and watch how it decreases as you become fitter. Observe the health improvements like lower blood pressure or cholesterol level. Set longer term goals such as participating in a community Fun Run and enjoy your achievements as they accumulate.

All these changes can serve as a motivational tools. But most importantly it keeps us connected with our exercise and helps to enhance the experience, which is what slow solutions are all about.

WALKING PROVIDES MANY OF THE BENEFITS OF AEROBIC EXERCISE, AND SHOULD NOT BE OVERLOOKED AS AN IMPORTANT PART OF ANY HEALTH AND FITNESS PROGRAM.

IT IS NEVER TOO LATE TO START EXERCISING

If you are currently inactive, do not despair. You may have missed out on the benefits from regular physical activity yesterday, but there is always the rest of your life. There is still time. It is truly better late than never. Adopting a regular exercise routine for the first time reduces your future chances of disease and disability. Even if you already have disease and disability, exercise will improve your outcome (from any cause and from cardiovascular disease in particular) when compared to remaining sedentary. But the best outcomes start today.

WALKING TO SLOW AGEING

Simply walking provides many of the benefits of aerobic exercise, and should not be overlooked as an important part of any on-going health and fitness program. It is an enjoyable exercise that most people can easily and safely perform at any time of the day, all year round. Taking every opportunity to walk a bit further and/or a bit harder, soon adds up to better health outcomes. A regular brisk walking program will improve your aerobic fitness, lower your blood pressure improve your blood lipid profile and your lower your blood glucose levels. All of these physiological changes will reduce your future risk of having heart attack or stroke, developing diabetes, and some cancers by between 30-50%.

Like any slow solution, walking should have specific targets and outcomes. A pedometer provides a simple way of quantifying your daily walking program. They count each step by registering impacts as our feet hit the ground. It also provides a simple method to assess our current activity level, as well as a motivational tool to increase our activity further. Sedentary individuals will accumulate less than 5,000 steps/day, although everyone should have their own target based on their age and level of fitness, a general goal should be to walk at least 10,000 steps every day.

Based on an average step length of 0.8 meters, walking a kilometre means taking about 1,200 steps. If you do not have a pedometer, a distance-based or a time-based goal may also used as an alternative to a step count. For example, to get another 2,500 steps into a sedentary day at work, park the car 1 km or 10-15 minutes walk further away from your place of work.

Every exercise session should be started with a brief warm up. Start your walking program by walking at a gentle pace. Over the coming few weeks, increase the number of steps or the distance covered in each session so that you are achieving a daily minimum of 10,000 steps. Remember to include some variety in your program to make it fun, such as walk along the beach or in the hills as appropriate. Include

A MODEL WALKING PROGRAM

Beginner (no recent physical activity) Current step count averaging less than 5,000 steps/day						
Monday	Tuesday	Wednesday	Thursday	Friday	Saturday	Sunday
Minimum of 5,000 additional steps	Alternate activity or rest	Minimum of 5,000 additional steps	Minimum of 5,000 additional steps	Alternate activity or rest	Minimum of 5,000 additional steps	Longer walk in the hills (6,000 additional steps)
Daily Target						
10,000		10,000	10,000		10,000	11,000

Intermediate (some recent, but possibly infrequent, physical activity) Current step count averaging more than 5,000 steps/day						
Minimum of 7,000 additional steps incorporating some hills	Alternate activity eg. swim or cycle	Minimum of 7,500 additional steps	Minimum of 7,000 additional steps brisk	Alternate activity or rest	Minimum of 7,500 additional steps	Longer slow walk in the hills (8,000additional) steps
Daily Target						
12,500		12,500	12,500		12,500	14,000

Advanced (regular exerciser) Current step count averaging more than 6,000 steps/day						
Minimum of 8,000 additional steps incorporating some hilly terrain	Alternate activity eg. swim or cycle	Minimum of 9,000 additional steps Brisk walking	Minimum of 8,000 additional steps incorporating some hilly terrain	Minimum of 7,000 additional steps of walk-jog interval	Minimum of 8,000 additional steps brisk walking	Longer walk in the hills (10,000 steps)
Daily Target						
15,000		15,000	15,000	15,000	15,000	16,000

some longer walks on the weekend when you may have more time. After each walking session, undertake a brief 'cool-down', where you undertake some slower walking for 5 minutes and undertake your stretching program, as described below.

Once you are routinely achieving 10,000 steps/day, try to increase your walking speed or include some hilly terrain in your walk or aim for 15,000 steps. By increasing your walking pace or effort you can aim to increase your heart rate to keep most of the session within your target heart rate zone. As you become fitter include some intermittent jogging as part of your daily walking program. Keep challenging yourself, it's the only way you will improve!

AN AEROBIC EXERCISE PROGRAM

There are lots of other ways to add aerobic exercise to your day, including jogging, cycling, swimming, circuit training and sports, such as soccer, squash and tennis. To stimulate adaptations in our body and reap the health benefits, it is important to progressively challenge ourselves by changing the program's Frequency, Intensity, Time and Type of activity (known as the FITT principles).

F = Frequency - exercising more often is better. To improve aerobic fitness, we should aim to progressively increase our exercise frequency from a minimum of 3-4 times/week to 5-6 times/week. However, it is a good idea to plan one day each week as a recovery day.

I = Intensity - to improve your level of aerobic fitness you need to place sufficient stress on your cardiovascular system to produce the body's adaptive response. This means maintaining your exercise heart rate within the aerobic training zone.

T = Time - aim to exercise for a minimum of 30 minutes per day on at least 5 days per week. This may be accumulated in small blocks or intervals throughout the day, or in one 30 min session. As you get fitter, plan to progressively increase your exercise sessions by around 5 minutes per week, up to a total of 60 minutes per day.

T = Type - the type of exercise you undertake should be geared towards your interests and goals, but generally plan to include different types of exercise. Your current health and any musculo-skeletal injuries may also need to be taken into consideration. The best health outcomes will be achieved from a balanced program of regular aerobic activities combined with strength and flexibility

STARTING YOUR STRENGTH TRAINING PROGRAM – 10 KEY POINTS

Muscle strength is an important asset for health and independence as we get older. Resistance training offers a very important way of maintaining, and even improving our muscle mass and strength, which tends to decrease as we age.

1. Ensure you have proper guidance in developing an individualised program that is right for your abilities, enjoyment and mindful of any health or injury limitations. If you have not undertaken a weight training program before, seek professional advice before starting. Membership of a local gym or personal training studio will provide some level of supervision, advice and safety, as well as access to a larger range of machines. This will also increase the scope of the exercises that can be included in your resistance training program. A qualified personal trainer will better be able to assist you in your initial session(s) and to get you underway. However, individualised personal training will come at an additional cost of between $60 and up to $120/hour.

2. Always warm up prior to undertaking a weights program. Begin with a walk or slow jog, or perform your activity at a lower intensity for the first 5 to 10 minutes of your workout. If you start your physical activity while cold, you are more likely to be injured. Stretching is best done after the warm-up and as part of the cool-down phase after exercise. When your muscles are warm, they are more pliable so as to increase the range of movement. Stretching is important for injury prevention and joint flexibility, and maximising exercise performance.

3. At the start of any weights program obtain, some initial instruction on the correct 'form' for each exercise. This not only ensures the exercise is doing what it is was designed to do, but using good form also reduces the chance of injury. Perform your exercises in front of a mirror to check your exercise form is correct, or ask a trainer or partner to provide feedback.

AT THE START OF ANY WEIGHTS PROGRAM, OBTAIN SOME INITIAL INSTRUCTION ON THE CORRECT 'FORM' FOR EACH EXERCISE.

If you are a beginner, it is often advisable to start with specifically designed, pin loaded machines, if these are available. These machines have the advantage of being highly specific, isolating the muscle to be worked and supporting the other muscles. Whilst these machines might look intimidating, they have the advantage that the weight or resistance applied can be easily changed. Most also have the added advantage that a trainer is not required to 'spot' you to ensure your safety. As you become more experienced however, barbells and dumbbells, called free weights, are often preferred, as these also engage the muscles that stabilise the joint. As these movements are not restricted to one plane, joint stabilisation becomes an important component of the exercise.

4. When starting your program, begin with a weight that enables you to complete the required number of repetitions for each exercise, without compromising form or with undue fatigue. The focus must be on good exercise form, rather ensuring the weight lifted is near maximal.

5. All joints have different muscles that work in opposing directions, such as flexion and extension. An example is the biceps, which flexes the elbow, and its antagonist muscle, the triceps, which extends the elbow. When designing a program, it is important to ensure that muscle strength and the range of movement are kept in balance. Part of an initial individual assessment should determine the strength, postural and flexibility priorities of any exercise program. Many weights programs often neglect the stabilising muscles of the upper back, spine, and shoulder joints.

6. Work through your resistance program. Allow yourself a brief rest of 30-60 seconds between each exercise. On completion of each exercise, record the weight lifted and the actual number of repetitions you have completed on your program card. At the initial session aim to perform one set of each exercise and focus on becoming familiar with the correct exercise form. At the next session, which should be approximately 48 hours later, perform two sets of each exercise, using the same weight or resistance as the initial session. Allow 60 to 90 seconds rest between each set and again focus on performing each exercise with good form. For the third session, complete the target 3 sets of each exercise. For subsequent sessions slowly begin to increase the weight so that the last few repetitions of each set of each exercise are near maximal. Ensure you continue to maintain correct form for each exercise while slowly increasing the weight lifted.
To increase your strength you must progressively overload your muscles by increasing the resistance they are required to work against. As soon as you accomplish the specific goal for each exercise (e.g. 3 sets of 12 reps), you should increase your weights.

7. Ensure you provide adequate opportunity for rest, regeneration and growth for your muscles. Don't work the same muscle group two days in a row. You will achieve better results if you allow your muscles to fully recover between workouts.

8. You should aim to strength train 2 to 4 times a week. By alternating the days on which you strength train with your aerobic exercise, this will provide you with a well balanced exercise program.

9. A weights program can be conducted at a gym or it can be designed so it can be completed at home with minimal equipment and expense. A pair of variable dumbbells with up to 20 kg of weights, 2-3 therabands (these consist of a length of rubber tubing of varying thickness), a fitball and a basic horizontal bench or equivalent, is all that is required to undertake the home resistance training program outlined further on. Make it a habit and part of your lifestyle. Significant improvements in strength can be achieved within 6 weeks and these benefits can be maintained even with 1 to 2 sessions per week.

10. Always include a stretching program at the completion of your weights program to ensure you maintain your joint and muscle range of movement. On completion of your weights session also perform a brief cool down of 5-10 mins walking to assist your recovery.

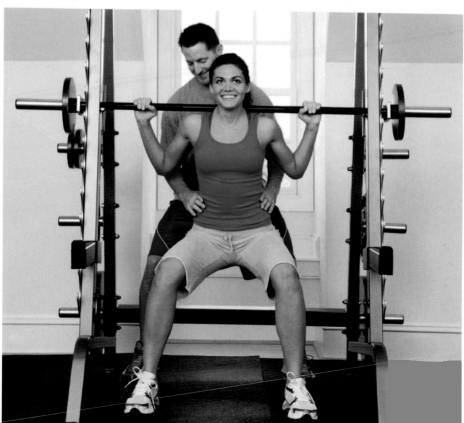

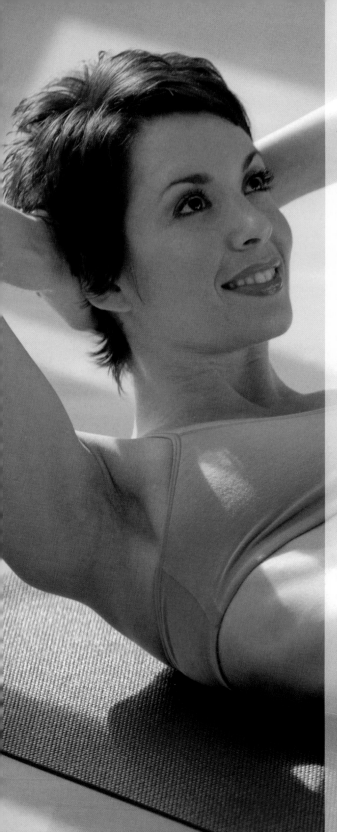

THE ABDOMINAL 'CORE' MUSCLES AND BACK PROBLEMS

The abdominal core muscles stabilise and support the lower spine and pelvis. They consist of three integrated layers. The most important of these is the innermost layer which includes the transverse abdominis (TA), which wraps horizontally around the trunk, lumbar spine and pelvis. This muscle acts like a corset to stabilise the lower back and pelvis. Strengthening the TA is important for the prevention and management of back pain, a common problem as we grow older.

To learn how to activate the TA, lie on the floor with the knee and hips flexed. Place your fingertips on the front of your lower abdominals just above the pelvic bone and SLOWLY draw in your lower abdominals. Imagine your navel is being drawn closer to your spine. Do not hold your breath as this means you are also (incorrectly) activating your upper abdominals. You should be able to feel the increase in the muscle tension underneath your finger tips. Alternatively, you can imagine you are trying to stop your urine flow, as this cue will also activate the TA muscles. Individuals with a history of back injury may have difficulty activating their TA, and some professional assistance from an exercise physiologist or physiotherapist may be required.

Once you have successfully activated the TA, you can include a number of exercises that require you to stabilise your abdominal core. Try activating your TA as above and then slowly extend one leg and return it to the starting position. Repeat with the opposite leg and then repeat 10-15 times while keeping the TA activated. When performing your strength training program, or in daily lifting tasks, always focus on initially activating your TA to ensure the lumbar spine and pelvis are stabilised. This will reduce the possibility of a back injury.

YOUR RESISTANCE TRAINING PROGRAM

Name of exercise (muscles exercised)	Sets and repetitions weight (as required)	Key form elements
1. Step ups onto a 40 cm bench or step (quads, hamstrings, glutes)	3 x 20 reps lead with each leg Carry 3-5 kg DB as required	Keep torso upright and tighten 'core'. Stand up to full height on top of step. Take care not to trip while stepping.
2. Prone plank (on elbows toes, or knees) (abdominal core muscles)	Hold initially 20-30 secs Repeat 3-5 times with 60 secs rest between repeats	Draw in and tighten your core muscles. Lift body and off floor and keep body straight. Stop exercise if any back pain develops.
3. DB bench press (pectorals, anterior deltoids and triceps)	3 x 12 reps Weight 2-5 kg	Lie on bench, fitball or floor With DB resting on front of shoulders, push DB directly vertical in a controlled manner until arms are fully extended Return to starting position.
4. Seated rowing (posterior deltoids rhomboids, trapezius, latissmus dorsi and biceps)	3 x 12 reps Use theraband	Sit with back upright and chest high. Link the theraband around feet. Pull shoulders back and then pull ends of theraband to armpits. Do not lean back.
5. Curl-ups with twist (rectus abdominus, obliques)	3 x 15 reps each side	Lie on back arms crossed on hips. Tuck chin into chest and twist to one side to touch hands on outside of knee. Repeat both sides.
6. Static lunge (quads, glutes and calf muscles)	3 x 12 reps with both legs Carry 3-5 kg DB as required	Stand astride with one foot forward. Place hands on hips, keep back upright, lunge forward to take weight on the front foot, hold for a few seconds and then return to starting position.
7. Inclined chin ups (latissimus dorsi, biceps, deltoids and pectorals)	3 x 12 reps No weight	Find a sturdy bar at chest height. Hang on the bar with legs extended to the floor. Keeping body straight, pull your chest up until it touches the bar. Lower body to starting position.
8. Half squats using fitball support against wall (quadriceps and glutes)	3 x 12 reps Carry 3-5 kg DB as required	Place a Fit ball against the wall and in the small of your back. Leaning against it with feet slightly in front of hips. Lower your body until your upper thigh is horizontal to floor. Keep back upright and chest high.
9. Seated DB overhead press (deltoids, trapezius & triceps)	3 x 12 reps Weight 3-5 kg	Sit on a bench or chair with DB's in front of shoulders. Push ups up so DB's are directly above the shoulders. Return to start.
10. DB curls (biceps and anterior deltoids)	3 x 12 reps Weight 3-5 kg	Stand astride with back upright and arms extended. Curl DB up to chest by only flexing elbows. Do not swing your trunk as part of the lifting movement. (If this is required, the DB's are too heavy and the weight needs to be reduced).

YOUR BASIC STRETCHING PROGRAM

Optimal exercise is not just working hard. To get the best muscle performance and reduce the risk of injury, a program including stretching exercises may also be helpful. In these activities, a limb is slowly moved to the end of the range of movement until tension is felt in the muscles to be stretched. This end position is then held for 10-30 seconds while the muscle or joint structure is held on stretch, before returning the limb to its starting position. Repeat 3-5 times.

It is recommended that you perform a stretching program on completion of both your walking and resistance training program.

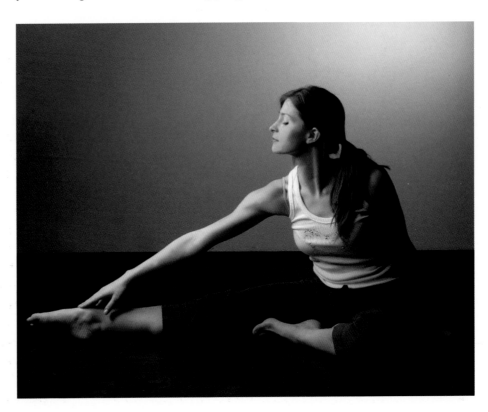

Stretching exercise	Exercise description
Hamstring stretches	Lie on your back with knees flexed. Place your hand behind your knee and lift one leg as high as possible, making sure your knee is kept straight. Hold this position for 10-30 secs, then return to the starting position. Repeat 3-5 times with each leg.
Quad stretch	Stand on one leg, holding an upright for stability. Grasp one foot and flex one knee to pull your heel to your buttock. Return to the starting position. Repeat 3-5 times with each leg.
Knee roll side to side	Lie on your back with knees and hips flexed. Draw in your core muscles and slowly rotate both knees to try to touch the floor. Hold this end position for 10-30 secs and slowly rotate your knees to the other side. Again hold for 10 secs and repeat 5-6 times.
Supine knee across chest	Lie on your back with legs straight. Lift one leg to your chest. Using your opposite hand, push your knee down towards the floor. Hold this end position for 10-30 secs, then return to the starting position. Repeat 3-5 times with each leg.
Back arch	Lie prone with hands placed on the floor under your shoulders. Push upwards with palms against the floor and arch your back. Push hips down towards the floor. Hold for 10 secs and return to starting position. Repeat 3-5 times. (If any back or leg pain is experienced during this movement, avoid this exercise and seek professional advice).
Corner shoulder stretch	Using the corner in a room, place your hands against opposing walls, shoulder-width apart. Lean into the corner, keeping your chest high. You should feel the stretch across your chest and at the front of your shoulders. Hold this position for 10-30 secs. Repeat 3-5 times.
Calf stretches	Lean against a wall with one foot in front of the other. Bend your front knee and take your weight on your front leg. Keep the heel of your back leg on the ground. You should feel the stretch in the calf of your back leg. Hold this position for 10-30 secs. Repeat 3 times.

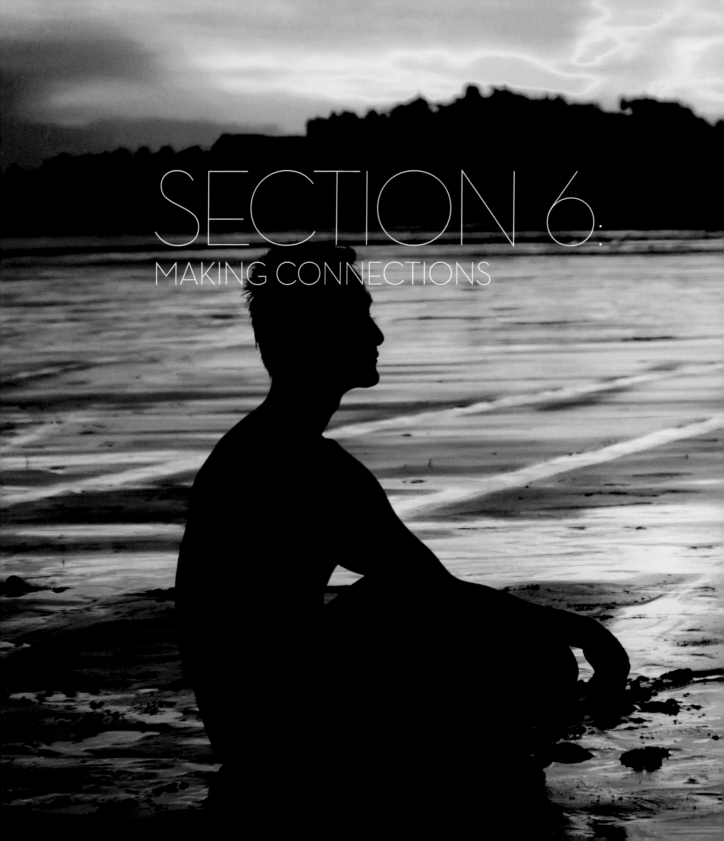

SECTION 6:
MAKING CONNECTIONS

Health resides in the totality of being human - mind, body, emotions and spirit. These are not separate elements, they are intimately interconnected. Everything we think, feel or enact has a consequence on our bodies and our ageing. While the close links between mind and body can drag you and your health down, this connection can also be harnessed to heal, renew and transform. It is often said that ageing is part body and part attitude! In this section, we examine some tools to retrain our body's physiological processes and look at ways to take care of our mind, so it takes care of us.

KATE'S EXPERIENCE

Living in the fast lane, I became desensitised to the stress I was under. I just told myself it was normal to feel tired and run down. Then one day I opened my eyes and noticed I wasn't going where I wanted. We all have the ability to slow down if we want to. Try different techniques to discover which ones are most comfortable and powerful for you; ones you can make a regular part of your lifestyle. I'm a bit extreme and like to fast-track things, so I'm possibly more aggressive than some in searching out new tools and techniques for self-improvement, so in this section you will find some tools that you may not have been exposed to before. There is a whole body of work around biofeedback, for example, which means re-training your body's physiological processes. I've tried all the tools in these sections and found them amazing as they have really accelerated my capacity to de-stress and improve my brain function. Meditation makes you feel GREAT and is definitely one of the 'magic bullets' for healthy ageing, however a Zen-like state can be hard for some people to access. In search of the brainwave activities of Zen monks, I've also used currently using heart rate variability training and audio-visual entrainment as an alternative, as this better suits my fast living brain!

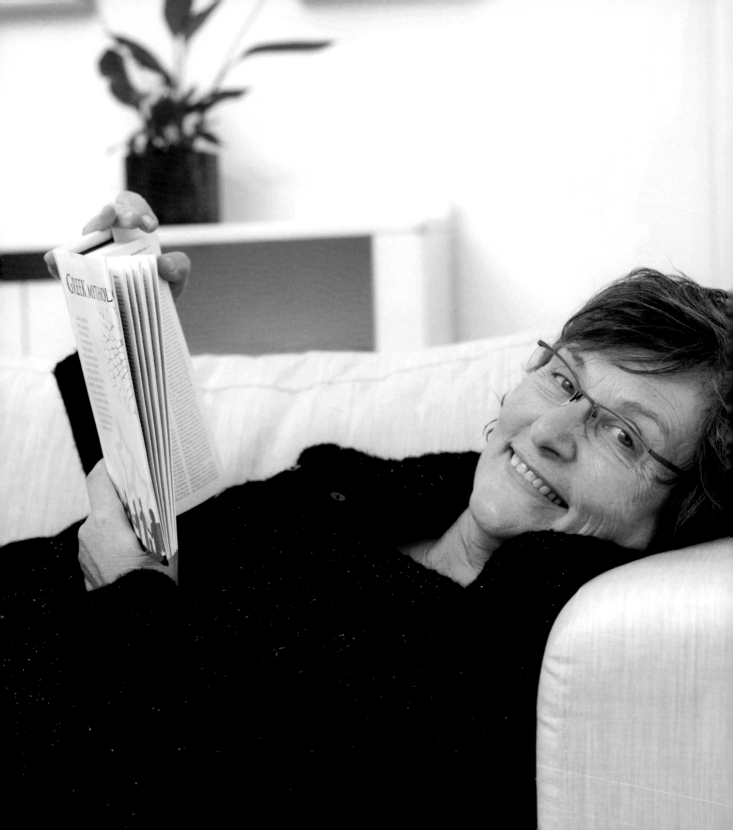

CHAPTER 23
KEEPING YOUR MARBLES
[COGNITIVE FUNCTION
& THE AGEING BRAIN]

If life was a game, the winner would be the one with the most marbles at the end. Even in the absence of brain diseases such as Alzheimer's or Parkinson's, as we age we all experience some decline in our cognitive skills - our ability to think, remember, calculate and learn. But one trick to slow ageing is holding on to your cognitive functions when all about you seem to be losing theirs.

Age-related decline in cognitive function occurs for a number of reasons. There is a progressive loss of brain cells (grey matter), so that by the time you reach the age of 90, on average, one in every 10 brain cells is gone. More important is the loss of nerve fibres and connections (white matter), which may result in you ending up with less than half of what you had in your prime.

More marked changes are seen in some areas of the brain, reflecting local mismatches between supply and demand, protection and overload. And this means that some functions, such as processing speed, attention span, working memory and learning, are affected more significantly than others. For example, as you age, it may take you longer to think through a problem or make a calculation. It may become more common for you to forget the simple things, such as where you left the car keys. At the same time, other things, such as vocabulary, past knowledge and skills, remain relatively intact. These things are appreciated as 'wisdom'.

In some individuals, cognitive deficits are more severe and widespread, and the ability to function independently is compromised. This is known as dementia and can be the result of accelerated, age-related processes, or of superimposed brain damage due to degenerative diseases, such as Alzheimer's or Parkinson's, or a stroke.

A number of factors influence the rate at which we may lose our marbles:

> The elements of ageing, oxidative stress, calories, advanced glycation and inflammation are all associated with cognitive decline and can be influenced by the choices we make (see earlier chapters).

> Atherosclerosis: the same process that narrows the large arteries in the heart also starves the active brain of oxygen, so the things we can do to prevent heart attack (lowering 'bad' LDL cholesterol and systolic blood pressure, controlling weight, preventing diabetes, quitting smoking will also help to keep our brains working better for longer.

> Physical activity: Individuals who remain fit and active appear to retain their cognitive faculties better throughout life.

> Chronic stress: has been shown to shrink those parts of the brain important for working memory and is unequivocally linked to cognitive disorders. So find time to relax and make constructive lifestyle changes that help prevent stress.

> Equally, cognitive enhancements can help you deal better with stress.

> Genetic predisposition: some genes are associated with a higher risk of dementia. Although you can now test for many potential genetic disorders if you have a family history, the tests are not 100% reliable and most of your options for prevention can be undertaken regardless.

> Quality sleep: poor sleep doesn't just make you tired the next day. We need quality sleep to function during the day and build the brain connections that we need for tomorrow.

> Nutrition: our diet may play an important role in slowing rates of cognitive decline and dementia. Especially beneficial are diets naturally high in:

☑ Omega-3 fatty acids, found in fish, fish oils, nuts and omega-3 supplements. By contrast, a high intake of trans fats and saturated fats is asociated with increased rates of cognitive decline.

☑ B vitamins, especially Vitamins B9 and B1

☑ Antioxidants. Including Vitamins E and C, carotenoids, flavonoids and enzymatic co-factors; a. In particular, berries containing high levels of anthocyanins (such as blueberries, blackberries and raspberries) have been shown to have useful effects on cognitive function

None of the associations listed above have been validated in clinical trials. This does not mean interventions are ineffective, but it does indicate that at present the safest way to replicate the findings is to adopt the dietary and lifestyle habits that have been shown to result in these benefits (such as regular exercise, weight control and diets high in fruit, vegetables, cereals and fish).

A number of herbs, including ginkgo biloba, rosemary, ginseng, sage extract and Bacopa monniera (Brahmi), have been shown to have positive effects on working memory and other aspects of cognitive functioning in some individuals, but their long-term impacts on cognitive decline remain to be established.

BUILDING BRAIN RESERVES

As discussed in chapter 3, the manifestations of ageing depend not only on the ageing process itself, but also on the reserves we have accumulated to help our body withstand time's inevitable losses. This is no different in the brain department. It seems that the chances of dementia are lowest in those with bigger brains and better education and in people whose work has required more mental activity.

Although most of these important neural connections form when we are young, it is never too late to build additional brain reserves. Even in ageing adults, the brain can adapt to form new connections and generate new cells. A long-term commitment to keeping active - both mentally and physically - can delay the impacts of ageing on the brain and give us a good excuse to have a lot of fun! By contrast, each additional hour of watching mind-numbing television seems to make dementia more likely as you age.

Again, there is no one answer for everyone. Some will prefer solving crosswords, playing chess, bridge, Sudoku or other mind-games. Crafts, reading, learning new languages or skills can all be stimulating activities. Join a club or society and stay socially active as well as mentally active. The trick is to find something challenging that you can enjoy and commit to it. Try to avoid fads, which may look like fun, but are rarely sustainable.

A number of simple exercises are available that will help give you a mental edge in the short term, regardless of your age. Whether any of these can keep you from developing dementia is unknown; what is probably more relevant is such exercises increase your chances of reaching old age with as many marbles left as possible. As the number of marbles you have appears to determine the threshold of almost every degenerative problem, it's surely worth giving your brain a regular workout.

A LONG-TERM COMMITMENT TO KEEPING ACTIVE - BOTH MENTALLY AND PHYSICALLY - CAN DELAY THE IMPACTS OF AGEING ON THE BRAIN AND GIVE US A GOOD EXCUSE TO HAVE A LOT OF FUN!

ASSESSING BRAIN FUNCTION

☑ Questionnaires - batteries of cognitive tests of thinking power are widely used to examine the impact and rate of ageing. There are many simple standardised tests now available, many of them computerised, with alternate forms to allow accurate follow-up over time. The most comprehensive tests assess emotional intelligence, depression, anxiety, stress, trauma (head trauma and emotional trauma), sleep, neurological disorders, substance use and personality, and then compares your results with others of the same age and gender.

☑ Brain imaging techniques - in use today such as Computerised Tomography (CT), Magnetic Resonance Imaging (MRI), functional MRI (fMRI), Single Photon Emission Computerised Tomography (SPECT), Positron Emission Tomography (PET). Each can tell you about both structure and function.

☑ Quantified electroencephalogram (QEEG) - assesses brainwave activity using small electrodes placed on the scalp, which it compares to healthy people of the same age and gender. This can identify the extent and location of abnormal brain function or brain disease. QEEG has the advantage of being non-invasive, painless, safe and dynamic (brain function is seen in real time). It is also quick, usually requiring no more than 90 minutes to prepare and administer.

RE-TRAINING YOUR BRAIN

There is much we can do to enhance our brain's function. One of the most important parts that can be built up is working memory – the part of our brain used for temporarily storing and manipulating information, such as mental arithmetic, attention span, remembering instructions and following through on them. Working memory is important for a wide range of cognitive functions and is especially vulnerable to ageing. Recently, a number of exercises have been developed to train and enhance working memory in the short-term. Although the long-term impacts are less clear, significant and measurable improvement in the cells that determine the threshold for Parkinson's disease have been recently shown. Another approach to enhance the ageing brain is biofeedback - skills that help you self-regulate your brain activity are acquired by way of immediate feedback and positive reinforcement.

One example is neurofeedback, where feedback is achieved by hooking you up to an electroencephalogram (EEG), which painlessly records spontaneous electrical activity (brain waves) through your scalp.

Skilled neurofeedback therapists monitor these patterns, then feed back information about changes in your brain activity via displays on television monitors or radio signals. This 'biofeedback' can be used to develop self-reliant techniques for controlling and redirecting the dominant electrical rhythms of your brain. A QEEG taken first can also be helpful in identifying the best focus for your brain retraining and reduce training time.

In healthy individuals, neurofeedback techniques can improve performance in exams, sport and artistic expression. How the methods actually work is a matter of ongoing research. It has been argued that biofeedback training, an attention-demanding task, simply serves to improve attention and concentration through repetition. Neurofeedback techniques, however, also seem to have specific and long-lasting effects on brain physiology and metabolism, apparently stimulating the development of new neural pathways, improving blood flow in the brain and even the generation of new brain cells. These effects may also be beneficial, in the context of our ageing brain, to memory, reaction time, processing speed and general cognitive functioning. In addition, some individuals report improvements in everyday functioning, including writing, playing card games, actions involving short-term memory as well as sound, restful sleep.

An alternative (and less expensive) way to regulate the brain's function is via Audio Visual Entrainment (AVE). AVE uses displays of sound and light to guide the brain toward specific frequencies. The brain will essentially 'join in', following a flicker of light, the throbbing of a sound or even a tactile stimulus such as stroking: like a carriage pulled behind a locomotive (hence the term entrainment), the brain is carried 'up' or 'down', increasing or decreasing its dominant frequencies in response to particular stimuli. For example, when a setting on the AVE device designed to 'up-train' the brain is selected, neural activity will follow the stimulus into the 'fast wave' range – and most people will experience a growing sense of focus, energy and concentration.

In individuals with impaired function, AVE can produce sustained improvements. This is possibly because the methods prevent inattention, but there is also evidence that repeated stimulation of brain cells actually promotes brain growth, blood flow and formation of new neural connections, the latter of which may be important in slowing the effects of ageing. So find some way to stimulate your brain and turn it on.

OPTIONS TO KEEP YOUR BRAIN ACTIVE

☑ Increase physical activity
> Try a cardio class at your local gym
> Have a session with a personal trainer or exercise physiologist
> Walk to the shops or to work instead of driving
> Go for a weekend bike ride with your family
> Throw a Frisbee in your local park

☑ A high intake of trans-fats and saturated fats is associated with increased rates of cognitive decline, so increase your intake of omega-3 fatty acids (fish, fish oils, nuts and omega-3 supplements). Go to chapter 12 for a comprehensive list of options

☑ Eat a 'rainbow' of fresh fruits and vegetables daily to ensure your brain gets access to valuable antioxidants. Go to chapter 8 for a comprehensive list of options

☑ Try a new recreational pursuit — go camping if you are typically city-bound

☑ Keep challenging your brain — do the crossword, a puzzle, start a Bridge course, read regularly, play word association games – whatever mental activities you choose, keep your brain working on a daily basis
> Keep engaging in new activities
> Learn a new language
> Read up on a novel subject
> Enrol in a TAFE or university course
> Do crosswords, Sudoku or brain puzzles

☑ Manage stress — find time to relax and make constructive lifestyle changes that help prevent stress
> Try a yoga class
> Start meditation — 5 minutes morning and evening is a positive beginning

OPTIONS TO KEEP YOUR BRAIN ACTIVE

- ☑ Get quality sleep — if your sleep habits are poor make changes to improve them (see a comprehensive range of options at the end of chapter 26)

- ☑ Take up gardening. Even if you live in an apartment you can do gardening in a pot

- ☑ Book in for a series of neurofeedback sessions to enhance feelings of wellbeing

- ☑ Buy an AVE system and give your brain a boost- www.mindalive.com for a reputable brand

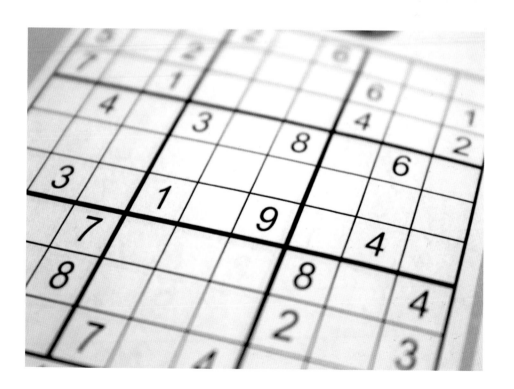

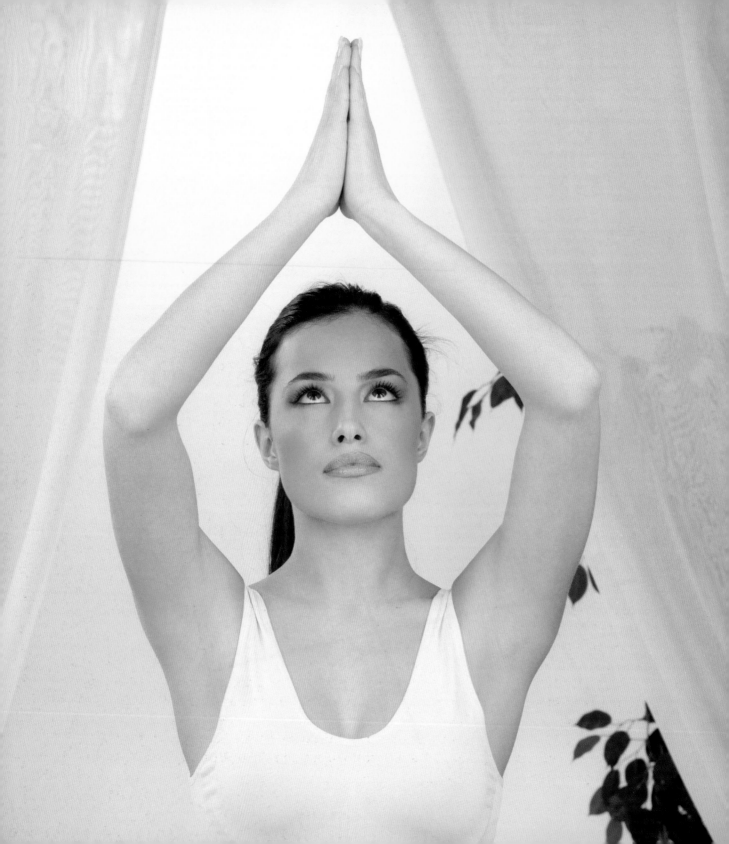

CHAPTER 24
CHANGING YOUR THINKING
[MIND BODY TECHNIQUES TO SLOW AGEING]

Mind-body medicine, or what is known as psycho-neuroimmunology, focuses on ways we can harness the healing capacities of our mind-body communication channels. It recognises the impact of emotional, mental, social and behavioural factors on our health. Health resides in the totality of being human - body, mind, emotions and spirit. If our emotions are not in balance, our physical body suffers. We can exploit these connections to support optimal health and quality of life as we age.

In this chapter we look at proven ways to harness the healing capacities of the mind-body connection, and examine the impact of mental, emotional, spiritual and behavioural interventions on our health and ageing. Mind-body practices have been shown to have powerful and direct effects to slow ageing. The potential benefits of mind-body practices are many, including relaxation and the successful management of stress, which we cover in the next chapter. Some of the benefits of mind-body practices come about simply by making us feel better about ourselves and our lives. And with happiness comes all its benefits: enhanced feelings of creativity and improved concentration, alertness and vitality, as well as the confidence to make better lifestyle choices.

Today, we recognise that a wide variety of mind-body techniques can affect our health. Breathing techniques, biofeedback, meditation, guided imagery, yoga and mindfulness practices are just some of the many different methods we can use to focus our minds and bodies and bolster our resilience. The following pages cover the principles and practices of some of these more common methods.

While mind-body techniques can produce profound and lasting change, they are slow processes. To make an impact in our lives, they each will take time and require engagement, goal setting, willingness, long-term commitment and most importantly individualisation. As with all slow things, if regular mind-body practices become embedded in the fabric of our lives, they will become progressively more sustaining and invigorating as the years go by.

THE ANATOMY OF THE MIND-BODY CONNECTION

The links between mind and body have been known for thousands of years and they form an important part of many traditional healing techniques. Until recently, we have known very little about how this mind-body communication occurs.

We know one rotten apple can spoil the whole barrel. It was originally thought that this was through mystical forces transferred through the ether into the other apples. We now know that it is not magic, as bad apples produce an array of hormones and other chemical signals. Although originally regarded with scepticism as a similarly mystical phenomenon, the complex connections between the mind and body are also grounded in fact.

Some mind-body connections are hard-wired, like the nervous system, through which the brain receives and sends signals that control the health and function of our tissues.

Some connections between our mind and body are soft-wired. Our brain controls the release of hormones and chemicals that influence the growth, function and ageing of almost all organ systems. At the same time, our body sends chemical signals to our brain about the state of its health and any pressing needs. One example is the release of inflammatory cytokines - protein messengers secreted by our immune system that affect the way our brain functions. Another example is how the release of chemical signals from excess fat can affect our appetite, mood and desire for physical activity.

The full nature of all the interconnections between mind and body are only now being discovered and many - probably most - remain uncategorised. As in the apple barrel, this does not make these connections any less real.

INTERVENTIONS TO HARNESS THE MIND-BODY CONNECTION

1. BIOFEEDBACK

Biofeedback is a conditioning or training technique in which we develop and learn ways to gain self-control over some of our body's functions (including muscle tension, breathing and heart rate) that are not normally controlled – or even, for the most part, noticed.

This self-control is achieved by continuously monitoring and measuring specific bodily functions, then feeding back this information in real time as a visual or acoustic signal. The process of biofeedback allows us to identify, then practice our own ways to modify our physical parameters, as changes made in the desired direction are immediately 'fed back' to us, observed and reinforced.

By achieving a degree of control over our key physical functions, we feel more in control of our emotions and thought processes, which in turn may improve our attitudes, health and sense of wellbeing. Ultimately, these skills are so well honed that we can employ them in the absence of feedback and in real-life situations.

Various biofeedback techniques have been developed, including those that measure and feedback data on body temperature, sweat production, breathing rate and depth, muscle tension and heart rate variability (HRV).

HEART RATE VARIABILITY (HRV)

☑ HRV measures the beat-to-beat variations in our heart rate. Variability is an indicator of good health, adaptability and longevity.

☑ In healthy young individuals, the interval between consecutive heartbeats is not metronomic, but oscillates dynamically, with peak heart rates often 20 or 30 beats faster than rates at their low point.

☑ A loss of HRV is often seen in the ageing heart, with as little as 3 to 5 beats between their highest and lowest heart rates.

☑ HRV can be targeted directly through biofeedback methods. This approach entails teaching ourselves to control our HRV instantaneously by changing our thought processes and behaviour. This is usually achieved through breathing techniques, constructive thinking such as mindfulness, recalling memories of tenderness with loved ones, and other relaxation techniques. The biofeedback allows us to identify and fine-tune the techniques that are best for us.

☑ HRV monitors, such as the Resilience Builder™, are widely available for purchase. This easy-to-install, computer-based tool includes a breathing pacer that allows you to identify the breathing rate at which your heart-rate variability is the greatest. This is known as your resonance frequency. For most of us, this frequency is around six breaths per minute and six cycles of heart-rate change per minute. Once we have established our own frequency, we can then practice breathing at the desired rate, recalling moments of tenderness and practicing constructive thinking, such as mindfulness, without needing the feedback monitor, because we know it works.

2. MEDITATION

Meditation is a widely-used mind-body technique in which relaxation and focused attention (contemplation) are combined to produce a heightened state of self-awareness. This is often achieved by concentration on an object, such as a flame, beads, a thought or visualisation, or a process, such as breathing, a repetitive prayer or mantra, a sound or an exercise. This concentration serves as an anchor to prevent our thoughts from drifting off into the 'busyness' and 'noise' of our minds, and keeps us focused on the present.

There is no best way to meditate. Many different meditative disciplines exist, encompassing a wide range of different practices, often with specific goals. Some can do their meditation when they are out running, when they sit by the sea or in a church. What will work for one individual may be inappropriate for the next. Yet once found, a means to meditate can be an important step to transform our lives and find the stability and confidence we need to live and age well.

A meditative state has effects on both the mind and the body. Like many successful relaxation techniques, meditation reduces stressful brain activity. Depending on the depth of the meditative state, it can also increase the brain activity normally associated with deep sleep, essentially rewiring the circuitry of our brain, albeit temporarily. Recent research even shows that meditation can produce some structural thickening in the cortex of the brain, and reduce the age-related thinning of brain tissue. A meditative state is also associated with improved balance of the autonomic nervous system, increased heart-rate variability and improved release of beneficial hormones, such as melatonin and DHEA, which decline with age. Cortisol levels, which increase during periods of stress and in the ageing body, are also normalised by meditation.

Meditation is an important tool for relaxation. Yet it has also been shown to have a number of independent actions in promoting physical and mental health, as well as longevity. For example, meditation has been shown to lower blood pressure, improve glucose metabolism, weight control and immune function. Improvements in hearing and vision have also been documented with meditation.

3. FOCUS ON THE HERE AND NOW: THE ART OF 'MINDFULNESS'

When we first see or hear something, there is a fleeting instant of pure awareness just before we conceptualise or 'think' about the thing – before we identify it. That moment is known as 'mindfulness'. It is the mental equivalent of what we see with our peripheral vision, as opposed to the hard focus of our normal or central vision.

A common malady of our fast-paced world is that we are so intent on understanding things that the moment of mindfulness is passed over. Rather than always having to

CHANGING YOUR THINKING

234

evaluate our cognitive and emotional experiences, mindfulness teaches us simply to notice them. This increases our openness to experience and reduces our tendency to label some experiences negatively.

Mindfulness reflects only what is happening in the present moment. It is the ability of our mind to pay deliberate attention, in a particular way, to the present moment, and to do so in a non-judgemental way.

The concept of mindfulness has its origins in many cultural and philosophical traditions, which recognised that these moments of unfocused awareness contain a very deep kind of knowing. In modern psychological practice, mindfulness techniques are being used as a powerful tool to reduce our stress levels and heal our psyches.

We can cultivate mindfulness using a variety of techniques, including yoga, mindful walking, mindful breathing, listening to music (music therapy) or spending time outdoors (eco-therapy), all of which have a meditative component.

It is important to distinguish 'mindful' meditation from 'concentration' meditation, which entails restricting the focus of our attention to a single stimulus, such as a word, object or thought. If our attention wanders, it is redirected back to that anchor. No attention is paid to the nature of the distraction.

In contrast, mindfulness meditation involves observation of constantly changing internal and external stimuli as they arise. Rather than shutting out the world, mindfulness meditation entails practicing being receptive to any and all stimulation that may arise.

Mindfulness training can help us gain greater awareness of many aspects of our personal beings, rather than simply paying attention to those that seem most emotionally pressing. Enhanced awareness leads to an increased sense of mastery over mental processes. This improves our mood and lowers the likelihood that we will brood on our past failures, which can lead to loss of confidence in our health-related choices.

4. BREATHING TECHNIQUES

Almost all mind-body therapies include focused breathing techniques. Traditional Chinese Medicine teaches you that a tranquil mind produces regular breathing, and conversely that regular breathing produces a concentrated mind. By consciously mimicking the unconscious 'relaxation response' in our body, we gain some of its benefits, as well as greater mastery over ourselves.

Breathing techniques are among the simplest forms of self-regulation, freely available to anyone wanting to reduce the effects of stress on body and mind.

The great thing is that we don't need to do it in a special environment or even sit in a specific way. Once we know how to breathe correctly, we can practice our breathing techniques wherever we are.

Most techniques involve slow-paced, steady breathing, using our diaphragm, rather than our chest muscles, and slowly increasing the volume of air as we inhale and exhale. Think of "LESS" -- LOW, EVEN, SMOOTH, SLOW and gain a growing awareness of the processes involved in our breathing.

A regular practice of slow, deep breathing has been shown to have a number of beneficial effects on human health, particularly when used in combination with other modalities. When we breathe slowly and deeply, we stimulate the relaxation response associated with calm, digestion and healing.

5. CREATIVE VISUALISATION

Imagery and stories have a dramatic power to heal and transform our lives. 'Guided imagery' uses directed thoughts, suggestions and mental imagery to evoke our senses and guide our imagination toward particular goals. One goal might be a state of complete relaxation, which is useful for reducing the impact of stress. Alternatively, guided imagery can be used to invoke feelings of youthful vitality that may help slow the ageing process.

In principle, if an image is strong enough, our concentration is focused and our disbelief is suspended. Our bodies and minds respond as if what we are imagining is real. For example, we may be able to achieve a relaxed state by imagining ourselves in a peaceful place, such as a garden. The more powerfully we can embrace and experience the imagery, the more effective the transformation is likely to be.

The process of visualisation can be self-guided or prompted by guided meditations delivered via scripts, CD, DVD or instructors. Guided imagery is often used in combination with relaxation, meditation and mindfulness practices, because we are more open to the power of imagery when we are deeply relaxed.

Guided imagery has become a popular approach to managing stress and enhancing energy, motivation, focus and performance. It has also been used successfully to treat a wide variety of disorders, including high blood pressure, chronic pain, anxiety and depression. Incorporated into a slow-ageing program, it can also be used to help us reach our goals. The power of imagery can also be a tool in rejuvenation. Some therapists use imagery to guide us as we are immersed in an experience of 'age regression' designed to carry us back via our memories to earlier stages of life associated with feelings of youthfulness and vitality.

Once we arrive back in our childhood, many images can be used to 'harvest' the vitality of youth. We can then bring this vitality back to the present, using it to help rejuvenate our bodies and lives. This kind of imagining may seem simple, but it can have profound effects on human physiology. In particular, studies have shown that imagery techniques can be used to modify the functioning of our immune systems, partly by reducing stress, thereby allowing our immune systems to function more effectively. Relaxation without an active imagery exercise attached appears to be less effective at reducing some physiological parameters, including inflammation.

More recently, these techniques have been used by a number of cancer researchers to assist patients in developing images of their bodies fighting killer cancer cells, helping them to boost their immune system function and enhancing their survival rates.

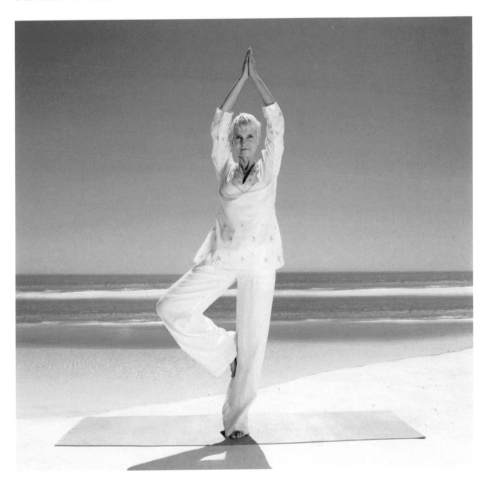

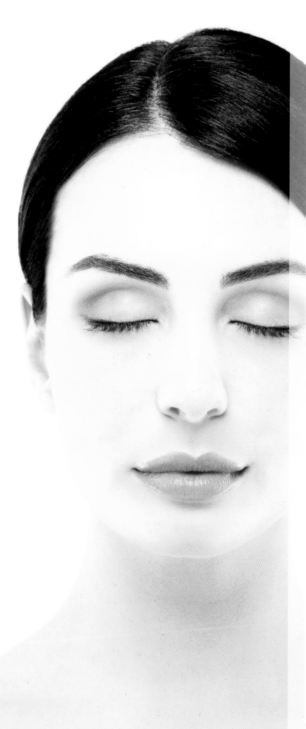

EASY BREATHING TECHNIQUES

> Breathe in slowly and deeply through your nose, concentrating on the diaphragm. The aim is to feel your abdomen rise, not your chest. Feel it rise as you inhale and fall as you exhale. The key is to observe, rather than to engage your thoughts. Keep returning your focus to your breathing.

> When your breathing speeds up, slow it down by extending the duration of your exhalation (anywhere from one-third to double your inhalation time). Relax your body, especially the stomach and abdomen, allowing it to swell outward and relax back inward, or follow the stream of breath from the moment of inhalation until you have fully exhaled.

> Posture is also important: if you slump forward, your diaphragm cannot move freely. It also helps to close your eyes and lie on your back with your arms at your sides, palms upward. If you're sitting, place your feet flat on the floor. After several minutes of practice, you can move to any comfortable position and continue 'mindful' breathing.

> Each time you inhale, take in as much breath as you think is possible through your nostrils, then a little more. Pause for a moment before you exhale. Exhale gently and slowly through your mouth, emptying your lungs as much as you can, then a little more! As you exhale, purse your lips to create a slight resistance to the flow of air, and enhance your awareness of this airflow.

> Each time you practice your breathing, you are stretching and exercising your diaphragm muscle, which is essential for better breathing. A 'breath pacer' can sometimes be helpful initially to guide your efforts, until it becomes natural to breathe in a smooth and regular fashion.

6. YOGIC PRACTICES

No discussion of mind-body techniques would be complete without mention of yoga, the ancient Indian philosophy of living that includes physical postures, breathing techniques, meditation, relaxation, moral codes and other practices. Together, these practices provide a path to self-realisation.

Although their roots and practices are intertwined, there are two main philosophical branches in yoga - Hatha (to do with the physical and energetic body) and Raja (known as the eight-fold path, or the path of meditation). Each of these branches offers a method by which we can come to better understand who we really are and what our life purpose is. In practice, we tend to blend these philosophies into one that is just right for us.

Sometimes these blends become popular 'styles' of yoga, such as Iyengar, which focuses on correct postural alignment; Ashtanga, which emphasises dynamic, flowing sequences; Satyananda, a contemporary, classical, integrated form of yoga; Bikram, a sequence of postures practiced in a heated room; and Kundalini, which focuses on the movement of energy.

In the West, a yoga class commonly involves a blend of three practices, mostly asana (postures) and pranayama (breathing techniques), which are stepping stones to acquiring the physical and mental discipline needed to practice the third component, meditation, effectively.

There is good evidence that repeated and sustained yoga has a range of beneficial effects on health and wellbeing, from lowering blood pressure and stress levels to improving sleep and mood. The trick is to find what works for you and stick at it. Attending a yoga class can also increase social contact and provide an increased sense of meaning or spirituality.

THE SUM OF THE PARTS

For many years, the connections between our mind and body were viewed with scepticism, even derision, and those who believed in their significance were looked on by many as mystical pseudo-scientists. While charlatans do exist, as they have for centuries, the existence and importance of both hard-wired and soft-wired connections are recognised by almost all health practitioners today. There are many ways to utilise these connections for health and ageing. This chapter has touched on just a few of the more commonly practised mind-body techniques. While all of these have been shown to be effective when looking at groups of people, not everyone will work for all of us. There will, however, be one that is right for each one of us, one that each of us can incorporate effortlessly into our daily routine to strengthen, support and renew. It may be a slow process, which takes a long-term commitment.

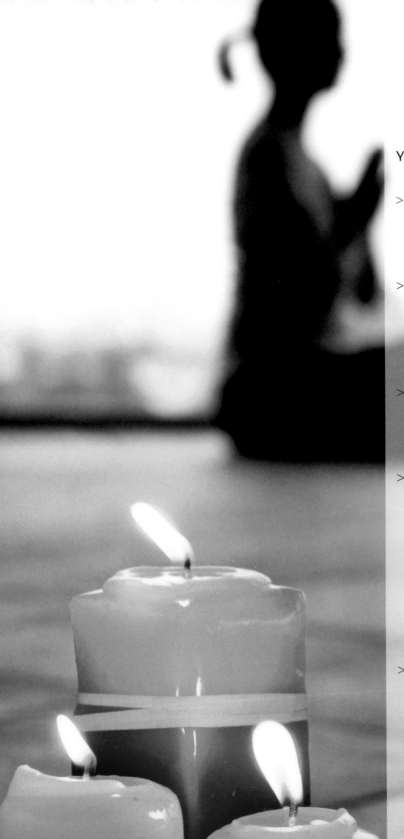

YOGA IN THE FAST LANE - FIVE TIBETANS

> This rejuvenation technique has long been practised by Tibetan Buddhist monks to slow ageing, increase energy, calm the mind and strengthen the body.

> The story goes that in the 1930s, retired British Army officer Colonel Bradford discovered a remote Tibetan monastery where the resident monks were very old, yet appeared amazingly healthy and 'ageless'.

> The monks claimed that the secret to slowing ageing lay in the five special movements they performed daily, which stimulated the flow of a natural life-energy throughout their bodies.

> T5T is a modified version of the original Five Tibetan rites. Ten minutes per day of practice is all you need. It was developed by Carolinda Witt to take into account how our very different, modern, sedentary lifestyles are from the traditional, more menial lives of the Tibetan monks. The integrity of the original five rites remains intact, but T5T makes the practice simple to perform.

> T5T takes these ancient movements and boosts their power by combining them with an energy-boosting breathing method and core stability training to strengthen our belly and protect our spine. T5T makes us strong from the inside out.

OPTIONS TO OPTIMISE YOUR MIND BODY CONNECTION
☑ Book in to a meditation class
☑ Learn the breathing technique outlined in this section and practise it at least three times daily
☑ Buy an HRV training tool, such as the Resilience Builder - go to innate-intelligence.com.au/resilience
☑ Get eight hours of sleep a night
☑ Go for regular walks in the park
☑ Join a 'laughter club' - go to www.laughterclubs.com.au
☑ In situations of conflict, take a deep breath before you respond
☑ On a daily basis, practise a creative visualisation in which you see yourself happy and in peak condition as you age
☑ Enjoy yourself: those who laugh, love and live better tend to live longer, too
☑ Find a quiet place at lunchtime to collect your thoughts
☑ Cultivate mindfulness - buy a CD that teaches mindfulness or do a class
☑ Join a yoga course or do regular sessions (as a group or solo). Embrace T5T (www.t5t.com.au) as a simple starting point with real benefits

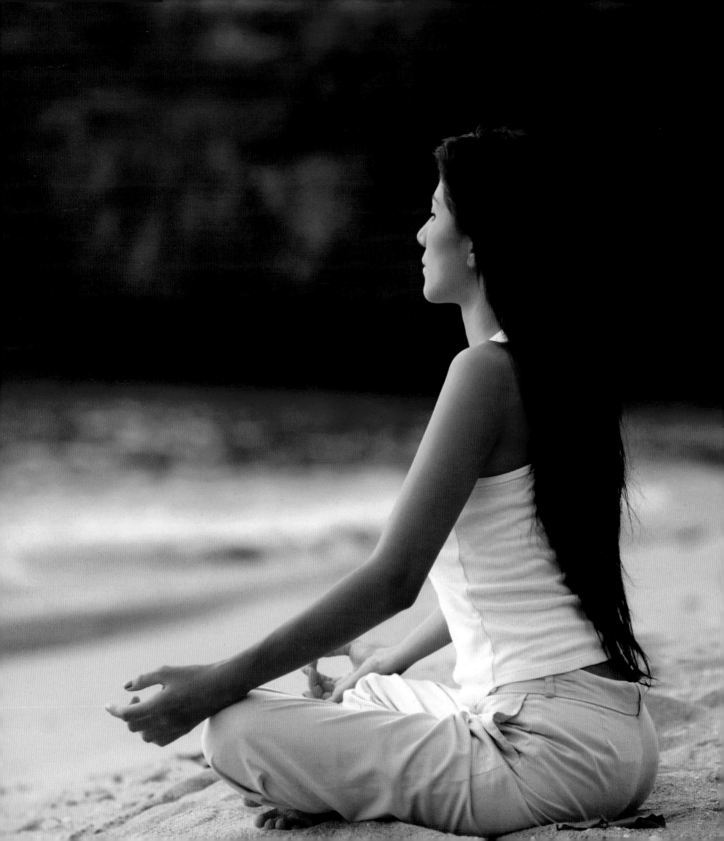

CHAPTER 25

AGEING AND STRESS

Every day, our lives are filled with challenges. Each triggers a range of protective responses that work to help us defend ourselves, cope and adapt. Our brains are the main drivers of these stress responses, as well as their main target. They decide when there is a problem and act automatically to give our body the tools needed to fight, survive or quickly run away (the 'fight or flight' response).

The intensity of our stress responses are determined not only by the intensity of the threats, but by a host of other factors, including context, genes, gender, previous experiences, coping skills and personality traits, as well as age itself.

A stress response that is inadequate leads to problems - either too much stress or an inefficient response. Equally, a stress response that is excessive or lacks regulation can sometimes be as harmful as the stress itself. In fact, stress can be a killer. Even single periods of stress in our past, such as mental illness, abuse or suffering, can cast long shadows and may be associated with shorter life expectancy.

This chapter will look at the stress response and how it influences, and is influenced by, ageing.

THE STRESS RESPONSE

The key players in the stress response are the autonomic nervous system (ANS), inflammatory cytokines and stress hormones.

The ANS provides balance through regulating its two opposing arms: a sympathetic nervous system that controls our responses to stress and a parasympathetic nervous system that controls relaxation. Too much sympathetic activation, as occurs with ageing, means our response to stress is exaggerated. Reduced parasympathetic tone, associated with being overweight, inactive or lacking quality sleep, also augments the effects of stress.

A number of inflammatory cytokines – the signalling molecules of our immune systems – are released as part of our stress response. These sensitise our brains to further stress. Our levels of cytokines increase progressively with age. This increase is faster in people suffering from chronic stress, diabetes and obesity, who also age faster.

Cortisol is our major stress-response hormone. It acts to mobilise resources to protect and repair our bodies. For the same stress, older individuals tend to produce more cortisol, and this response persists for much longer, making any stress more damaging.

MEASURING STRESS LEVELS

You can measure your stress levels in a number of ways:

1. QUESTIONNAIRES

A variety of questionnaires have been designed to evaluate stress. Given that measurement of stress is subjective, most of these rely on a degree of openness and self-awareness.

Other questionnaires record stressful life events, such as deaths and divorces, over a period of time, then add their scores together. Each event's score is based on how stressful that event is deemed to be for most people. More specific surveys have been developed for certain professions and populations. Although imperfect, all have been shown to predict poor health outcomes.

2. HEART RATE VARIABILITY

This measures the beat-to-beat variations in our heart rates. It is one useful indicator of the balance between our sympathetic and parasympathetic nervous systems. The stressed heart is too steady, with less beat-to-beat variation than normal, indicating impaired regulation of our cardiovascular system, stressed systems and increased risk of death. Conversely, increased variability is an indicator of low stress, adaptability and longevity.

3. CORTISOL LEVELS

Repeated blood tests taken at regular intervals over a day or 24-hour urinary-free cortisol give a good picture of our changing patterns of cortisol release. Salivary cortisol tests are a simple and popular tool, but cannot determine our cortisol production over the course of a stressed day.

4. SKIN TEMPERATURE

When we are stressed, more blood flows to vital organs, such as our brains, while blood flow to our skin surface is reduced. This is partly how lie detectors and 'mood rings' detect stress or strong emotions. It is a simple way to get biofeedback on the success of any relaxation techniques we practise (which, by increasing activation of our parasympathetic nervous system, raises skin temperature).There are many ways to handle stress, including relaxation, hypnosis, exercise, disclosure, conditioning and interventions. Many of the most successful strategies fit with the seven principles of slow ageing:

A SLOW GUIDE TO STRESS MANAGEMENT

1. AWARENESS AND ENGAGEMENT

Identifying the source of stress in our lives is the first step in controlling it. For example, time management comes partly from identifying the burden of our workload. Equally, conflict resolution comes from recognising both the impasse and the fact that something can be done to resolve it. In other cases, our disclosure of stress (such as abuse) can be an important initial step in its management.

Another key component is to identify those factors that are central to controlling our stress levels. But this is not easy. We may feel relaxed, but are we dealing effectively with the stressors in our lives? How can we tell whether the stress management strategies we adopt are working for us? All these questions should be adequately addressed in a good stress management program. The most important component of any such program is that it helps us become aware of how our choices can positively influence our health and wellbeing, leading to a sense of control that, in itself, helps reduce the stress in our lives.

From self-awareness comes self-control and other forms of mental discipline that help us cope with stress. Just reflecting on what's good in our lives can help because, through this action, we can discover where we need to go to find the things that make us feel happy and energised.

While some support can be found inside ourselves, external support systems are also important. People who age well (and are less stressed) are those who have stayed connected with their world. It may be that a lack of stress allows this to occur, or that robust support allows some of us to cope with stress better than others.

2. GOAL SETTING IS ESSENTIAL AS PART OF A STRATEGIC PLANNING PROCESS

It is important to formulate individual goals that denote progress to each of us. Some of these can be established through feedback techniques; other goals are more personal. It's helpful to record the things we like in our lives and do what we can to improve anything we aren't quite happy about. Making our intentions clear ensures we are in greater control of where our lives are going. Just by doing this, our stress loads are lessened.

3. ELIMINATE THE NEGATIVE; ACCENT THE POSITIVE

Changing the way we perceive potential stressors can modify the impact of stress on our bodies. If we think we are stressed, we are, but when we think we have resources that will enable us to cope, stress is no longer such a threat.

Some of this 'stress-resilience' lies in our confidence and coping skills. Some lies in our ability to maintain a positive outlook. All these capacities can be cultivated and fostered. People who are stress-resilient can experience the same stressors, such as gridlocked traffic, yet interpret them more positively, expecting that everything will be fine, rather than a problem. They are better able to deal with stress because they believe they can.

A number of studies have shown that simply learning to 'accentuate the positive' is associated with reduced stress and a lowered risk of heart disease. With practice, optimism can be learned and become part of our (longer) lives. Simply changing our attitude and outlook can slow ageing.

4. SEEK LONG-TERM SOLUTIONS FOR LONG-TERM HEALTH

The best long-term health and wellbeing strategies are powered by the force of habit, so integrating helpful practices into our lifestyle is one of the keys to healthy ageing. Some common examples include exercise, taking quality time out and employing mind-body techniques. When used routinely, each can serve to build our resilience to stress.

Some of the most common herbal stress-fighters are the 'adaptogenic herbs', such as ginseng and rhodioloa, which can increase our body's resistance to stress, possibly by improving our mood and boosting physical and mental performance. Various pharmaceutical drugs are also available. Each of these agents has its side-effects and limitations, and are best used for limited periods when stress is most acute, with other techniques taking over as we attain greater control.

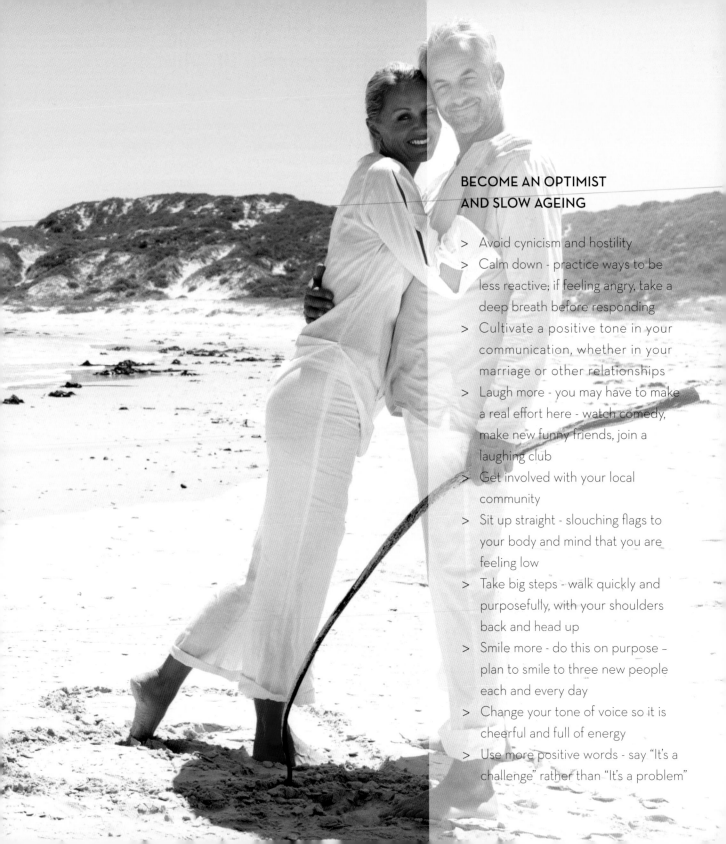

BECOME AN OPTIMIST AND SLOW AGEING

> Avoid cynicism and hostility

> Calm down - practice ways to be less reactive; if feeling angry, take a deep breath before responding

> Cultivate a positive tone in your communication, whether in your marriage or other relationships

> Laugh more - you may have to make a real effort here - watch comedy, make new funny friends, join a laughing club

> Get involved with your local community

> Sit up straight - slouching flags to your body and mind that you are feeling low

> Take big steps - walk quickly and purposefully, with your shoulders back and head up

> Smile more - do this on purpose – plan to smile to three new people each and every day

> Change your tone of voice so it is cheerful and full of energy

> Use more positive words - say "It's a challenge" rather than "It's a problem"

5. THERE IS ALWAYS MORE THAN ONE ANSWER

All sorts of stress-intervention programs have been shown to be effective, from formal psychotherapy, time-management training, relaxation techniques and meditation to diet, sleep and regular exercise. But there is never just one answer: many of the best programs incorporate a number of components. Complex problems require complex solutions.

6. SUPPORT IS OUT THERE, SO GET HELP

Some stresses cannot be managed by ourselves, alone, no matter how hard we try. Sometimes our fruitless efforts become sources of major stress. If we are unhappy, we must talk to friends or consult counsellors, coaches or people who understand and care for us.

This is so important, yet ironically the very times we most need the help of others are often the times we tend to 'shut down', not wanting to burden the people who can help. The more competent we are, the more likely it is that we won't want to 'bother' others. We are then at risk of becoming progressively unhappier and less able to cope. There are many professionals who can help us find ways to relieve or combat our specific stressors, while treating us as individuals. So get some professional help.

7. BE SELECTIVE - FIND A SOLUTION THAT IS RIGHT FOR YOU

Each of us needs to find what works best for us by connecting with our own sense of intuition, rather than with someone else's experience. We need to try new things and choose those that seem right for us.

Just as stress affects each one of us differently, effective stress management must fit our unique needs. One size never fits all and this is particularly the case when we're dealing with the subjective experience of stress.

For some of us, exercise is the best stress release; for others, classical music or gardening does the trick. To suggest that all of us must do the same thing to manage our stress is to display ignorance about the nature of stress, and about the potential each of us has to find our own method for its management.

UN-STRESS AS WE WOULD UNDRESS

Our stress responses are common companions in our modern lives. Most of us wear them like heavy coats to keep us warm and dry. They can get a bit heavy after a while, but our 'coats' need not be black. Nor do we need to wear them every day.

NOT ALL STRESS IS DAMAGING

Intermittent or low-level exposure to stressors can sometimes make us stronger: this is known as hormesis. Obvious examples are the stresses and strains of exercise and intellectually challenging activities. By promoting stress resistance, the hormetic effects of mild, repetitive stress may have a beneficial impact on our longevity. For example:

> heat stress (such as that induced by jumping into a hot Jacuzzi every day)

> cold stress (such as the stress of taking a cold shower)

> periodic partial fasting (such as consuming 80% of our usual kj intake one day per week)

> regular physical activity

> acupuncture

These trigger the release of natural molecules, called hormetins, that stimulate our stress response pathways and help them to adapt. Some examples of hormetins include celasterols and paeoniflorin, present in some medicinal herbs; the isothocyanates in broccoli; allicin, found in garlic; and curcumin, in turmeric. Each of these hormetins has been shown to have a range of biological effects, depending on the dosage. In each case, too much exposure is damaging (eg. extreme cold stress results in hypothermia), but just enough can make us more resilient.

OPTIONS TO HELP BUILD STRESS RESILIENCE

☑ Pay attention to your stress and its sources

> Write a journal and jot down what stresses you and what makes yo feel good over a week or month. Take note and make changes to increase 'feel-good' activities and to reduce stressful activities

> Get a coach or councillor

> Make sure you have 'me' time

> Book a weekly massage or facial

> Take time to read a non-work-related book

> Organise time off from your household – have one day a week where you don't do cooking, cleaning, management or household chores

> Join a book club

> Go to the movies – in the middle of the day!

> Find out what makes you happy and do this regularly

☑ Improve your time management skills

> Buy a yearly planner or diary and USE it

> Map out the things you need to put your attention to so you are clear on priorities

> Plan the things you need to do in life and prioritise in the same way you would when developing a business plan

> Delegate, delegate, delegate

☑ Allocate time purely for relaxation

> Make a list of possible weekend or short getaways and work your way through it

> Exercise is a great release – go for a walk, go to the gym or find someone to go to a salsa class with

> Listen to music

> Take up gardening

OPTIONS TO HELP BUILD STRESS RESILIANCE

> Try volunteering

> Call a friend each week – old or new

☑ Make an appointment to see your doctor or stress management consultant

☑ Do the simple things well to optimise your health your wellness – this will help to improve your body's resilience

> Increase physical activity – regular exercise will lower your stress levels and improve stress responsiveness. Go to chapter 22 for guidance on how to do this

> Fight weight gain – being overweight is not only a source of stress but it also increases sympathetic activity and reduces your resources to deal with day to day stress. Go to chapter 9 for a comprehensive list of options

> Eat a healthy diet – go to chapter 19 for helpful dietary guidelines

> Get quality sleep – poor sleep compounds the effects of stress. For a co prehensive list of options go to chapter 26

> Get sex into your life! Go to chapter 27 for a comprehensive list of options

> Join a social group

> Plan regular holidays or breaks if yours is a pressured lifestyle: don't hang out for a time when you feel you can afford that 'big trip'

☑ Try some new techniques to bolster your stress resilience

> Try yoga, pilates, tai chi or a similar class (T5T only takes 10 minutes)

> Take a weekly meditation class or listen to a meditation CD before bed each night

> Practice mindfulness during the day. If you don't know much about this, then go buy a book or CD and learn about it.

> Use an AVE system - tune for relaxation before you go to sleep or for peak performance in the morning

> Deep-breathe whenever you remember to do so (taking 6 to 8 breaths per minute). Set an alarm or a visual cue that reminds you to do it hourly. Adopt the breathing guidelines, detailed in the last chapter

> Buy a HRV tool to build stress resilience. Using biofeedback tools like HRV can help to boost parasympathetic nervous system activity

> Go to http://www.innate-intelligence.com.au to learn more about building stress resilience

☑ Cultivate optimism

> Reframe your language to give it a positive, not a negative spin: what you say about things affects how you feel

> Write a daily or weekly gratitude journal

> Give compliments – you'll most likely start to receive more as a result!

☑ Cultivate your social support network

> Join a sports club, a book club or social network

WHY IS STRESS KILLING US?

> Heart attacks and strokes - up to a third of all heart attacks may be attributable to chronic stress.

> Infections and cancer - when we are stressed, we seem to pick up every bug going around. These stressful times are also when cold sores and shingles tend to raise their ugly heads. Chronically stressed individuals are at highe risk of some cancers and have worse survival rates.

> Cognitive decline - prolonged stress can actually cause some areas of our brains to shrink. In susceptible individuals, chronic stress can trigger depression and other mental illness.

> Sexual dysfunction, including erectile dysfunction and difficulty in maintaining sexual arousal, are common complications of stress.

> Impaired intestinal function – diarrhoea, constipation, irritable bowel, ulcers, etc.

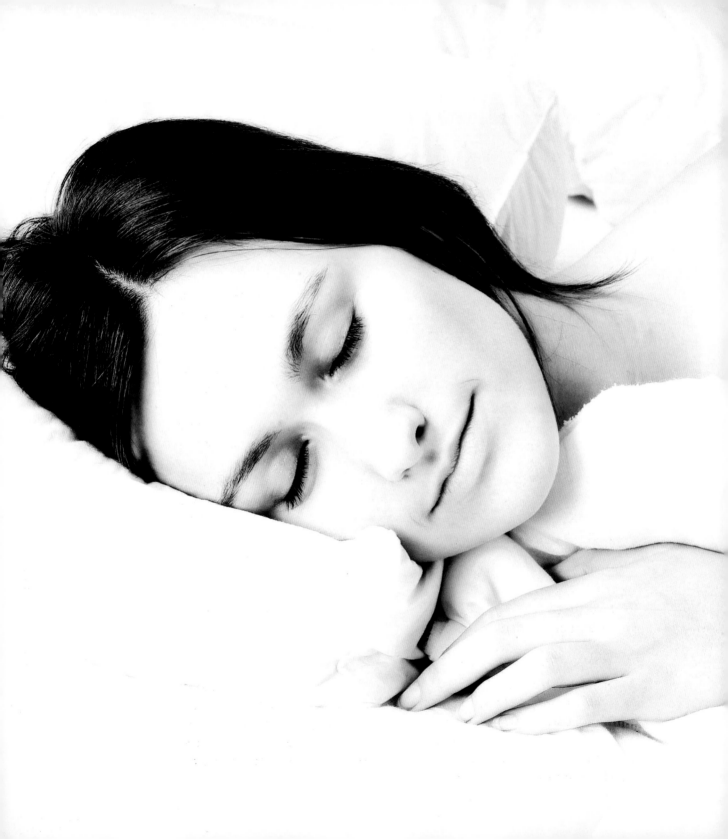

CHAPTER 26

A GOOD NIGHT'S SLEEP
[SLEEP & AGEING]

It is often said: "there is nothing like a good night's sleep". Anyone who has experienced nights of broken sleep knows how true this is. The third of our life most of us spend asleep can significantly affect the two-thirds of our lives that we spend awake.

Sleep brings many benefits, just as there are hazards associated with reduced sleep quality and quantity. So if we can improve our sleep, we can also impact our health, ageing and longevity.

Sleep is more than just conserving energy: it serves a number of essential functions we simply cannot do without. Sleep really does have restorative qualities for our body's growth and rejuvenation.

Sleep also affects our capacity to build memories, rewiring our brains to ensure that newly-gained knowledge is effectively organised and stored for future use. Getting more 'quality sleep' helps us to remember, process and understand things better.

On the flip side, too little night-time sleep doesn't just mean daytime sleepiness; it also makes our brains less efficient. Sleep deprivation can also lead to weight gain as our tired bodies think they have too little energy and try to compensate with food. In fact, both too little sleep and too much sleep are associated with reduced life expectancy.

HOW MUCH SLEEP DO WE NEED?

A common myth is that we all need eight hours of sleep every night. The amount of sleep we need to feel good varies among individuals, seasons and even over the course of the working week. Some people need nine hours, yet others function very well on six hours. There is no magic number that suits us all, Goldilocks. The most important determinant of our sleep needs is simply how well we function during the day on the amount of sleep we get.

As we age, we tend to need less sleep. Our sleep also becomes lighter and we experience more awakenings. These are absolutely normal and should not be a concern. Worrying about these awakenings can lead to the development of insomnia.

WHAT MAKES US FALL ASLEEP?

Sleep itself is straightforward; the difficult part, sometimes, is getting into that state. Many things tell us that it's time to sleep.

Obviously, the longer we stay awake, the sleepier we become: this is called homeostatic regulation. Usually, we are awake for 16 hours or so before we get sleepy.

Another regulator of sleep is our body clock (circadian rhythm), which links sleep with other bodily cycles, such as temperature, growth and levels of various brain chemicals, including serotonin, cortisol and melatonin (see chapter 27).

These two basic instincts can be used to our advantage when we are trying to send ourselves to sleep. Getting strong homeostatic sleepiness means going to sleep no earlier than 15 to 19 hours after waking up. Optimising circadian sleepiness means going to sleep when we start to feel drowsy in the evening – neither earlier nor later.

Our clock is usually timed so that we fall asleep around 11pm and wake up at 7am. Some of us (often referred to as 'night-owls') have later-timed body clocks and may not be ready to fall asleep until around 2am, preferring to sleep until 10am. Others (the 'larks') have early-timed body clocks and can fall asleep quickly in the evening – often by 9pm – but then wake early.

Unless we use alarm clocks, the timing of our waking is determined primarily by circadian rhythms, so even if 'larks' are sleep-deprived, they are unlikely to sleep in. These different timed body clocks do not pose a problem. However, sleeping 'out of sync' with our body clocks, even if we have been awake for a long time and feel sleepy, is relatively inefficient. Trying to fall asleep too early, in relation to our natural rhythms, is simply ineffective.

An example of how this works is seen when daylight and darkness patterns fail to gel with our body rhythms. This is generally experienced as jet-lag, but is also seen in shift workers and following even small changes in our circadian rhythm, such as at the beginning or end of daylight savings periods. This mis-timing can make it difficult for us to fall asleep or wake at the right time for a number of days.

The good news is that we can usually reset (entrain) our body clocks each day by means of cues such as light, noise and activity. For example, a dark, quiet room helps to promote sleep. Taking a hot bath, shower or sauna in the late evening sometimes helps us to fall asleep, as our temperatures tend to drop post-bathing, so our bodies think it must be 'sleep time'.

By contrast, exposure to bright fluorescent light in bathrooms, or emanating from computer screens or televisions, will prevent sleep. Another way to synchronise our body clocks is to expose our bodies to bright light, which is usually obtainable for free, without a prescription. For those troubled with early-morning waking, exposing ourselves to bright natural light in the evening can delay our body clock by a few hours. Equally, delay in getting to sleep can sometimes be helped by getting some bright morning light to bring the clock forward.

For those who need to reset mis-timing body clocks, melatonin is available on prescription. This is designed as short-term therapy and most preparations contain large amounts of melatonin (1-3mg), usually several times more than are our bodies' normal circadian rhythms in order to clonk us back into cycle. The melatonin available over the counter in many pharmacies contains little active ingredient and is usually ineffective at correcting insomnia (although it may have antioxidant benefits – see chapter 32).

SLOW SOLUTIONS FOR BETTER SLEEP

Bearing in mind the slow principles detailed in chapter 2, a number of simple things can be done to improve our sleep patterns and, with them, our health.

1. UNDERSTANDING AND CONTROLLING OUR SLEEP

The first part of SLOW is always awareness. It's not 'just sleep', in the same way that it's not 'just food' or 'just sex'. Sleep is a major part of of our lives and must be nurtured as we get older. The best way to do this is to pay more attention to it.

Just because sleep is an unconscious activity, this doesn't mean we have no control over it. The things we do while we are awake can greatly influence the quality and quantity of our sleep.

2. STRATEGIC PLANNING AND TARGETING OF APPROPRIATE GOALS

If we are busy people, it is important we give ourselves adequate time at night to sleep. If we habitually come home in the evening and work quite late into the night, we usually reduce our overall sleep time. So whenever we are able, we should plan to go to bed a little earlier. Relax, listen to our body, then when we feel sleepy, toddle off to bed.

Sometimes more sleep is not the answer. For example, if we do start to experience long night-time awakenings, we should not simply spend more time in bed. Just the opposite, we should reduce our time in bed. For example, if we are lying in bed for eight hours, but only getting seven hours sleep, we should only stay in bed for seven hours, thus spending almost all of our time in bed asleep. This will give us better quality sleep and help associate the bedroom and the bed with sleeping, not being awake.

3. ACCENT THE POSITIVE OF SLEEP, ELIMINATE THE NEGATIVE

Sleep is not a punishment (as it sometimes seems to be for young children). Along with appropriate scheduling and pacing of our days, establishing 'sleep routines' – whether they involve sex, reading bedtime stories or simply slipping between a clean set of sheets – can be an enjoyable part of the process, as well as a very healthy one.

> WHENEVER WE ARE ABLE, WE SHOULD PLAN TO GO TO BED A LITTLE EARLIER. RELAX; LISTEN TO OUR BODIES, THEN, WHEN WE FEEL SLEEPY, TODDLE OFF TO BED.

We can also make waking a positive experience. There are few things more stressful (or irritating) than an alarm clock so loud that it scares us awake. This sort of rude awakening can damage our memory, learning, attention and mood. An established sleep pattern is almost always accompanied by a healthy waking pattern.

Although sleep is important, it is better not to unnecessarily worry about sleep, especially while in bed, where it will strengthen the association of the bed with worry. This can lead to anxiety that will prevent sleep and lead to feelings of fatigue the next day.

4. MAKING CHOICES THAT ARE SUSTAINABLE FOR THE LONG-TERM

Slow solutions are those that can be incorporated into our daily routines and become good habits. Our body clocks will love us for employing them as they make it easier for us to keep to time. Where possible, we should attempt to go to sleep when we normally feel gathering drowsiness, not earlier or later. We should try to maintain the same 'wake-up time' and morning light exposure every day, and resist sleeping in to attempt to 'catch up on sleep', as this can delay the timing of our body clocks for the first few days of a new week and lead to those 'Monday morning moody blues'.

IMPACTING YOUR SLEEP

ALCOHOL	Alcohol is a sedative often used as an aid to sleep (as a 'nightcap'), but the effect is short-lived. Not only does alcohol tend to fill up our bladder, it also disrupts healthy sleep patterns. It is better not to drink alcohol for at least two hours before bedtime.
FOOD	The release of hormones when we eat can also delay the onset of sleep, which is why it is unwise to snack just before going to bed.
CAFFEINE	Caffeine stimulates our brains for up to six hours after we have our last shot of coffee, tea, cola or energy drink.
EXERCISE	Often we see people out walking or running in the morning. Far from indicating insomnia, morning exercise is one of the best ways to promote sound sleep. In fact, exercising early in the day can significantly enhance the quality of our sleep at night. Not only is it a great way to absorb sunlight and re-set our body clocks, physical activity also works to enhance deep sleep. However, exercising within three hours of bedtime is not recommended as it releases stress hormones that keep us awake. For sleep to happen, we need to wind down so our brains can give over to the sleep cycle. They cannot do this if they are trying to do something else, whether that be coping with stress or engaging in mental or physical activity.
WORK	Where possible, we should put work away at least an hour or two before bedtime.
STRESS	One of the most important influences on our modern sleep patterns is daytime stress. This can be emotional, physical or environmental stress, such as a noisy workplace, but the result is almost always a bad night's sleep. When stress is the culprit, the cause, not the symptoms, must be treated. Evenings can be the best time of day to practise relaxation, breathing and other mind-body techniques.
ENVIRONMENT	Getting good sleep is easy if you have a good place to get it. You may think you can sleep anywhere, but a dark, cool and quiet room, clean sheets and a decent mattress that allows us to maintain anatomical neutral positions comfortably makes a difference. Use the bed only for sleeping, sex and very relaxing activities such as reading. You may be asleep, but your days will thank you for it.

5. DON'T BE EXCLUSIVE - COMPLEX PROBLEMS REQUIRE COMPLEX SOLUTIONS

There are many different programs designed to improve our sleep by helping us deal with our daytime issues. There is little point (and rarely any joy) in trying to fix our sleep problems directly when stress, inactivity or other issues during the day are the real culprits. Equally, stress management, mind-body techniques, exercise and getting an optimal diet through the day tend to make things run more smoothly at night.

A variety of sedatives can help us get to sleep. These include herbal and over-the-counter preparations and prescription drugs. Although many of these are effective in the short-term, they are not slow solutions; they are not tailored to our individual needs; they help us to avoid our problems, rather than address them; and they can be detrimental to our health and wellbeing in the long-term.

6. SUPPORT IS OUT THERE, GET HELP

Sometimes getting a good night's sleep can seem like an impossible task and we get into such deep ruts that it is difficult to get out. Fortunately, there are many professional therapists out there who can help us get our sleep rhythms back in sync.

7. BE SELECTIVE - DO WHAT'S RIGHT FOR YOU

One of the keys to getting a good night's sleep is finding a plan we like and can adhere to in the long-term. As Goldilocks learned, it is important to lie on each bed and find the one that best suits our individual needs. The amount of sleep we need in order to feel (and be) well rested varies among individuals, seasons and even over the course of the working week.

So find out about yourself and listen to the feedback. See how you are performing by keeping a log or journal. Do you tend to feel better on Mondays? Are you making it through to the afternoon without flagging?

Follow your progress and set new goals as you go. It is important to follow up your successes and failures. Not everything will work, but when something does and you wake up feeling refreshed, it is worth bottling.

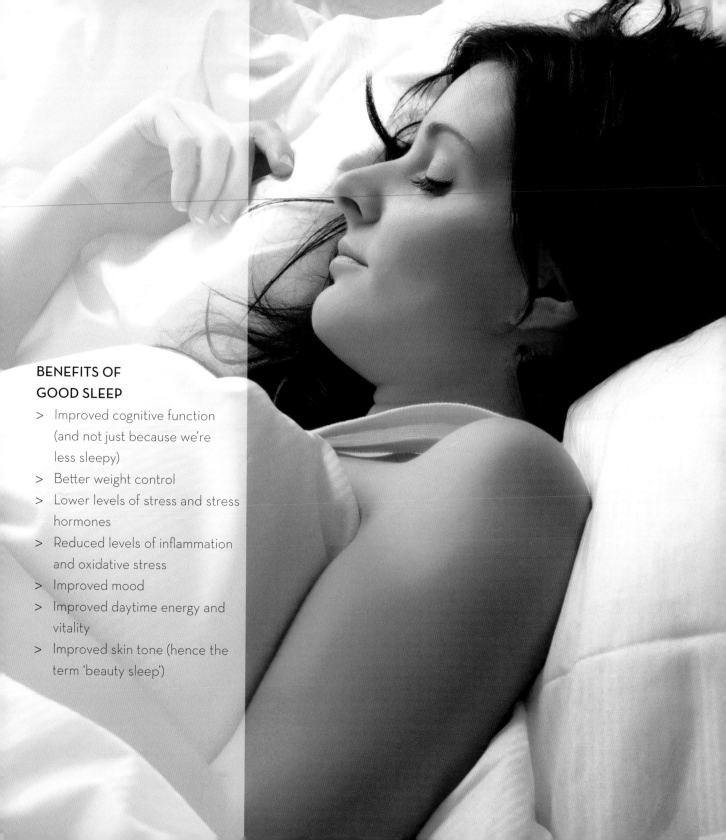

BENEFITS OF GOOD SLEEP

> Improved cognitive function (and not just because we're less sleepy)

> Better weight control

> Lower levels of stress and stress hormones

> Reduced levels of inflammation and oxidative stress

> Improved mood

> Improved daytime energy and vitality

> Improved skin tone (hence the term 'beauty sleep')

OPTIONS TO HELP YOU GET A GOOD NIGHT'S SLEEP

☑ Establish a pattern that suits your body and stick to it
> Go to bed and wake up at the same time every day, even on weekends
> Limit the time you spend in bed
> Only go to bed when you're sleepy
> If you don't fall asleep within 15 minutes or wake up and can't fall back to sleep within that amount of time, get out of bed and do something relaxing until you feel sleepy again

☑ Use your bed only for sleeping or sex

☑ Get more exercise
> Do exercise first thing in the morning exercise; apart from getting it out of the way before you get sidetracked, it is a great way to bolster your spirits
> Get out of your office and take in some bright light during the day. This is a great chance to exercise your body and your brain and as a bonus you sleep better too

☑ Deal with stress – this is one of the biggest causes of insomnia and must be managed head on if you want to get a good night s sleep. Many stress management techniques have been shown to improve your quality and quantity of sleep
> Get a meditation CD and listen to it before going to bed
> Invest in an audio visual entrainment system and use this before going to sleep to enhance your quality or sleep and so you get to sleep faster

☑ Keep out the light from the street or the next room

☑ Keep the TV and the computer out of the bedroom

☑ Block-out street noise with the right choice of window, garden planting or other simple tricks

OPTIONS TO HELP YOU GET A GOOD NIGHT'S SLEEP

☑ Replace your worn-out or uncomfortable mattresses with one that allows you to maintain an anatomically neutral position

☑ Avoid drinks containing caffeine after 2pm (or noon, if you're caffeine-sensitive)

☑ Don't drink alcohol for at least two hours before bedtime

☑ Don't eat just before going to bed

☑ Put work away at least a couple of hours before going to bed

☑ Talk to your doctor about hormonal deficiencies that may be affecting your sleep (see chapters 28-32)

☑ Forgo naps, especially close to bedtime

☑ Ask your doctor to prescribe a melatonin supplement

☑ See a practitioner if you continue to have sleep problems

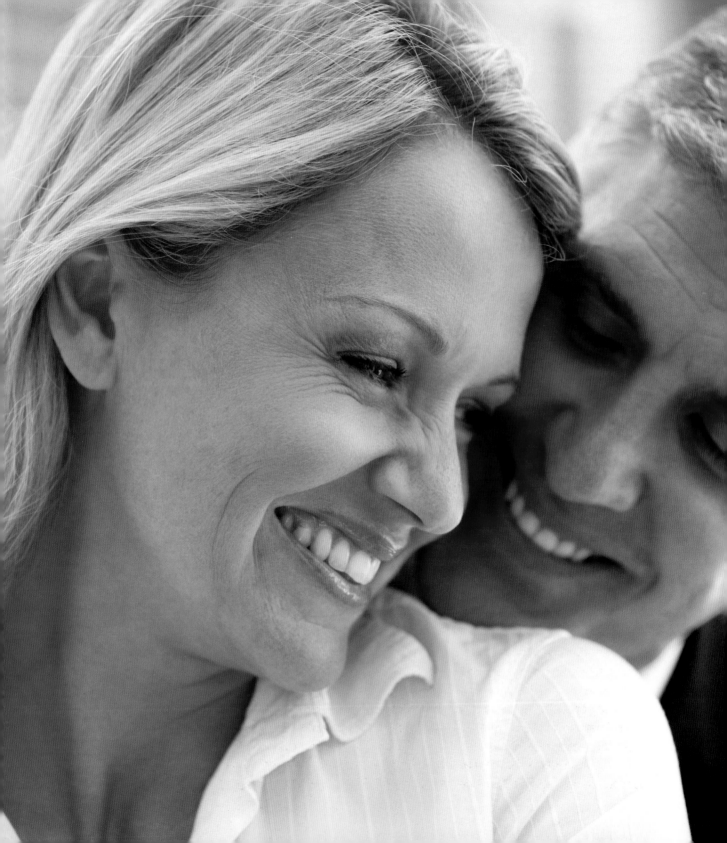

CHAPTER 27

INTIMATE CONNECTIONS
[LOVE, SEX & AGEING]

When it comes to living a long, healthy and happy life, one thing is crucial. "All you need is love," sang The Beatles – and they may be right. What seems to be most important to our ongoing good health is making and retaining significant personal connections in our lives. Many of us achieve this by finding compatible men and women and forming lasting intimate partnerships.

As part of a strategy to slow ageing, it makes sense to put aside time and energy to foster and maintain our key relationships. These connections offer health benefits at least as important as those that flow from adopting healthy diets. Better still, combine the two: share a slow meal with a loved one or take a long walk with a friend.

Social isolation can lead to mental stress, depression, decline and disease. Loneliness is a killer. Lonely hearts suffer twice as many heart attacks and are four times less likely to survive them. Cancer, stroke and other diseases are also more common in those with fewer social and personal connections.

Intimate connections also play their part, enhancing both the quality and quantity of our lives. It is often said that sex makes us younger. This is not just about having the kind of relationship or vigour that makes frequent sex possible.

Sex itself has effects that may be considered life enhancing. Indeed, traditional Tantrism doctrines speak of sexual ecstasy as a path to rejuvenation. However, the number and frequency of orgasms are not the only factors that determine how beneficial physical intimacy is to our health.

Think of holding hands or sharing a hug, and how these intimate gestures make us feel. Think how physical affection can reinforce the bonds between us and make us feel connected to something bigger than ourselves. This is not just a psychological sense of confidence, warmth and wellbeing. Intimacy has real, physiological effects on our bodies, helping to reduce stress, prevent disease and slow ageing.

KEEPING THE SEX ALIVE

In the eyes of many people, youthfulness is synonymous with our ability to express our sexual desires, while ageing is the process through which these capacities decline.

This need not be the case; older people have sexual desires too. On average, they have sex as often as younger folk. Yet while age is no obstacle to good sex, it does impact significantly on our sexual functions.

As women age, for example, they may take longer to attain the vaginal lubrication needed to make sexual intercourse comfortable and set the stage for climax, and their orgasms may decrease in number and intensity. In ageing men, it can take longer to obtain and maintain erections sufficient to enable satisfactory sexual intercourse.

But our decline in sexual function need not be a barrier to sexual enjoyment, provided our specific needs are recognised and met (with lubricants, topical creams and sufficient stimulation or foreplay, etc).

There are a number of reasons for our so-called 'age-related' changes. Declining levels of sex hormones, especially testosterone, can impact on our level of desire and sexual interest, as well as the functioning of our sex organs.

Physical and mental diseases can also contribute to our sexual problems, while relationship factors and the impacts of stress are heightened as we age. Declining sexual function as we age is also linked to reduced sexual activity. And this can set a vicious cycle in motion because with sex, it seems, it's a case of 'use it or lose it'.

Fortunately, all the factors mentioned above are modifiable. What happens depends partly on the choices we make today in relation to improving and maintaining our health and our sexual functions.

For example, exercise helps us to maintain our sex organs in peak condition. Rewarding sexual experiences serve to bolster our levels of arousal and make sex better for us in the future. In fact, frequent sexual activity when we are younger is associated with a slower rate of decline in our sexual functions as we grow older.

CAN'T GET NO SATISFACTION? (SLOW SOLUTIONS FOR BETTER SEX)

Sex is a major part of our lives that must be nurtured as we grow older. Those of us hoping to improve our sex lives can adopt a number of short-term approaches. Although many are effective temporarily, they are rarely slow solutions. There are, however, various 'slow' and simple principles that we can adopt to improve our sex lives and, with them, our health.

1. UNDERSTANDING AND ENGAGEMENT

Sex on 'autopilot', emotionally disconnected and disengaged from our partner, is a lesser experience, just as 'fast' lives are often wasted. Take the time to slow down and enjoy the ride. Learn when your body begins to feel excited and what it takes to make you feel satisfied. It's also important to be aware of the things that get in the way of sex. Problems with sex (sexual dysfunction) are more common as we age, but they are not an inevitable consequence of ageing, in the same way that getting heart disease and cancer are not givens. Similarly, we can help to prevent sexual dysfunction by the actions we take today.

Erectile dysfunction is the most common sexual problem in ageing men and one of the main reasons women say they stop having sex. A man's inability to maintain an erection can be the result of many factors. Coordinated function among nerves and blood vessels and the right stimuli are always required to get it up. If any or all of the necessary components aren't functioning optimally, an erection will fail.

Ageing, along with many of its associated diseases and the drugs used to treat them, may cause erectile dysfunction. It has been estimated that more than 50% of men with diabetes have difficulty achieving erections. So one of the most effective ways to avoid problems with our penises tomorrow is to do all we can to prevent diabetes and other age-related diseases today.

Reduced levels of desire and arousal are the most common sexual issues for ageing women. These problems are usually the result of complex changes in body chemistry, particularly sex hormones, as well as barriers to sexual enjoyment and relaxation, including stress, anxiety and, in some cases, our partner's sexual dysfunction.

Its management therefore usually involves modulating both chemistry and behaviour. For example, DHEA may be useful in restoring testosterone levels and libido, and is most successful when combined with strategies to improve emotional closeness and communication.

As women age, we experience another pitfall: our failing ability to reach climax. There have been many books written on the female orgasm, but little is known about what stops it being triggered in some women. Consequently, there are no simple pills we can take to prevent this problem.

In many cases, older women must develop a different relationship with their bodies and partners. The best protection against losing the ability to climax appears to be frequent good sex. Increased intensity and duration of genital stimulation, particularly of the clitoris, can also enhance our ability to experience more rapid arousal and stronger orgasms.

2. STRATEGIC PLANNING AND TARGETING OF APPROPRIATE GOALS

Achieving satisfying sex means satisfying the goals and targets we set for it. We often put undue focus on a single performance goal (such as one partner's orgasm, or mutual orgasms), whereas the whole is probably more important to our overall satisfaction – and orgasms are far more likely when we feel a general sense of wellbeing.

One slow way to better sex is changing our conceptualisations. One of the common slow themes in this book is our emphasis on quality over quantity. For example, traditional Tantric practices advocate non-goal-oriented sexual experiences, in which foreplay is prolonged and performed for its own sake, rather than as a means to an end.

Plan time just for you and your partner, away from kids, friends and family. Schedule 'couple time' so that the demands of your life don't interfere with intimacy and sex doesn't start to feel like a chore that has to be fitted in between taking out the garbage and falling asleep. Sex can mean a long, sensuous session or a satisfying quickie. Discuss with your partner what works for you both and mix it up.

It is important that we give ourselves adequate time to enjoy sex. Try setting aside special times and creating a sense of place and purpose for sex, evoking all our senses. Sex should take its time and may require us to engage in more, not less, foreplay as we grow older. That does not mean avoiding spontaneity, but just as we take time to prepare a meal or enjoy life in general, we should be willing to take our time having sex Why rush a good thing?

3. ACCENT THE POSITIVE OF SEX, ELIMINATE THE NEGATIVE

Sex is not a chore, nor is it a requirement for a loving relationship. For it to be 'slow', it must be a positive experience. If we let our expectations of failure or other negative emotions drain the joy from sex, we also lose many of its potential health and wellbeing benefits. In fact, the health benefits of physical intimacy are closely linked to the degree of satisfaction we get from the experience.

4. MAKING CHOICES THAT ARE SUSTAINABLE IN THE LONG-TERM

Slow solutions are those that can be incorporated into our daily (or nightly) routines. That does not mean we should avoid spontaneity; rather it means we need to facilitate it. We can do this very simply, or in more elaborate ways, but good sex almost always stems from good habits.

There are many exercises we can do to improve and maintain our sexual functions. Of course, sex is the best exercise for maintaining our sexual organs (and the relationships that sex reinforces) in peak condition.

Pelvic floor exercises, for instance, entail us rhythmically contracting, holding and releasing muscles in our pelvic regions as if to stop the flow of urine.

5. DON'T BE EXCLUSIVE - COMPLEX PROBLEMS REQUIRE COMPLEX SOLUTIONS

Many different programs are available to help us improve our sex lives. But the magic comes not from the little blue pill, but from what we do with it. Moreover, interventions to improve our sex lives are unlikely to last unless they are combined with additional measures to keep us healthy.

Those of us who stay physically fit, keep our brains stimulated and remain interested in a variety of activities are likely to feel more attractive and self-assured and are more likely to maintain our libido.

Managing stress in our lives, optimising our diet and doing all we can to prevent disease are actions we can take to keep us healthy – and robust health is the best prescription for a pleasurable sex life as we grow older. Smokers might want to bear in mind that every cigarette makes their (sex) life shorter!

A number of 'aphrodisiacs' are available that claim to enhance sexual functioning and enjoyment. All are known to have strong placebo effects - perhaps just knowing they have something to do with sex puts our mind in the right place. Many have real, measurable effects on sexual functioning in some individuals (see following table).A number of foods are also alleged to have aphrodisiac qualities, although it is unknown whether they really do or people simply think they do. But since sexual desire is all in the mind, it probably doesn't matter!

6. SUPPORT IS OUT THERE, GET HELP

When problems arise (and they will, in most of us, at some time), they affect both partners. We may try to pretend otherwise, but we know! Most of us feel uncomfortable disclosing our sexual problems and this serves to compound our difficulties.

The biggest barrier to overcoming sexual problems is our reluctance to share our feelings and ask for help. Being open and honest with our partners about needs, interests and desires is the key to overcoming problems. If there is anxiety, shame, lack of interest or dissatisfaction around having sex with your partner, talk about it.

Effective communication is as critical to our sexual lives as it is to our everyday lives. The act of communication itself can be seductive, enticing and sexual. Many sex therapists have success simply by improving couples' emotional closeness and communication, in and out of the bedroom.

Getting help also sometimes means talking to your doctor or health care provider. A number of effective drug treatments are now available. It may be that the simple step of seeking help can improve your ability to maintain intimate relationships, as well as your quality of life and longevity.

7. BE SELECTIVE - DO WHAT'S RIGHT FOR YOU

There have been many books written on the subject of good sex, just as there are thousands of books claiming to describe 'the perfect diet'.

But there is never one perfect solution. We are all different, especially when it comes to what turns us on. One of the keys to good sex is finding patterns that we like and can be maintained in the long-term. It really doesn't matter what these patterns are, as long as they are well matched with who we are and they give us the satisfaction and intimacy we need for our emotional, mental and physical health.

Many concepts will not work for you and others may seem too difficult, but just as Goldilocks sampled every bed and bowl before deciding where to sleep and how much to eat, it is useful to try different sexual styles and positions to find those that best suit our individual desires.

Try practising different thoughts and behaviours in relation to sex, and learning new sexual patterns. Chocolate body paint, anyone?

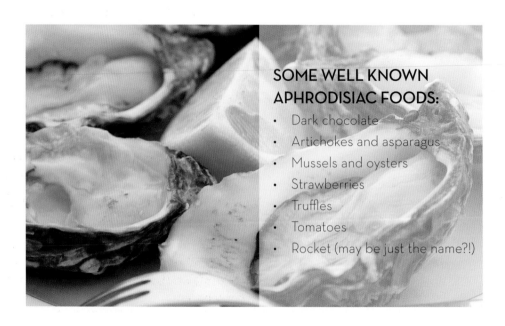

SOME WELL KNOWN APHRODISIAC FOODS:
- Dark chocolate
- Artichokes and asparagus
- Mussels and oysters
- Strawberries
- Truffles
- Tomatoes
- Rocket (may be just the name?!)

APHRODISIAC	FOR MEN, WOMEN OR BOTH	HOW IT IS SUPPOSED TO WORK
Extract of Yohimbe Bark, Yohimbine	For men	This is prescribed for the treatment of erectile dysfunction. Some users also report a cumulative improvement in their sexual function and libido over time. Low dose preparations of yohimbe bark are also available over-the-counter, but should be used with caution as many contain toxic alkaloids besides yohimbine. Side-effects can include rapid pulse, sweating and panic reactions in some people.
Nettle Root	For both sexes	Extracts of nettle root can boost active testosterone levels in both men and women.
Asian Ginseng (Panax)	For both sexes	This can increase sexual performance and libido, as well as reduce stress. This effect is not seen with American or Siberian Ginseng.
Withania	For men	This Indian herb can maintain vitality and improve sexual performance in older men.
Ginkgo	For men	This can have a positive effect on sexual function and erectile dysfunction in men.
Horny Goat Weed	For both sexes	This traditional Chinese herb that boosts sexual performance, possibly by modifying hormonal signalling. In the long-term, these may have some negative effects in men, such as breast enlargement.
Tribulus Terrestris	For both sexes	Supplements containing Tribulus Terrestris (also known as Yellow Vine, Caltrop or Goathead) are widely used to increase libido. It probably acts by increasing active testosterone levels, but may also have direct effects on erectile function.
Arginine	For men	This may improve erectile function by increasing blood flow to the stimulated penis in much in the same way as Viagra does, although its actions are less selective.

OPTIONS TO KEEP THE SEX ALIVE

☑ Involve your partner – this may seem the most obvious thing written in this book, yet sex and sexuality are often kept too private, so that success comes by accident or telepathy, rather than effective team work

☑ Be aware of the health (or otherwise) your sex life - you don't need to be paranoid. But neither do you need to pretend that everything is all right

☑ Create an environment of trust with your partner so that you can explore your sexuality:
  > Set ground rules e.g. If sex in a public space is your worst nightmare, tell your partner that you don't feel comfortable
  > Choose to be non-judgemental when discussing sexual issues
  > Avoid playing the blame game
  > Tell your partner what you really want…or show them
  > Know your limitations and feel free to express them

☑ Recognise the different needs of sex as you age – both women and men may need more stimulation, foreplay or lubrication
  > Start with kissing…it will often lead to more
  > Buy a bottle of lubricant and keep it by the bed. Use it if you need it and make it part of the fun
  > As a couple, find out what sex toys you are both interested in and try them out
  > Try 'sexy talk' or phone sex to get in the mood
  > Realise that for each of us the time to orgasm will vary so take the time and allow the process to happen without pressure
  > Discuss your sexual fantasies with one another. Know that this doesn't necessarily mean playing them out; discussing them might be enough to get you in the mood

OPTIONS TO KEEP THE SEX ALIVE

☑ And remember: sex isn't all about the sex act – it can include romance and intimacy, too
> Start with a massage or intimate touch
> Plan time together without family or friends – go on a date!
> Choose not to have sex tonight and extend the intimacy with the promise of things to come

☑ Don't stop! It doesn't have to be perfect the first time or even every time Increase physical activity and stop over-consumption - these are the main preventable cause of erectile dysfunction and sexual dysfunction in women. See previous chapters for guidance

☑ Optimise your hormones - low hormonal levels will reduce your libido. See your doctor to check that your hormones are within optimal ranges

☑ Manage stress - stress gets in the way of good sex. Stress management techniques have been shown to improve sexual function and satisfaction

☑ Try yoga, meditation rhythmic breathing or other relaxation techniques

☑ Stop smoking - see previous chapters for an extensive list of options

☑ Make an appointment to see a health care professional about sex problems. Sex therapy has a high success rate in helping couples solve their sex-related problems through guided discussion and negotiation. There are also a number of medical solutions, apart from the little blue pill!

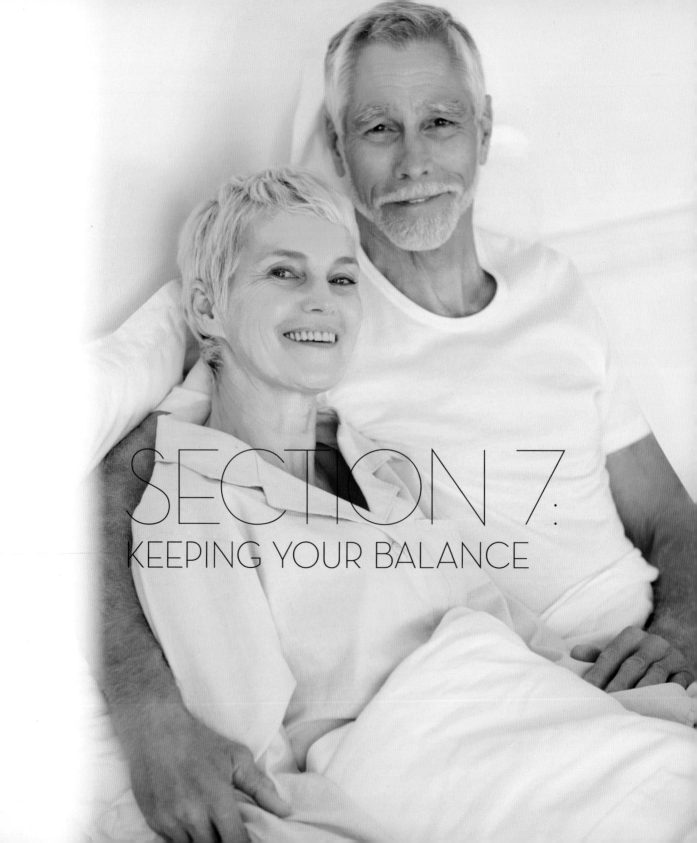

SECTION 7:
KEEPING YOUR BALANCE

Successful ageing is all about achieving and maintaining balance. When walking along a narrow log, it is the signals of our senses, their adaptation and coordination that tell us how best to make the next move. In the ageing body, this is the job of the neuroendocrine system, with hormones as the chemical signals, including sex hormones, growth hormone, cortisol and melatonin. This section looks at the important changes in our hormones as we get older and the potential role of hormonal replacement as a means of modifying the ageing process.

KATE'S EXPERIENCE
My initial exposure to a doctor with nutritional and hormone-related qualifications was a key plank in my quest for wellness. He started me on DHEA and this gave me a completely new lease on life. I was on fire! When I first started, I remember getting out of bed in the morning with the feeling that my whole body had woken up – there was no more creakiness and I felt completely energised. I started sleeping better, lost fat and developed more lean muscle, had lots of energy and my old friend - libido - came back to my life!

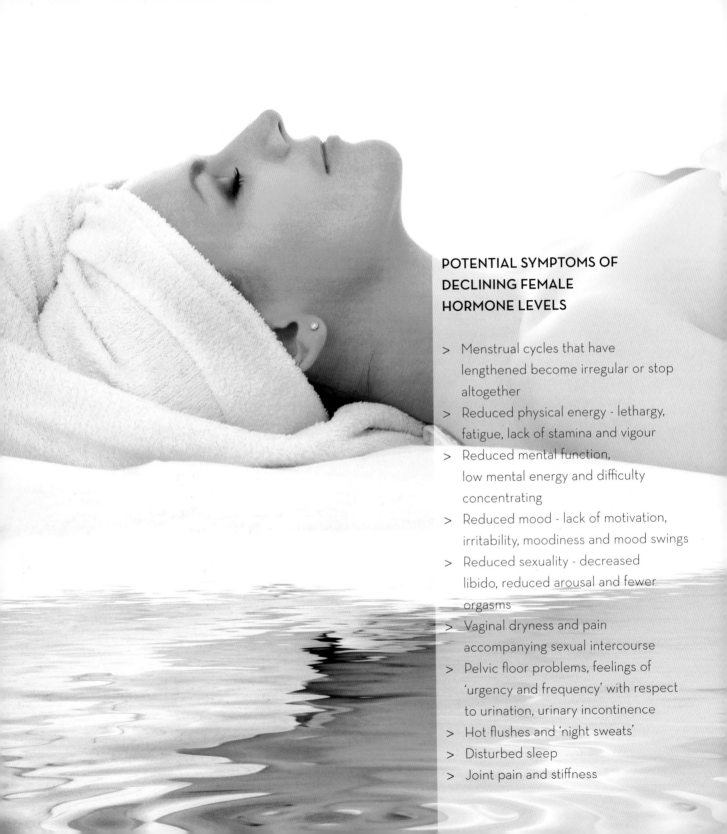

POTENTIAL SYMPTOMS OF DECLINING FEMALE HORMONE LEVELS

> Menstrual cycles that have lengthened become irregular or stop altogether
> Reduced physical energy - lethargy, fatigue, lack of stamina and vigour
> Reduced mental function, low mental energy and difficulty concentrating
> Reduced mood - lack of motivation, irritability, moodiness and mood swings
> Reduced sexuality - decreased libido, reduced arousal and fewer orgasms
> Vaginal dryness and pain accompanying sexual intercourse
> Pelvic floor problems, feelings of 'urgency and frequency' with respect to urination, urinary incontinence
> Hot flushes and 'night sweats'
> Disturbed sleep
> Joint pain and stiffness

CHAPTER 28

FEMALE SEX HORMONES

Every woman in her mid to late forties experiences a natural transition in the way her major female sex hormones are produced and released. Over the next five to 10 years, the production of major oestrogens (estradiol and estriol) and progesterone slows, becomes erratic and eventually shuts down altogether due to the exhaustion of hormone-producing reserves in the ovaries. During the latter part of this transition, menstrual cycles lengthen, become irregular and eventually stop, signalling the end of fertility – known as menopause.

The process of ovaries shutting down involves not just an end to reproductive functioning, but changes in almost every aspect of a woman's body and life. Individual experiences vary, but many women also experience distressing symptoms including hot flushes (hot flashes), mood changes, disturbed sleep and concentration, urinary incontinence, joint pain and stiffness, vaginal dryness, sexual dysfunction and reduced quality of life. Severe menopausal symptoms, such as hot flushes, are more common in those who are overweight, inactive or smokers.

Other changes that occur with the menopause are more subtle, though equally important for health and wellbeing. Oestrogens are key regulators of growth and function in many tissues, from our bone to our skin, our pelvic floor to our brain. As oestrogen levels decline, these structures also undergo significant changes. Loss of oestrogen, for example, triggers accelerated bone loss, making bones more fragile and pushing many women closer to the threshold of osteoporosis (see chapter 34). At the same time, our skin becomes drier and less flexible, contributing to the development of wrinkles. Increased levels of bad (LDL) cholesterol, together with reduced clotting capacity and impaired vascular function in post-menopausal women, contributes to an increased risk of heart attack and stroke.

A history of menopausal symptoms is all that health professionals usually need to determine whether our hormone levels are declining. Blood tests to check levels of various hormones can also be done, which can be useful to establish whether young women are going through menopause prematurely.

Hormone replacement therapy (HRT) is widely used by women wishing to manage their menopausal symptoms. In addition, many believe that delaying the loss of oestrogen levels by up to 10 years through HRT may also delay various complications of ageing by a similar length of time.

Certainly, HRT is an effective treatment for hot flushes, vaginal dryness and other distressing menopausal symptoms. Most menopausal women on HRT also report less sleeplessness and tiredness, a restored sense of mental focus, greater energy, improved mood and heightened libido, with all these improvements continuing for as long as they stay on HRT.

The same can be said for preserving the architecture and strength of our bones. Those women who start HRT in their peri-menopausal years appear to have a lower risk of fracture in later life. Some studies also suggest that if women take HRT during peri-menopause, they have a slightly lower risk of dementia.

However, recent data raises the possibility that using HRT for five or more years may have a number of negative health consequences, particularly with respect to heart disease and breast cancer.

Where it is indicated, HRT should be started in the critical window before, or around the time of, the menopause to reduce the risk of heart disease. However, the magnitude of this effect is small when compared with other ways to prevent heart disease, such as working to lower 'bad' cholesterol levels and blood pressure or quitting smoking (see chapter 5).

But if we start HRT late, more than 10 years after reaching the menopause, the risk of heart disease is increased by HRT. This is possibly because the receptors through which oestrogen would normally signal its protective effects have also long since disappeared. Certainly, HRT should not be used by women who are at risk of heart disease or clotting, as its actions in these situations may be detrimental.

Another potential concern with HRT is the suggestion that it may slightly increase our risk of breast and ovarian cancer. Again, this risk is very small compared to smoking, or eating and drinking too much, which we would happily do every day. Nonetheless, those with a family history of breast cancer or other conditions linked

THE OTHER POTENTIAL CONCERN ABOUT HRT IS THE SUGGESTION THAT IT MAY SLIGHTLY INCREASE OUR RISK OF BREAST AND OVARIAN CANCER. AGAIN, THIS RISK IS VERY SMALL.....

BENEFITS AND RISKS OF HORMONE REPLACEMENT THERAPY (HRT)
Potential Benefits
☑ Prevent and treat menopausal symptoms – hot flushes, vaginal dryness, pelvic floor discomfort, sleeplessness and tiredness, a lethargy, low mood and following HRT
☑ Significantly lower rate of bone loss that leads to thin, weak bones (osteoporosis) and an increased risk of fracture
☑ Slightly reduced risk of heart attack and stroke
☑ Slightly reduced risk of cognitive decline and dementia
☑ Slightly reduced risk of colon cancer and age-related vision loss associated with macular degeneration
Potential Risks
☑ Slightly increased risk of breast and ovarian cancer
☑ Slightly increased risk of heart attack and stroke (if HRT is started well after the menopause, or in those with established heart disease)
☑ Intermittent vaginal bleeding
☑ Increased risk of gallbladder stones, especially if overweight

with increased risk of breast cancer should consider non-hormonal methods of managing menopausal symptoms and bone loss.

No woman should continue using HRT for more than 10 years as many of its benefits disappear after this time, while the risks to those using it may increase.

HRT is available in a number of different forms, delivered via oral, transdermal or vaginal routes. Women who have not had hysterectomies are usually given a 'combined' regimen, in which oestrogen is combined with progestogen. This combined therapy can be taken on a cyclical basis (like the contraceptive pill) or on a continuous, daily basis. Women who have had hysterectomies can take daily doses of oestrogen without progestogen.

Generally, the choice of dose is determined by the reasons for starting HRT. To control unwanted menopausal symptoms, the lowest effective dose is preferable. Low doses also reduce the chances of experiencing side-effects such as breast tenderness and intermittent vaginal bleeding.

There is no data to indicate which is the best HRT formulation. In most comparisons, the benefits turn out to be roughly the same, so we should take the one that works for us and ignore the advertising.

Proponents of bio-identical hormone replacement therapy claim it is superior to HRT as it uses hormones that are chemically identical to those found in our bodies. In addition, compounded troches or lozenges of bio-identical hormones can be tailor-made based on individual symptoms and the result of blood tests.

However, at this time, there is no evidence to suggest that bio-identical hormones have any special advantages over those used in conventional HRT. And with the controversies surrounding old fashioned HRT still ringing in our ears, it may be wise to treat this new form of HRT with some caution. Most compounded preparations have not been through clinical trials large enough to confirm their relative safety.

A number of natural alternatives to HRT have proven popular for managing menopausal symptoms. These include:

> Plant-derived isoflavones (from soy, clover, flax, hops or other sources) that are able to bind and partially activate oestrogen receptors – so-called phytoestrogens. Foods naturally high in phytoestrogens, such as soy products including tofu, tempeh and soy milk, flaxseed and linseed, provide too little to effectively treat menopausal symptoms. However, high dose supplements are widely available.

> Herbs such as Tribulus Terrestris and Vitex are used to increase natural hormone levels by inhibiting the enzymes in our livers that metabolise oestrogen.

> Other herbal products, including Black Cohosh (cimicifuga), are promoted as offering 'hormone-free' relief for menopausal symptoms, although they probably act by modifying our levels of the brain hormone serotonin.

THERE IS NO EVIDENCE TO SUGGEST THAT BIO-IDENTICAL HORMONES HAVE ANY SPECIAL ADVANTAGES OVER THOSE USED IN CONVENTIONAL HRT.

On the whole, small clinical trials with these supplements have failed to confirm replicable benefits, although some women will experience improvements in some menopausal symptoms.

More selective non-hormonal solutions to menopausal symptoms, including gabapentin, SSRIs and clonidine, are available on prescription. Overall, however, conventional HRT is far more effective for the relief of severe menopausal symptoms.

OPTIONS TO HELP COMBAT THE MENOPAUSE

☑ Be aware of your symptoms - don't suffer in silence or pretend it isn't happening

☑ Keep a menstrual diary - note any changes in your usual menstrual cycles, reduced physical and mental energy, low mood, mood swings, reduced libido, disturbed sleep, pelvic-floor problems, joint pain and stiffness

☑ Make an appointment to see your doctor to see what your options are if symptoms impact on your life (and don't procrastinate about doing it)

☑ Get more omega-3s – omega-3 fatty acids have a number of positive actions on mood, inflammation and vascular function
   > Eat more cold-water oily fish, flax seed (linseed), purslane, kiwifruit, lignon berries, black raspberries and walnuts
   > It is recommended to take a gram of EPA and DHA each day, or 2-3 g/day of alpha-linolenic acid from plants. This is the equivalent of an oily fish meal 2-3 times every week

☑ Increase your physical activity
   > Take up swimming, dancing or bike riding
   > Join a flexibility class
   > See previous sections for an extensive range of options. Also go to chapters 21 and 22 for a look at exercise and ageing

CHAPTER 29

MALE SEX HORMONES

In both men and women, blood levels of the major male sex hormones (called androgens) decline by about one per cent a year, from our mid-thirties. This decline is called the andropause.

Many of the symptoms of low testosterone levels are non-specific, and are often readily attributed to ageing or disease, without looking for the real cause.

By the age of 70, at least one in every 10 men experiences the 'androgen deficiency of the ageing male' (ADAM), in which low testosterone levels are associated with a reduced quality of life and symptoms that include reduced libido, erectile dysfunction, fatigue, disturbed sleep and a reduced capacity to concentrate.

Women in their 40's have on average half the testosterone level they had in their 20's. In women, this decline can make a major difference to libido, mood and general wellbeing. Low testosterone levels also contribute to skin wrinkling, pelvic-floor problems and 'middle-aged spread'.

The effects of testosterone are not confined to quality of life. Testosterone levels also play an important role in maintaining strong bones, cognitive function, and metabolic and cardiovascular health.

Although ageing is the most important player, the risk of symptomatic androgen deficiency appears greatest in those with diabetes, smokers, those who are overweight or obese, alcoholics and those suffering from chronic stress (which disrupts almost all hormonal pathways to some extent). All of these conditions can be prevented if we make the sensible dietary and lifestyle choices.

In women, androgen levels may also be modified by oral HRT, which decreases the amount of testosterone that is available to keep us at peak function. This effect is not seen in transdermal estrogens (patches), which should be considered in women on HRT with sexual dysfunction or unexplained fatigue.

For men who think they may be low in testosterone, a number of screening questionnaires are available that identify those most likely to be at risk. Any abnormal score can then be followed up by blood tests. Usually, testosterone blood tests are taken as early in the morning as possible, as this is when testosterone levels tend to peak and this peak tends to flatten out with ageing. Salivary testosterone can also provide a reasonable approximation of free testosterone levels. Adult men with abnormally low levels of total testosterone (less than 8nmol per litre) or with low free testosterone levels (of less than 10nmol per litre) and symptoms that suggest low levels are generally said to be suffering from ADAM.

There is no good reason for men to check testosterone levels or take supplements in the absence of symptoms. Moreover, using testosterone in the absence of deficiency is problematic, as prolonged use can have negative effects on health and mood (such as 'roid rage' – the aggression that often accompanies ongoing use of steroids).

For women, there are no standardised screening questionnaires for low testosterone levels. However, women with adequate oestrogen levels who have significantly diminished sexual motivation and/or desire, persistent unexplainable fatigue or a decreased sense of well-being should consider having their testosterone levels tested or a trial of androgen supplements, once other possible causes of their symptoms are excluded. Treatment thresholds for women are unclear. Many clinicians advocate just treating women based on symptoms, as most tests are only standardised for male levels of testosterone, and quite inaccurate at the 10–20 times lower levels of testosterone found in healthy women.

For symptomatic men and women who have low levels of testosterone, supplementation can improve their quality of life and their sexual, mental and physical functioning. This is hardly surprising, as all androgens are performance-enhancing drugs.

Testosterone treatment now comes in many forms, including capsules (Andriol), patches (Androderm), gel (Testogel), short-term injections administered every one to three weeks (Sustanon), long-term 'depot injections' every four to six months (Renadron) and testosterone pellet implants that contain only testosterone extracted from plant materials. The best formulation for men depends on how much they need to restore testosterone levels and reduce their symptoms.

› Reduced mental and physical energy: lethargy, fatigue, daytime sleepiness, lack of vigour and stamina, low mental energy, difficulty concentrating.
› Reduced sexuality: decreased libido, erectile dysfunction, reduced levels of arousal and number or strength of orgasms.
› Flattened mood, irritability, lack of motivation.
› Decreased sense of wellbeing.
› Weight gain – 'middle-aged spread' or 'beer belly'.
› Thinning or loss of pubic hair.
› Reduced muscle bulk.
› Skin-wrinkling and flabby, 'tuckshop' arms.

For women who need very little testosterone to restore healthy levels, transdermal patches and topical gels are preferred. For post-menopausal women, testosterone should be administered in combination with HRT due to a lack of adequate safety and efficacy data on testosterone alone.

Prohormones such as androstenedione, androstenediol and DHEA, each of which is partly metabolised into testosterone, can also be very effective in increasing testosterone levels in women. DHEA also has other beneficial actions, which are discussed in the next chapter.

Some herbal formulations work to inhibit liver enzymes, thus increasing the bodies' natural testosterone levels: these include Tribulus Terrestris, Eurycoma Longifolia and Vitex. None of these herbs can be considered effective methods of treating androgen deficiency and have their own risks.

BENEFITS AND RISKS OF TESTOSTERONE SUPPLEMENTS
Potential Benefits
☑ Treat symptoms – improved energy, strength, mood, and feelings of well-being
☑ Increased arousability, desire, frequency of sexual activity, frequency of orgasm and sexual satisfaction
☑ Lower rate of bone loss and muscle strength that lead to an increased risk of fracture
☑ Small reduced risk of diabetes, heart attacks and strokes
☑ Small reduced risk of cognitive decline and dementia
☑ Small reduced risk of breast cancer in women
Potential Risks
☑ Side-effects of testosterone supplementation include acne, increased in facial hair weight gain (muscle, rather than fat), breast enlargement and changes in mood (including increased levels of aggression at high doses)
☑ Some prostate cancers may be sensitive to testosterone, so men taking testosterone supplements should be repeatedly screened for prostate cancer
☑ When used in appropriate doses, testosterone does not cause women to look and behave like men, though transgender women have used very high doses of the hormone for this purpose

OPTIONS TO HELP COMBAT THE ANDROPAUSE

☑ Be aware of your symptoms – don't just assume it is just getting old and suffer in silence

☑ Take note - do you have a diminished libido, persistent unexplainable fatigue or a decreased sense of well-being?

☑ Increase physical activity - this will help slow the declining testosterone levels by maintaining weight control, taking actions to help prevent the onset of diabetes and obesity
> Take up weight training 2 to 3 times per week – get a trainer or go to a class at your local gym
> Develop your own stretching program – buy a book that shows you how

☑ Get quality sleep. Inadequate sleep is associated with reduced testosterone levels and makes the symptoms of low levels all the worse. See the options outlined in chapter 26

☑ Manage stress. Try yoga, meditation, rhythmic breathing or other relaxation techniques. See chapter 25 for a full range of options

☑ Stop smoking. Even second hand smoke will reduce your testosterone levels

☑ Make an appointment to see your doctor about testosterone if symptoms impact on your life
> For men, take a simple screening test for low testosterone levels
> For women, consider switching to transdermal estrogens (patches) for HRT or ask about a trial of testosterone or prohormones like DHEA

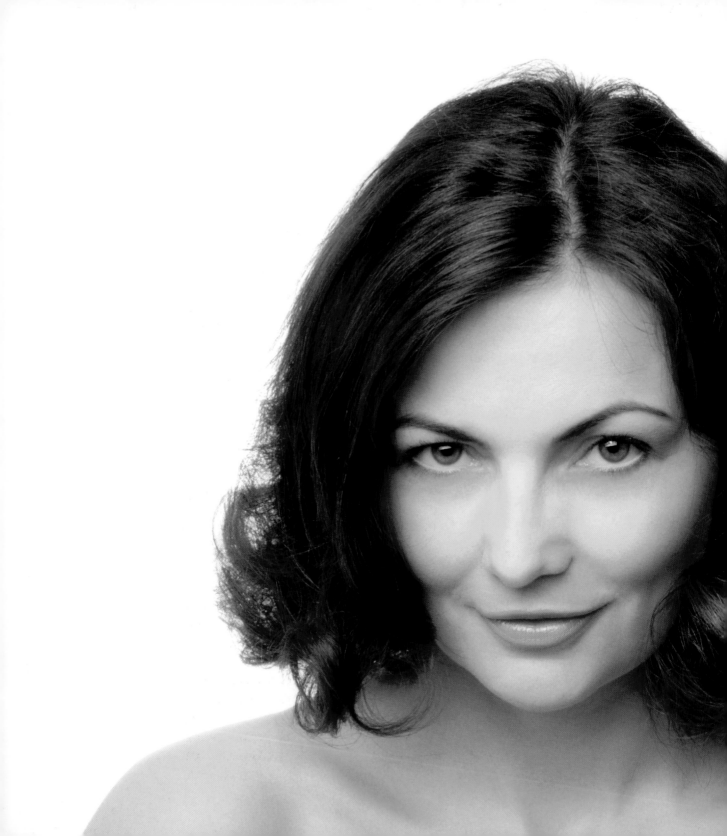

CHAPTER 30

DHEA

Dehydroepiandrosterone (DHEA) is one of the most plentiful steroid hormones in the body. It has a range of important effects on our health. DHEA is produced primarily by our adrenal glands, with smaller quantities also being produced by our ovaries, testes and brains.

In common with other hormones, DHEA levels decline as we age. Once most of us reach the age of 75, DHEA levels have dropped to about 15 per cent of those we enjoyed at twenty-five.

DHEA is an important buffer for our sex hormones. DHEA is a weak androgen that can be converted into the male hormone, testosterone, with which it shares some of its benefits as well as its side effects. In women, DHEA supplements can increase testosterone levels and help restore a flagging libido. DHEA can also be metabolised into the female hormone, oestrogen.

Other beneficial actions of DHEA include boosting our immune system, increasing the function of growth hormone and balancing the effects of the stress hormone, cortisol, on our bodies. Taking DHEA supplements can also reduce levels of 'bad' (LDL) cholesterol, AGEs, and oxidative stress and to improve low mood and cognitive functions, including memory.

Studies have also suggested that declining levels of DHEA in our body are associated with an increased risk of heart disease. Those with the highest levels of DHEA tend to have the lowest risk of heart disease and the longest life spans. In fact, many anti-ageing researchers believe that replenishing our DHEA stocks so as to maintain them at youthful levels is highly desirable for optimal health and wellbeing.

For any of us who think we might have low DHEA levels, a simple blood test is available that measures Dehydroepiandrosterone sulphate (DHEAS), a more stable circulating form of DHEA. Some doctors also use salivary testing, but these can be expensive and the results are laboratory-dependent and often require additional verification via blood tests. Urine testing of our total 17-ketosteroids can also give an indication of our levels of DHEA release over a 24-hour period.

In those with low levels, DHEA supplementation can significantly improve quality of life. Usually, the first things to improve are fatigue, libido and general wellbeing.

DHEA is available on prescription in capsule form from compounding pharmacies. This means an appropriate dosage can be individually formulated based on our levels and symptoms. This is important, as there is much variability in our responses to DHEA (such that anything between 10mg and 100mg might be needed daily) and any dose needs to be adjusted individually to improve our symptoms, without causing adverse reactions. DHEA supplements should never be taken without ongoing biochemical/clinical assessment and individualised dosing (hence, DHEA tablets should never be ordered over the internet or bought on an overseas trip).

Side effects do not appear or be noticed in everyone. However, if they occur they are generally dose-related and mild, such as oilier-than-normal hair and skin, acne, hair loss and increased facial hair due to increased testosterone production. Men may also can experience breast enlargement due to DHEA's stimulation of oestrogen levels.

Because DHEA modifies our levels of various sex hormones, those who have or are at a high risk of cancer should not take DHEA. In fact, higher levels of DHEA have been correlated with an increased risk of developing breast cancer in some studies.

In recent years, 17-keto DHEA has been promoted as a superior version of DHEA. As this form of DHEA is less readily converted to testosterone and oestrogen, its side-effect profile is reduced. However, this also means that 17-keto DHEA is less effective than standard DHEA at restoring female testosterone levels, which is one of the most common reasons why women feel stronger and sexier on DHEA.

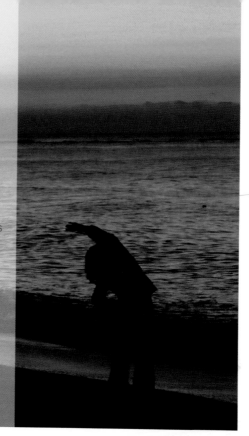

POTENTIAL SYMPTOMS OF DHEA DEFICIENCY

> Fatigue and lethargy
> Poor capacity to cope with stress
> Poor libido and sexual performance
> Dry skin
> Anxiety/depression
> Reduced muscle bulk
> Sparseness of body hair
> Weight gain

OPTIONS TO BOOST DHEA LEVELS

☑ Be Increase the amount of strenuous exercise you have in your exercise regime. This will help slow the slump in your youthful DHEA levels by keeping the pressure off your adrenal glands (which make DHEA) and preventing diabetes, which damages the adrenals. Take up running, swimming, football or weight lifting

☑ Manage stress. Go to chapter 25 for a variety of options to help build stress resilience

☑ Get quality sleep. Go to chapter 26 for a variety of options

☑ Keep a symptom diary - are you experiencing a persistent loss of stamina, strength, fatigue, lethargy, low mood, poor memory or reduced libido?

☑ Make an appointment to see your doctor about DHEA if symptoms impact on your life. Getting tested for low DHEAS is a simple way to know if it could be the cause

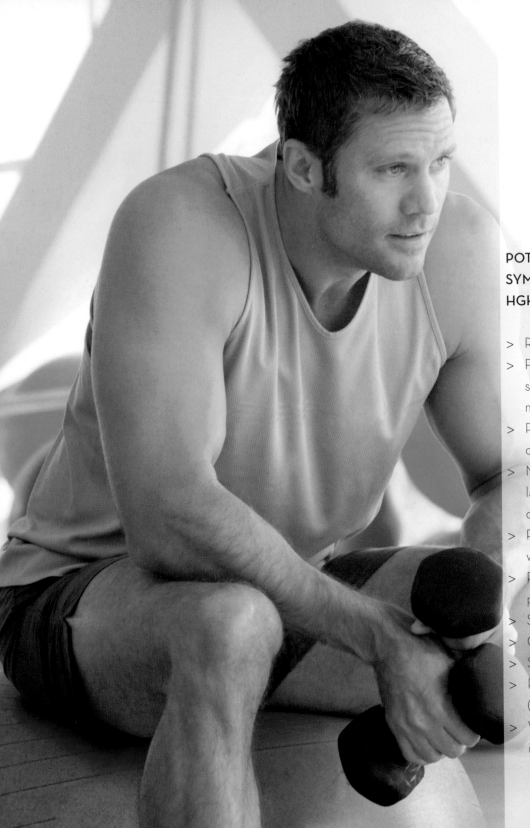

POTENTIAL SIGNS AND SYMPTOMS OF LOW HGH LEVELS

> Reduced vitality
> Fatigue, lethargy, loss of stamina, strength or muscle bulk
> Poor memory and concentration
> Mood changes, emotional lability, anxiety and depression
> Poor capacity to cope with stress
> Poor libido and sexual performance
> Sagging skin
> Cool dry extremities
> Sparseness of body hair
> Reduced bone density (osteoporosis)
> Weight gain (especially increased fat mass)

CHAPTER 31

GROWTH HORMONE

Human growth hormone (hGH) is a key regulator of growth in our bodies, acting to build and maintain structures and tissues from our toes to our hair. As we age, not only do our reproductive functions decline, but growth also slows and eventually stops. The decline in growth hormone as we age is known as the somatopause.

Levels of hGH fall with every year from puberty, with the sharpest declines seen in between 20 and forty, with a gradual ongoing decline thereafter. By the time we reach the age of 70 years, average levels have fallen to about 20 per cent of what they were when we were 20.

People who retain the highest levels of hGH have the lowest rates of dementia, depression, heart disease and some cancers. The potential importance of hGH to ageing is demonstrated by the fact that many of the signs and symptoms of ageing are seen in individuals efficient in hGH; including heart disease, bone thinning, expanding waistlines, cognitive decline and shortened life expectancy. Moreover, restoring healthy hGH levels in deficient individuals can prevent many of these degenerative changes. This finding has led the 'anti-ageing industry' to suggestion that all of us may also benefit from rejuvenating our hGH to levels seen when we were young. Again, the signs and symptoms of growth hormone deficiency are very non-specific and may be easily attributed to stress, disease or ageing. If we think that growth hormone levels may be low and impacting on our lives, there are several blood tests that can estimate the effective hGH levels in our bodies.

> Insulin-like growth factor (IGF-1) – this is the most widely used test of growth hormone activity. If you have low hGH levels, the manufacture of IGF-1 (which is partly growth hormone dependent) also falls.

> Insulin-like growth factor binding protein-3 (IGF-BP3) – like IGF-1, the manufacture of IGFBP-3 is growth hormone dependent, and levels fall when hGH is low.

> Growth hormone — measurements of hGH itself are unreliable as it is released in bursts and there may be little serum GH at any given time. However, many stimulation tests are available which tests the ability the brain to release hGH. Two examples are the intravenous arginine and oral L-DOPA stimulation tests. This test is easily performed in a doctor's office and is becoming more widely available.

Those with low levels of growth hormone and who are suffering their effects may benefit from supplements. It is illegal and dangerous to use growth hormone in adults outside of this indication.

BENEFITS AND RISKS OF SUPPLEMENTS IN THOSE WITH HGH DEFICIENCY
Potential Benefits
☑ Performance enhancement – Improved resilience, mood, sleep, memories and body composition as well as our cognitive, cardiac and physical performance.
☑ Lower rate of bone loss and improved muscle strength - Growth hormone is important for bone growth and turnover. For those with thin bones and low hGH levels, supplements can improve bone density and reduce the risk of fracture.
☑ Improved mood and ability to cope with stress - Growth hormone regulates the balance between sympathetic and parasympathetic tone in our bodies. Reduced levels of hGH are associated with increased sympathetic nervous system activity, which in turn is linked with stress, depression and anxiety. Restoring human growth hormone levels has been shown to have a calming effect, engendering an improved sense of wellbeing and reduced mental stress.
☑ Small reduced risk of heart attacks and strokes - Heart disease and stroke are more common in those with low levels of hGH. Restoration of our healthy levels helps us to reduce 'bad' cholesterol levels, inflammation and tendencies to suffer from clotting, while improving other parameters such as our body (fat) composition and vascular function. Replacement of hGH may also reverse early changes in our arteries that lead to strokes.
☑ Small reduced risk of cognitive decline and dementia.
Potential Risks
☑ Dose-related side effects are usually mild, but may include fluid retention, joint pain, carpal tunnel syndrome and dysregulation of sugar levels. These side-effects are minimised if dosing starts at low levels.
☑ Standard doses of hGH are not linked with any increase in cancer risk. Nonetheless, hGH should not be taken without appropriate cancer screenings prior to starting treatment (see chapter 5); nor is it suitable for those with a history or high risk of cancers (for instance, having a strong family history of cancers and/or being a smoker).

Treatment starts with a low dose and is adjusted according to each individual's clinical response until IGF-I levels normalise, significant side effects develop, or the benefits plateau. Women may require a slightly higher dose than men. The success of growth hormone replacement is enhanced if it is combined with other interventions to reduce cardiovascular risk factors (such as adopting a low-fat diet) and improving muscle strength and body composition (such as taking up regular exercise).

It should also be noted, however, that hGH injections cannot replicate the healthy hormone profile of young adults, which is 'pulsatile'. Interesting new data suggests that our ability to make and release hGH probably remains intact as our bodies age, yet imbalances between inhibitory and stimulatory signals in our bodies lead to declining hGH levels as we get older. New agents that restore pulsatile natural hGH secretion rather than trying to artificially replace it are likely to prove better options for managing deficiency.

OPTIONS TO COMBAT THE SOMATOPAUSE

☑ Increase physical activity
> Join your local gym - the increase in hGH is greatest with anaerobic exercise, like weights or resistance training

☑ Build stress resilience. See chapter 25 for a variety of options

☑ Get quality sleep. See chapter 26 for a variety of options

☑ Be aware of your symptoms - do you have a troubling and persistent loss of stamina, strength or muscle bulk, fatigue, lethargy, low mood, poor memory, weight gain and reduced libido?

☑ Make an appointment to see your doctor and get tested for low hGH levels if symptoms impact on your life

☑ Do not be tempted to buy or use growth hormone yourself – it is illegal and potentially dangerous

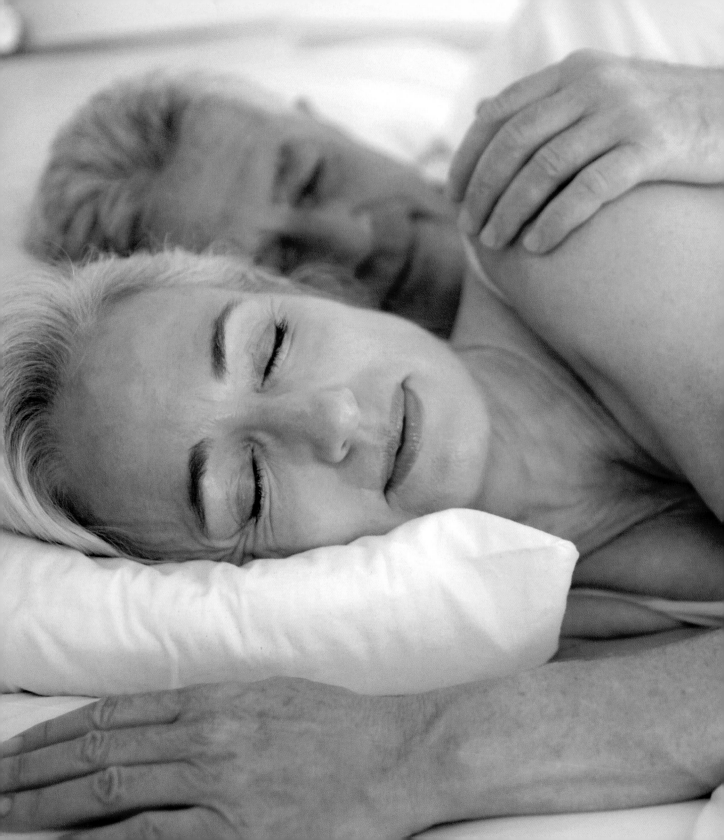

CHAPTER 32

MELATONIN & AGEING

Melatonin is a natural hormone released from our brains, as well as by the skin, intestines, bones and immune systems. Melatonin production in our brains is set according to our body clocks (circadian rhythms), with the highest levels seen at night (two to four hours after we go to sleep) and the lowest levels corresponding to maximal daylight hours (in the middle of the day).

When our eyes detect light, especially of short-wavelength light, such as that emanating from TV screens or fluorescent bulbs, the production of melatonin is suppressed. Longer-wavelength light (from the red or amber spectrum) is less inhibitory, which is why we find it easier to fall asleep by the glow of a fire or candlelight.

While this cycling of melatonin is important for the regulation of sleep cycles (see chapter 26) and aligning other parts of our circadian rhythms, melatonin also has a number of important, independent effects on our daytime health and ageing:

> Melatonin is an antioxidant, one of the few that is capable of reaching deep inside our cells into the mitochondria, the main source of free radicals inside our cells. By preventing damage to our mitochondria, melatonin may modify age-related loss of mitochondrial function, perhaps even affecting the ageing process.

> Melatonin can also prevent radical associated damage to lipids and cell membranes – membranes that exclude some other antioxidants. For example, melatonin can penetrate our brains, where it may help to combat free radicals that might otherwise contribute to our developing Alzheimer's and Parkinson's disease and other forms of cognitive decline.

> Moreover, melatonin may have important beneficial effects on our ageing immune systems. A number of studies have suggested that low melatonin alcohol intake, dietary habits and certain medications (e.g. levels are associated with the development of some cancers, particularly in those of us whose circadian patterns are disrupted, such as night-shift workers.

> Melatonin also interacts with and regulates the responses of our other hormonal signalling systems. For example, melatonin acts to reduce the effects of excessive stress hormones, such as cortisol, on our bodies, and sends signals through our oestrogen receptors that may modify hormone sensitive diseases such as breast cancer. In some women, melatonin supplementation may also improve thyroid function.

Our melatonin levels are not only victims of excessive time spent under bright lights and poor sleep habits. We can also modify our melatonin levels by changing a number of lifestyle factors, including our exercise, alcohol intake, dietary habits and certain medications (e.g. beta blockers). To make matters worse, the production of melatonin generally declines with age. In fact, some elderly individuals show little or no nocturnal increase in melatonin production. Obviously, this makes getting to sleep a problem, but it also may impact on their health and longevity.

IT'S ALSO IMPORTANT THAT WE SLEEP IN PROPERLY DARKENED BEDROOMS, AS DARKNESS IS THE MAIN STIMULANT OF MELA-TONIN PRODUCTION.

The simplest way to keep our melatonin levels up is by keeping our days light and our nights dark. If we expose ourselves to bright sunlight during the daytime, this serves to elevate our melatonin production at night, making the oscillations in our melatonin cycles bigger. So getting out and about not only helps us throughout the day but also at night. It's also important that we sleep in properly darkened bedrooms, as darkness is the main stimulant of melatonin production. Leaving televisions, computer screens or lights on – even with low-watt bulbs – near our sleeping areas significantly reduces our nightly production of melatonin.

Melatonin supplements are available on prescription as a way of resetting mistiming body clocks. These are designed as purely as short-term natural sleep aids and contain large amounts of melatonin (1-3mg), usually several times more than normally released during or body's natural cycles, in order to clonk us back into cycle.

Although melatonin is not a sedative, those starting out prescription-strength melatonin for insomnia might feel sleepy or irritable the next day, but dropping the dose can usually fix these problems. Some users report reduced libido (possibly because they fall asleep), while others experience disturbing or vivid dreams, especially when taken with Vitamin B6. Melatonin should not be taken in any form by pregnant women (or those trying to become pregnant), those with epilepsy or autoimmune conditions.

Melatonin available over the counter in pharmacies and health food stores contains very small amounts of melatonin. These are seldom enough to reset our body clocks or correct insomnia. Any sleepiness usually comes from other components that are included in the formulation. However, this does not mean that they don't have effects on oxidative stress and immune function, for which they are widely used by anti-ageing practitioners.

We can naturally get some extra melatonin from plants, including bananas, tomatoes, apples, cherries, walnuts, sweetcorn, oats, brown rice and rice bran. A fresh serve of these would generally contain as much or more melatonin that many OTC preparations.

OPTIONS TO MAINTAIN YOUR MELATONIN LEVELS

☑ Increase physical activity. This will help slow the declining melatonin levels by maintaining weight control, taking actions to help prevent the onset of diabetes and obesity

☑ Get quality sleep – go to chapter 26 for a variety of things you can do

☑ Learn to meditate – check out your local adult education centre or meditation centre for classes. Go to chapter 24 for details on meditation and mindfulness

☑ Go outside more often — If you expose yourself to bright sunlight during the daytime, this serves to elevate your melatonin production at night, making the oscillations in your melatonin cycles bigger. So getting out and about not only helps you throughout the day, but also at night. Better still, combine it with outdoor exercise!

☑ Sleep in a dark room — as darkness is the main stimulant of melatonin production. Leaving televisions, computer screens or lights on – even with low-watt bulbs – near our sleeping areas significantly reduces our production of melatonin

☑ Make an appointment to see your doctor about melatonin, if you have problems with your sleep cycle (such as early morning waking or difficulty getting to sleep)

SECTION 8:
QUALITY IS NEVER AN ACCIDENT

As a bottle of wine matures, it takes on a number of characteristics that add to the quality of the drinking experience. Its colour becomes deeper, its aroma more mellow, its texture more thick and its taste more refined. Sometimes it is the little things that make the biggest difference. In this section, we look at some of the little things that make a big difference to the quality of our ageing, including skin changes, fracture, continence and our senses of hearing and vision. Retaining each is an important part of savouring our own maturity and not allowing the ageing process to turn our wine into vinegar.

KATE'S EXPERIENCE

The key to slow ageing is quality. It is about enhancement of vitality. I don't want to live longer without quality, so I am taking steps when I am well. I've had annoying and sometimes major issues with eyes, pelvic floor and skin. In fact, I've had great joy in implementing interventions that have successfully fixed my appearance and function.

If not repaired after having babies, the pelvic floor can develop into a major issue in later life. Many women suffer incontinence, but allow it to go untreated. A small problem will become bigger, so do whatever it takes to make sure you don't allow even a tiny amount of incontinence be a 'normal' part of your life. When looking at fixing it (or any health issue), research your options carefully. Look outside the box for solutions too. I found that DHEA has been a 'magic bullet' when it comes to improving my skin. Hormone modulation using Chinese herbs cured my chronic dry eye, even though most doctors or optometrists don't realise there is a connection between hormone dysfunction and dry eye. Sometime as health system may fail us, but the benefit in the era we live in, most health issues have a solution. It's a matter of finding the one that works for you... and don't give up if the first one fails!

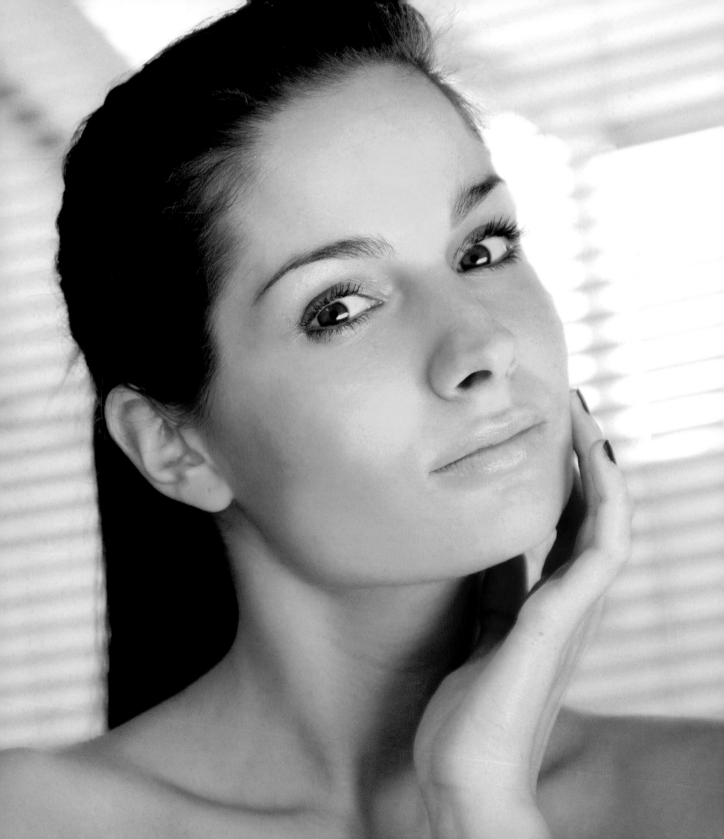

CHAPTER 33

KEEPING UPAPPEARANCES
[SKIN & AGEING]

The signs of ageing are most visible on our skin. We use it as an indicator of age, just as we judge a book by its cover. For this reason, there is an enormous industry whose aim is to reduce or mask the external signs of ageing. There are many products designed to cleanse, beautify, promote attractiveness or alter appearances, without affecting the skin's structure or functions (known as cosmetics). However, in this chapter we look at how ageing occurs and some of the effective ways to slow this process.

OUR AGEING SKIN

We all want better looking skin. We will get to this. First, it is important to know a bit about the skin itself.

Our skin is composed of multiple layers, all of which undergo some changes as we grow older. The outermost layer of our skin, the epidermis, is composed of a thick stack of skin cells. These cells are generated at the bottom of the epidermis. As they mature, they migrate toward the surface. The outermost part of the epidermis (the stratum corneum) consists of 25 to 30 layers of dead cells. These cells are eventually sloughed off as new cells push up from below. As we age, new cells form at a slower rate, making our skin thinner. Dead cells are not pushed off and instead pile up on the skin's surface, making it drier, rougher and duller in appearance.

However, the most significant changes in terms of our skin's appearance occur in the dermis. This layer is normally thick with connective tissue (mainly collagen, elastin and proteoglycans), which provides much of our skin's strength and resilience and some of its ability to retain water. With age, the dermis becomes thinner and drier. Instead of being a delicate scaffold, its main structural proteins deteriorate, leaving behind fragmented, thickened and disorganised fibres. These don't work as well as our better-organised, youthful matrix, either in maintaining the skin's support structures or providing healthy places for our skin cells to live. Over time, as our support tissues lose their ability to retain tension, our skin becomes less elastic (a condition known as elastosis) and more prone to sagging. Similar changes also lead to wrinkles. Another key component in ageing skin is reduced water content. However we might try to condition our skin with moisturisers (this is a good thing), our ageing skin gradually loses the ability to retain its state of hydration.

Finally, changes in the tissues underlying our skin also impact significantly on our ageing appearance. Although our waistlines tend to expand with age, there is a reduction in the deposits of fat under the skin on our cheeks, shins and the backs of our hands, making our skin look and feel papery. The loss of support tissue leads to sagging, with ageing faces looking more 'squared off' compared to the angular shapes of youthful faces.

OLD UNDER THE SUN (PHOTO-AGEING)

When we despair about the onset of lines and wrinkles, roughness and unwanted pigmentation, we need look no further than our time in the sun for its origins. Four out of five wrinkles, and most of the freckles on our faces, are due to sun exposure. Preventing excessive solar damage with the regular use of broad-spectrum, water resistant SPF30+ sunscreen, wide-brimmed hats and protective clothing is the most effective way to slow the ageing of our skin.

Exposure to UV, visible and infrared radiation from sunlight results in cumulative changes in the texture, colour and quality of our skin (known as photo-ageing). This can be appreciated when we compare the leathery, sun-exposed skin at our necklines with the skin on adjacent areas of smooth, unblemished non-exposed skin.

The effects of photo-ageing vary from person to person, depending on the duration and intensity of our sun exposure, skin type, genetic legacies and our diet. For example, a low-GI diet rich in vegetables, nuts, legumes and olive oil is associated with reduced rates of skin ageing, given the same cumulative exposure to the sun.

By contrast, increased skin ageing is seen in those with a high intake of meat, full-fat dairy and butter.

Early signs of sun damage to our skin may be difficult to see in the mirror or by looking at old photos. Imaging under UV light allows clinicians to look at superficial and deep pigments in our skin. An imaging test can give a score relative to our age. Repeat examinations can help track the effectiveness of treatment programs.

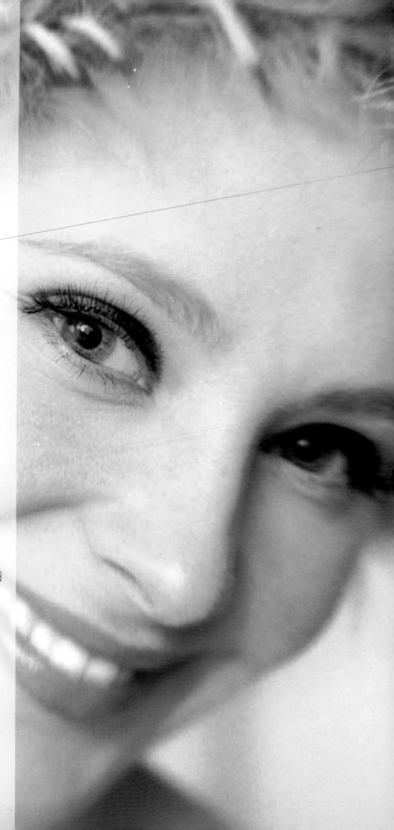

Antioxidants shown to improve the appearance of fine wrinkles and

skin elasticity when taken as oral supplements include:

> Vitamin E
> Vitamin C - higher doses may help reduce skin wrinkling
> Carotenoids, including lutein, lycopene and zeaxanthin
> Lipoic acid
> Soy isoflavones - regular oral supplements (40mg daily)
> Proanthocyanidins and flavonoids in grapeseed – these anti-inflammatory antioxidants reduce capillary fragility and inhibits the breakdown of connective tissue when used regularly (6g/day)
> Polypodium leucotomos fern extract
> Pycnogenol ® - extracted from pine bark, this potent antioxidant is often confused with pycnogenols, contained within grapeseed or other plants

ANTIOXIDANT DEFENCES FOR THE SKIN

Because of the important role of oxidative stress in skin ageing, almost every cosmetic now contains some antioxidants. The thing to look for is evidence that these products reduce the effects of UV damage (for example, by reducing the amount of damaged DNA) when used as the manufacturer intends, on the kind of skin it has been developed to protect – not just on the hides of lab mice. Don't believe every marketing claim and 'miracle in a jar'. We need to ensure the products we choose have sufficiently high concentrations of their purported active ingredients (where these are known). If this isn't stated, ensure the 'active' ingredients are listed in the top two-thirds of the ingredient list (preferably higher). Ingredients listed in the final third of the label list are probably present only in very small quantities.

Only a small number of topical antioxidants have been shown in clinical trials to reduce signs of skin ageing and wrinkles. These include:

☑ Retinoic acid, also known as tretinoin, is the most significant and well-researched topical anti-wrinkle agent. It is currently available only on prescription for treating established damage. Retinoic acid can also stimulate new collagen formation in the skin. The cosmetic effect of retinoic acid on skin is to reduce fine wrinkles, smooth rough skin and lighten brown spots. Retinoic acid also thins the top layer of skin, the stratum corneum, which leads to its smoothing effects, but it may result in increased water loss (dehydration). Tretinoin may also have a tendency to make skin light sensitive and should only be applied at night. It is essential that you use sunscreen and monitor skin dryness. Tretinoin should only be used under supervision.

☑ Retinol and retinal (Vitamin A) are widely used in OTC skin creams. To become active, they must be converted into retinoic acid. This is a very inefficient process, so the activity of products containing retinol is far less than retinoic acid. For best results, select a product with a high concentration of retinol, or one that has been specifically stabilised to prevent degradation with light and time.

☑ Vitamin C is an antioxidant that also stimulates collagen production in the skin. When used topically, Vitamin C provides a degree of photo protection from ultraviolet rays. For best effects, look for products with a Vitamin C content greater than 10% in order to penetrate to the deeper layers of skin. Stabilised forms, such as magnesium ascorbyl phosphate or ascorbyl palmitate, are preferred as they degrade more slowly. However, even in these forms, Vitamin C must be kept away from direct sunlight and used quickly once opened.

☑ Polypodium leucotomos fern extract (P. leucotomos) has been shown to help protect skin against UV rays. This extract has a number of beneficial actions: it inhibits free-radical generation and helps prevent DNA damage and UV-induced skin-cell death. The extract may also be a useful ingredient in sunscreens.

☑ Coenzyme Q10 (or Ubiquinione) is a potent antioxidant and also maintains cellular energy production. Reduced CoQ10 levels in ageing skin increase its vulnerability to solar damage and reduces its (energy-dependent) ability to repair and regenerate. When applied topically, a regular application of CoQ10 can improve wrinkles and elasticity. For best results, use a product with a concentration of at least 0.5%.

☑ Proanthocyanidins are antioxidants extracted from plants such as pine bark, grapes and apples. When used topically, they can reduce inflammation associated with sun damage and therefore improve healing and long-term appearance. Regular application can also lead to increases in skin hydration. Look for products with a 1% concentration of proanthcyanidins: these may be listed as grape-seed, flavonoids or Pycnogenol ® - extracted from pine bark.

☑ Polyphenols are potent antioxidants of plant origin. The best known include the catechins present in green tea; genistein, an isoflavone found in soybean; curcumin, found in the curry spice turmeric; and apigenin, present in many fruits and vegetables. When topically applied, these extracts can reduce the effects of ageing in the skin. However, the concentration required for these to have their optimal effects has not yet been determined.

SKIN MOISTURE

We all know how our skin looks and feels when we are dehydrated, such as after a long plane journey. Maintaining adequate levels of moisture becomes increasingly important as we grow older because ageing skin is less able to retain fluid, leaving it more vulnerable to dehydration.

The moisture retaining properties of our skin are mostly conferred by its glycosaminoglycan (GAG) content, which keep our skin looking full, soft and hydrated. Ageing is associated with a reduction in healthy matrix components, including less collagen and elastin, and reduced levels of some GAGs. This means the skin can no longer retain fluid as effectively.

Declining GAGs deep in our dermis cannot be replaced by topical applications, no matter what cosmetic companies say. They have to be delivered via injection or come from our inner (skin) health. Glucosamine supplementation (from 500mg of glucosamine daily) can also promote GAG synthesis in ageing skin and improve the appearance of fine lines and wrinkles.

Other simple tips for ensuring our skin stays moist include:
> Drink at least 2 or 3 litres of fluid per day. Drink more on long plane journeys, during heavy exertion and in hot, dry weather.
> Limit intake of caffeine, alcohol and salty foods, which increase fluid losses.
> Apply moisturisers morning and night to hold moisture in your skin.

Carefully select your soap and other skin cleansers to remove dirt, without removing the oils that prevent moisture loss. Use a gentle cleanser regularly, rather than harsh cleaning every so often. If your skin feels squeaky clean, dry and tight after washing, you may be doing more harm than good. Avoid strong detergents like Sodium Laurel Sulphate (SLS) and soap, which tend to disrupt the acid mantle, affecting your skin's protective barrier.

EXFOLIANTS AND DERMABRASION

Even after damage is done, there is much we can do to restore some of the qualities of our youthful skin. One of the most popular is skin resurfacing or dermabrasion, which removes damaged and disorganised outer layers of our skin and yields a 'polished' effect that is as much the result of better light reflectivity as it is of better skin quality.

This is usually achieved using a laser on the skin in short bursts, then allowing the skin to restore itself in a healthy way. This can be performed all at once, although better results are achieved by treating a small percentage of our skin's surface each time (called fractional resurfacing), so healing is quicker and we experience less downtime. Non-ablative lasers can also be used to reduce background skin redness, blotchy patches or the appearance of dilated or swollen blood vessels (erroneously referred to as 'broken' capillaries).

Microdermabrasion is a more gentle technique that removes only the outer layer of dead cells. This can be achieved by sanding the surface of the skin with crystals or a similarly abrasive surface.

Shedding and regeneration of the outer layers of the skin can also be achieved with a chemical peel. Some of the most common exfoliants include alpha hydroxyl-acids (AHAs), derived from sugarcane or fruit, and polyhydroxic acids (PHAs).

These clear the dead skin cells and stimulate collagen renewal and GAG synthesis. The net result is an appreciable reduction in the appearance of wrinkles and a reduction in signs of photo-ageing.

GETTING THE MOST FROM EXFOLIANTS

THE RIGHT DOSE:

Most over-the-counter AHA products contain concentrations of 8-15%. Products with concentrations lower than 8% do not result in significant benefits. Higher concentrations (25-50%) are more abrasive and should be administered under the supervision of a dermatologist.

THE RIGHT FORMULATION:

The response to products will be different in different individuals. It is worth trying a range to find what works for you. Older formulations, such as 'Jessner's solution', which relies on a combination of ingredients, still produce some of the best results, with a low incidence of side-effects.

THE RIGHT APPLICATION:

Whilst removing the top layer of dead skin cells does produce an 'anti-wrinkle' effect, it also removes valuable antioxidants, particularly Vitamins C and E, from the skin and increases sensitivity to sunlight. These side-effects can be minimised by applying exfoliants at night after cleansing your skin, then applying an antioxidant-rich moisturiser. Upon waking, wash your face and neck to clear away dead skin cells, then apply a moisturiser and sunscreen. Use exfoliants for six to 12 weeks at a time, then give your skin a chance to recover and become less sun-sensitive.

WHILE REMOVING THE TOP LAYER OF DEAD SKIN CELLS PRODUCE AN 'ANTI-WRINKLE' EFFECT, IT ALSO REMOVES VALUABLE ANTIOXIDANTS, PARTICULARLY VITAMIN C AND E, FROM THE SKIN AND INCREASES SENSITIVITY TO SUNLIGHT.

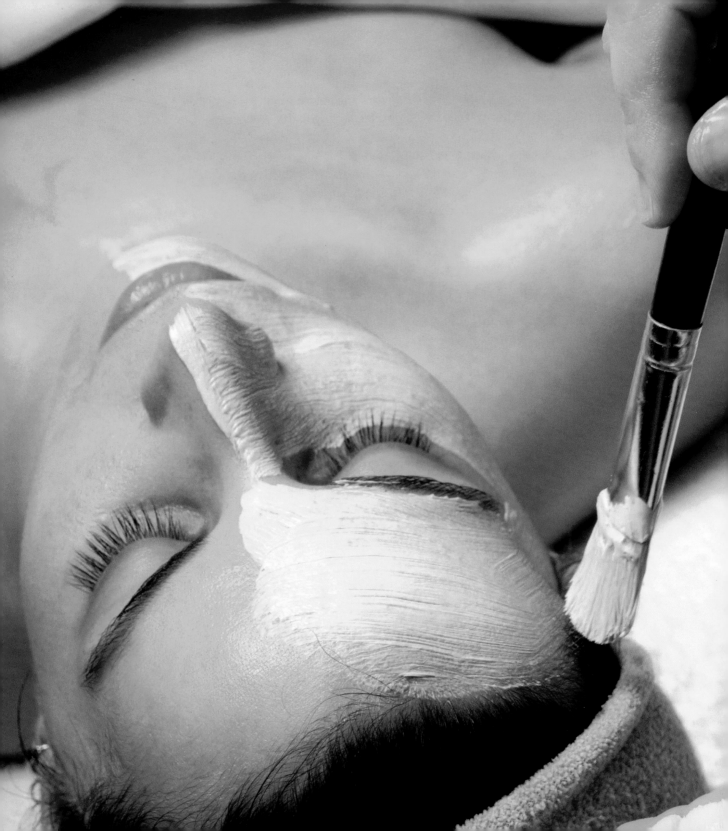

Don't use skin products containing AHAs or PHAs at the same time as using retinoic acid, as this may further increase your skin's sensitivity to the sun. For best results, alternate their use with products incorporating AHAs or PHAs on a monthly or six-weekly basis.

A BASIC REGIMEN FOR 'SLOW' AGEING OF THE SKIN

Our general health is reflected in the quality of our skin. If we want youthful, healthy-looking skin, it is important to first optimise our general health. This means managing our weight, nutrition, hormonal balance and hydration. Smoking, excessive alcohol consumption, a high fat diet, obesity and diabetes all impact negatively on the health and ageing of our skin, as well as on other parts of our bodies.

Whatever products we decide to use, we should make them a regular part of our ongoing skincare routine, not 'one-bottle wonders'. Chopping and changing among skincare products puts us right back at the start each time we change our regime. When you do try a new product, give it three months to work. Any less and you may not be giving a product a reasonable chance to have a significant effect on your skin. If you see no results in that period, it's likely that the product isn't working effectively for you.

We should remember, too, that no one product can stop the effects of time and sun. At best, we can use a combination of topical therapies, oral antioxidants, healthy diet and, most importantly, protection from excessive solar damage to slow the ageing of our skin.

OPTIONS TO HELP REDUCE AGEING OF YOUR SKIN

☑ Apply broad-spectrum, water-resistant SPF30+ sunscreen liberally before sun exposure and every two hours while you're exposed to the sun. Also wear wide brimmed hats and protective clothing and avoid tanning beds. Remember that UVA rays, visible and infrared light all have the capacity to penetrate glass, so even working near sun-drenched windows without protection can age your skin

☑ Drink more water - at least 2-3 litres of fluid every day. Drink more on long plane journeys, during heavy exertion and in hot, dry weather

☑ Cleanse, morning and night, every day to wash away excess oil, pollution, make-up and dead skin particles that build up on your skin's surface throughout the day

☑ Moisturise – morning and night - good moisturiser does more than merely keep your skin hydrated. Moisturisers protect and nourish your skin's structure and functions. Always choose moisturisers that suit your skin type. Make your moisturisers multi-task. Look for products that contain one or two key active ingredients to support collagen synthesis or those with added antioxidants

☑ Choose skin products high in antioxidants that reduce solar damage when used topically, like CoQ10, proanthocyanidins and polyphenols. Apply treatment products before moisturiser to ensure maximum absorption

☑ Eat a low-fat diet naturally high in antioxidants and omega-3 fatty acids. This will help moderate the deleterious impact of sunlight on our skin by preventing oxidative damage and inflammation

☑ Take antioxidant supplements for added efficacy – choose one that will get in to the skin like CoQ10, lipoic acid, and carotenoids, including lutein, lycopene and zeaxanthin

☑ Take 500-1000mg glucosamine daily to support collagen synthesis

☑ Stop smoking-see previous chapters for an extensive list of options

OPTIONS TO HELP REDUCE AGEING OF YOUR SKIN

☑ Optimise your hormones – low hormonal levels will impair your skins function and resilience. There are many things you can do to get your hormone levels up and keep them that way long term (see chapters 28-32)

☑ Get quality sleep as tiredness shows on our skin. When we are more rested, our skin is also more rested and the benefits are clearly apparent. They don't call it beauty sleep for nothing

☑ Make an appointment to get your skin assessed – the best way to look good when older is to deal with any changes in your skin early. It is not easy to spot these changes so get help and professional advice for choosing the right program that will work for you

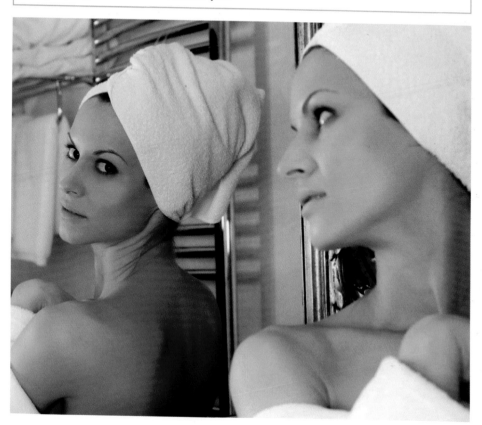

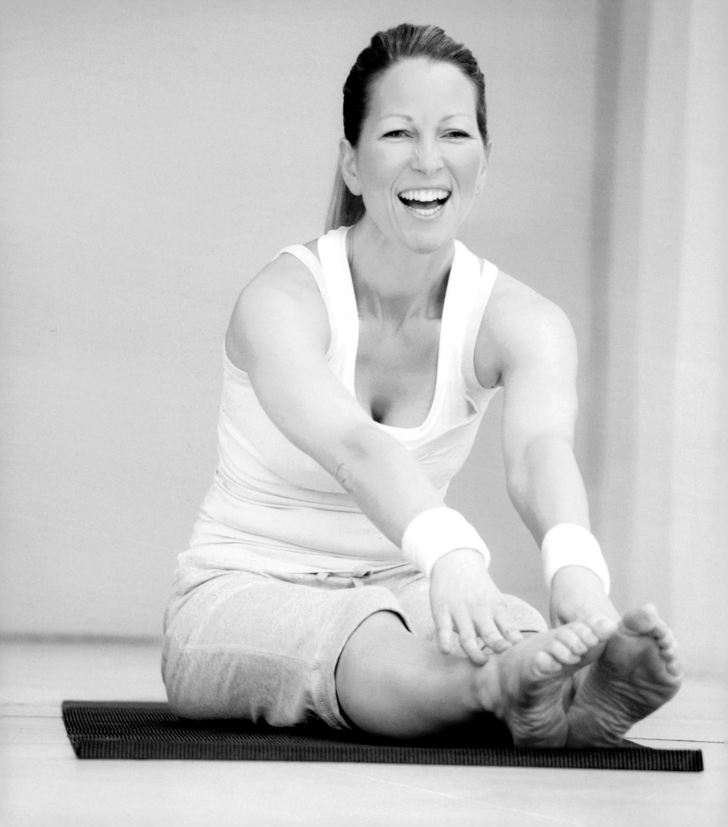

CHAPTER 34

HARD AND FAST
[BONES, JOINTS & AGEING]

Bone is not a lifeless skeleton, but rather a dynamic metabolic organ always on the go. On the outside, new bone is continuously built up, layer upon layer. On the inside, bone is continuously destroyed and reabsorbed. Continuous remodelling allows the body to replace tiny cracks before they weaken the structure, as well as adapt its shape and strength according to how it is being used. Like many ageing processes, this balance becomes more precarious as we get older, where increased reabsorption and slower formation of new bone leads to thinning of the bone, from the inside out.

In our early twenties, our bones are the thickest and strongest they will ever get. Subsequently, for every year that goes by, our bones become progressively thinner. Sometimes there comes a point where bone loss is so significant that the strength and integrity of the bone is compromised, leading to an increased risk of fractures. This threshold is called osteoporosis. About half of all women, and one in eight men, aged 50 years or older will have an osteoporotic fracture during their lifetime. While most of us have broken a bone at some time in our lives, when we are older, any fracture can have catastrophic effects on health and mortality.

Not everyone will develop osteoporosis or fractures. The stronger our bones are in our early twenties, the more time it will take before they are sufficiently thin to increase the risk of fracture, if at all. Although the major determinant of this peak bone mass is our 'thick boned' genes, maybe a quarter of all the variability is determined by nutrition and physical activity during the growth years of childhood and adolescence, as well as other factors like medication and illness.

Women are more likely to develop osteoporosis than men partly because they have a lower peak bone mass (by about 10%). In addition, the major female sex hormone, oestrogen, is an important regulator of bone formation and function. Loss of oestrogen associated with menopause leads to enhanced bone reabsorption and reduced bone formation. Low-dose oestrogen, as delivered in hormone replacement therapy, offers protection against bone loss, but only for as long as the oestrogen is taken. Oestrogens derived from plants (phytoestrogens), especially soy isoflavones, may have beneficial effects on bone health when used in doses much higher than can be achieved by dietary choices (ie. supplements). Declining testosterone levels associated with the andropause also have important consequences for our bones.

Apart from hormones, a number of other factors may tip the balance and result in fragile bones. Some of these factors include alcohol abuse, diabetes, smoking and prolonged bed rest. A number of prescription medications can also trigger bone loss, including chronic steroid therapy, Glitazones and those that suppress sex hormone production. In all cases, these factors bring ageing individuals closer to a threshold at which bone strength is compromised.

BY THE AGE OF 65, FOUR OUT EVERY FIVE PEOPLE WILL HAVE OSTEOARTHRI-TIS VISIBLE ON X-RAY AND TWO THIRDS WILL EXPERI-ENCE SYMPTOMS

It is recommended that everyone over the age of 65 have bone density measures performed to see how they are tracking. Even earlier tests may be warranted for those women with an increased risk of fracture, such as those with a small build, a family history of fractures, those with diabetes, steroid users and those who experienced premature menopause.

It may seem ages away, but small (slow) changes to make stronger bones today can make a big difference as to whether, or if, we develop osteoporosis. There a number of things we can do in our adult life to keep our bones stronger for longer.

Weight-bearing activities, such as walking, running and jumping, and strength-training exercises can reduce our risk of fracture in a number of ways. (See chapter 21). Exercise builds muscle strength and improves our coordination, which can reduce our risk of falling in the first place. Repeated pulling and pushing of muscle on bone also stimulates growth of stronger bone and slows bone thinning. By contrast, an inactive lifestyle means idle muscles and a faster rate of bone thinning.

Calcium is stored in enormous quantities in our bones. If calcium in our diet is insufficient to offset normal losses, bone is broken down to retrieve its stored calcium. Equally, if calcium intake is increased, bone reabsorption will slow and more calcium will be deposited as an insurance against hard times. Dairy products are usually suggested as the major dietary source of calcium. But calcium can also be obtained from low-fat sources, including seaweed, nuts, seeds, legumes and green leafy vegetables such as kale and okra.

Vitamin D is an important regulator of bone metabolism. The ability to get the most calcium from our diet is critically dependent on Vitamin D, so even if we consume lots of calcium in our diet or in supplements, they won't work if our Vitamin D levels are low. Most Vitamin D is synthesised inside the body in an inactive form. This is transformed in the skin by ultraviolet light and subsequently by the liver, before being stored in the fat for later use. Getting our stores up in the warm light of summer is how we get through a dark winter.

With changes in Vitamin D synthesis and less outdoor activities, our stores of Vitamin D often decline as we age. In fact, even in the sunny states, over half of all retirees have Vitamin D levels sufficiently low to denote vitamin deficiency. When Vitamin D levels fall to this extent, reabsorbtion of bone is sped up, while formation of new bone is slowed. This accelerates bone thinning, weakens muscles and contributes to bony aches and pains.

Keeping our Vitamin D levels optimal as we get older can be simply achieved by regular, sensible sun exposure. Vitamin D is also widely available in fortified products, such as cereals, bread and milk. A number of Vitamin D supplements are also available over the counter to help maintain healthy levels. These include Vitamin D2 (from plants or yeast), which is less potent than Vitamin D3 (from animal sources), so it needs to be taken in three times higher doses to achieve the same effect (ie. 10µg of Vitamin D3 is equivalent to 30µg of Vitamin D2). Vitamin D should always be taken in combination with calcium supplements or increased calcium intake for maximum effect.

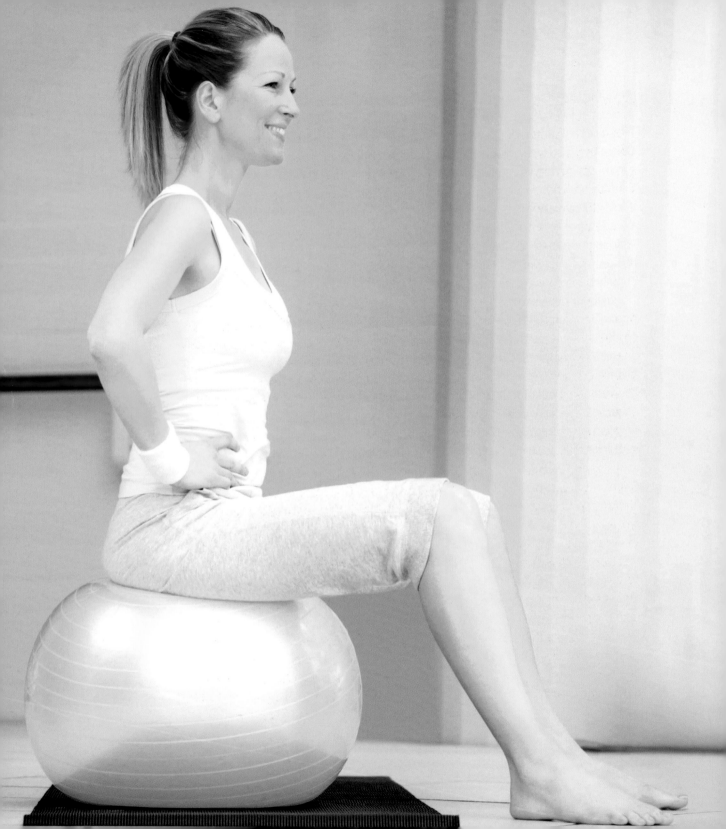

STIFF TIMES

Free-moving joints allow our skeleton and muscles to do the jobs that need to be done. These movements are facilitated by the flexibility of the structures surrounding each joint (tendons, muscles and ligaments), as well as internal lubrication and cushioning. The lubrication is provided by synovial fluid. Like oil in a hinge, this allows a joint to smoothly slide from one position to another. The cushioning is provided by cartilage, which covers the ends of the bones in a smooth, slippery surface, reducing friction and evenly distributing the load across the joint. A decrease of synovial fluid lubrication or the wearing down of the protective cartilage cover leads to pain and stiffness, known as osteoarthritis.

Osteoarthritis can affect any joint in the body, but is most common in the hands, knees, hips and spine. The processes that lead to osteoarthritis take a long time to develop, which is why it is most commonly seen in older individuals. By the age of 65, four out five people will have osteoarthritis visible on x-ray and two thirds will experience symptoms. These can vary in severity, from mild to totally incapacitating. Overall, arthritis significantly contributes to reduced independence and quality of life to a similar extent to heart disease and cancer, particularly in women.

Osteoarthritis is not the inevitable and unavoidable result of the years of moving and loading the joints of the body. Our joints are designed to be highly resistant to mechanical trauma. However, when extra stresses are placed on them, due to injury, overloading or instability, this can eventually lead to 'wear and tear'. Equally, if cartilage is abnormal, then even the normal stresses of daily use can grind the surface down.

With age, the surface of the cartilage becomes softer, while underneath its cushioning effects begin to lose their bounce. One factor involved in this change is the accumulation of AGEs, which make the cartilage structure more rigid (see chapter 10). Other factors that influence the resilience of cartilage include gender, genetic predisposition, diabetes and obesity. Weight loss reduces the impact and progression of arthritis, as well as that of diabetes, a major risk factor for arthritis.

Regular physical activity is the best way to prevent arthritis. This may seem strange as exercise theoretically puts more stress, not less stress, on our joints. However, regular exercise improves cartilage quality, reduces pain and builds stronger muscles, thus taking more of the stress off joints in the long run.

OPTIONS TO BUILD STRONG BONES

☑ Increase weight-bearing activities and strength-training exercises as will strengthen your bones and reduce your risk of fracture

☑ Get some sun - expose your skin on a daily basis to at least 10 minutes of sunlight in the morning or late afternoon. Vitamin D activation is greatest when the chest and back of the neck and shoulders are exposed. Better still, combine it with outdoor exercise!

☑ Choose fortified foods or Vitamin D supplements to maintain your levels of vitamin D, if you are not getting regular sun exposure or are over the age of 60

☑ Eat foods high in calcium but low in saturated fat - low fat milk and dairy, se weeds, nuts, seeds, legumes, and green leafy vegetables (like silverbeet, okra and spinach). Ensure adequate fibre intake at the same time, as this promotes calcium uptake from the bowel

☑ Take a calcium supplement (at least 1200-1500mg of elemental calcium daily). Few of us meet these target levels for calcium in our diet, so supplements are helpful for almost all women. Choose supplements that also contain vitamin D and K, magnesium and boron

☑ Make an appointment to get your bone density checked - if you are over the age of 65, or even earlier in women with an increased risk of fractures, such as those with a small build, a family history of fractures, those with diabetes, steroid users and individuals who experienced premature menopause

☑ Optimise your sex hormones - low levels of oestrogen and/or testosterone are associated with a faster rate of bone thinning, as well as other symptoms. There are many things you can do to get your hormone levels up and keep them that way long term. See Section 7 for details on hormone optimisation

☑ Stop smoking – smoking increases your risk and even second hand smoke will thin your bones. See previous chapters for various options to help you give up

OPTIONS TO STAY FLEXIBLE

☑ Stop over-consumption. Obesity and diabetes are associated with higher rates of arthritis
  > Eat smaller portions
  > Eat more slowly and chew your food thoroughly, so giving your body time to know when you have had a sufficient amount
  > Add fibre to your diet. If you have a problem with appetite control, take fibre tablets with a large glass of water 20 minutes before your meal
  > For further options to help with overeating, go to chapter 9

☑ Increase physical activity today and every day, any way you can. Regular exercise will strengthen your joints and reduce your risk of arthritis

☑ Take a flexibility class - good health is not just about being strong, but also staying supple. There are many simple exercises you can learn to stay flexible. Treat your self to a regular massage to stay even more supple

☑ Increase your intake of omega-3s - some studies have suggested a diet high in omega-3 fatty acids may be associated with lower rates of arthritis. In addition, omega-3 fatty acids may also help reduce stiffness of the joint and increase mobility
  > Eat more cold-water oily fish, flax seed (linseed), purslane, kiwifruit, lignon berries, black raspberries and walnuts
  > Consider taking omega-3 supplements

☑ Take glucosamine and chondroitin sulphate. Glucosamine is widely touted as an agent to treat and prevent osteoarthritis. Some studies have found that glucosamine sulphate may delay the development of arthritis or ameliorate its symptoms. Glucosamine is often sold in combination with other supplements such as chondroitin sulphate, another normal component of cartilage, which also stimulates cartilage health. For prevention take 500-1000mg of gl cosamine daily. For treatment between 1500-3000mg daily until symptoms lessen, and then reduce to 1500mg daily

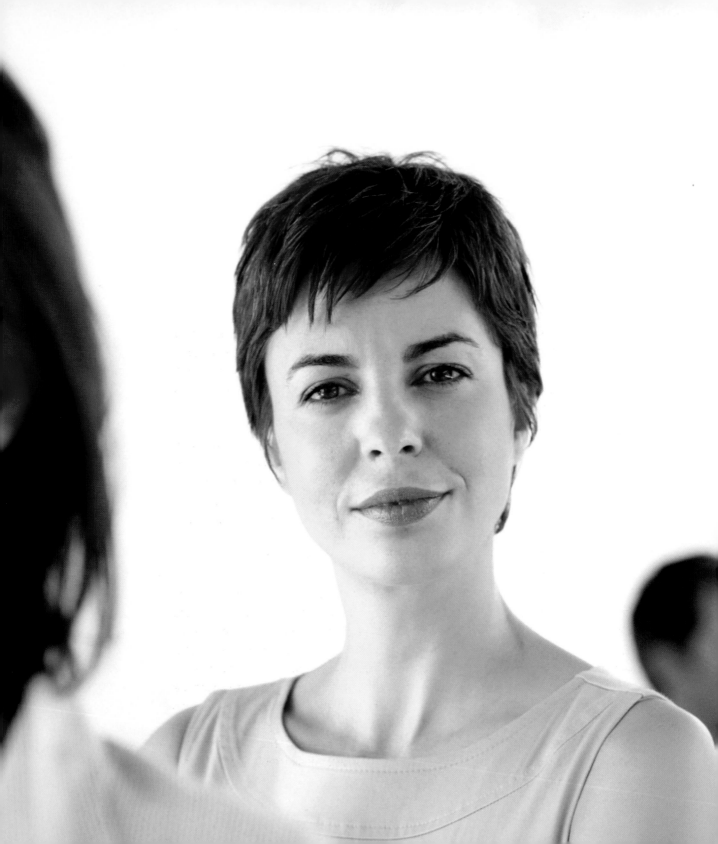

CHAPTER 35

HOLD TIGHT
[PELVIC FLOOR, PROSTATE & AGEING]

THE PELVIC FLOOR IN WOMEN

One of the keys to successful ageing is getting the best support in place and holding onto it for as long as possible. A good example of this is the pelvic floor, which provides vital support to ensure productivity and quality of life. Its muscle and connective tissues naturally form a hammock across the pelvis that holds its contents in place. These muscles also help maintain the functions of our bladder and bowels, and pelvic tone for satisfying sex.

Charged with holding things in place against the pressures of straining and gravity, the pelvic floor is vulnerable to the weight of time. There is also weakening of the connective tissues with ageing and damage to the nerves that control muscle tone. Reducing advanced glycation and supporting collagen synthesis with glucosamine and chondroitin sulphate can improve the mechanical properties of ageing connective tissue.

A number of other factors can accelerate the age-related decline in our pelvic floor or make its impact more significant.

The most important preventable factor is increased body weight. Other stresses on the pelvic floor, such as repetitive straining due to constipation, chronic coughing or regular heavy lifting, may also take their toll. Declining androgen levels contribute to a weakening of pelvic floor muscles. Oestrogen has limited effects on pelvic floor strength, but declining levels may contribute to an overactive or jumpy bladder.

Pelvic supports are also torn to a varying extent in most vaginal births, with the risk and extent of injury increasing with every additional delivery. Some women consider an elective Caesarean section (without experiencing labour) to limit this damage. However, this is only partly effective since considerable strain occurs prior to the due date. C-sections also have a number of other health implications for both mother and baby.

Some damage during labour may be prevented by pelvic floor muscle exercises, undertaken during pregnancy and continued after giving birth. It is thought that by increasing the strength of pelvic floor muscles, they are less prone to injury, recover faster and better support the downward pressure of the growing baby. We can become more aware of our pelvic floor muscles by using weighted vaginal cones. When individually introduced into the vagina, these devices are retained by active contraction of the pelvic floor. Essentially we teach ourselves to strengthen our muscles and follow our own progress. Pelvic floor strengthening may also prevent some of the weakening of the pelvic floor accrued as we age (and have benefits for preserving sexual function).

Yet even when maintaining a healthy body weight and performing pelvic floor exercises, many women experience some sagging of their pelvic floor supports during their lifetime. About every second woman experiences some urine leakage each month, with the frequency and severity increasing with age. The most common form is stress incontinence, where small amounts of urine unintentionally leak with coughing, exercising or other things that put pressure on the bladder. It is usually due to reduced support from the pelvic floor.

An overactive bladder is the second most common cause of urinary incontinence in women. It involves involuntary and inappropriate contractions of the bladder, frequently and suddenly making us feel the urge to urinate. Sometimes we leak before we can stop it or get to a bathroom (urge incontinence). The bladder can be jumpy like this if it is irritated, such as with an infection, or if it is too full. Caffeine is another common and avoidable trigger. Many women have symptoms of both stress and urge incontinence (known as mixed urinary incontinence).

At its most severe, sagging of the pelvic floor leads to prolapse, whereby pelvic organs (the bladder, rectum or uterus) protrude into the vagina. Up to half of all women will have some prolapse, which may go unnoticed without close examination. However, fewer will experience severe symptoms, such as bladder and bowel frequency, and incontinence problems, bulge symptoms or pain with intercourse.

Incontinence and prolapse should not be seen as an inevitable part of ageing. Rather than suffer in silence, it is important to seek help early, as there are now many simple options available to fix any problems.

For mild pelvic floor weakness, exercises and pessaries can be useful. Bladder retraining (behavioural therapy), biofeedback, electrical stimulation and a number of different drugs are also effective for urge incontinence.

For the woman who has a major reduction in her quality of life, it is possible to reinforce the pelvic floor with a sling of mesh tape, without needing major surgery or a destructive hysterectomy. During this minimally invasive procedure, a tape is inserted through tiny incisions in the abdomen and vaginal wall. No sutures are required to hold the tape in place, recovery is fast and the cure is effective for life. What good is a long life if it means long suffering too? If you have problems, get help today!

OPTIONS FOR A HEALTHY PELVIC FLOOR

☑ Do pelvic floor exercises.
  > While in the shower, perform an inner squeeze for 6 seconds and repeat this until you get out
  > Every time you finish emptying your bladder do 3 strong inner squeezes, holding for 5 seconds each
  > Practice pelvic floor muscle contractions as you make love. This has the added benefit of enhancing your sex life!
  > Put a note on your bathroom mirror and on the car dashboard to remind yourself to squeeze

☑ Keep up your androgens with DHEA and other interventions. Declining androgen levels with age contribute to weakening of pelvic floor muscles and can be corrected with good effect (see chapter 30)

☑ Keep up your oestrogens, if you have an overactive bladder – HRT or local application of vaginal oestrogens can be effective in some post-menopausal women

☑ Take glucosamine and chondroitin sulphate to support collagen synthesis

☑ Reduce exposure to AGEs in your diet to promote the flexibility and function of connective tissue (see chapter 10)

☑ Make an appointment to see your doctor about incontinence. What good is a long life if it means long suffering too? If you have problems, get help today!

THE PELVIC FLOOR IN MEN

The pelvic floor is less of a problem for ageing men, who have been spared the trauma of childbirth. Nonetheless, one in five men over the age of 60 have urinary incontinence. Many men suffer from an overactive bladder due to damage to the

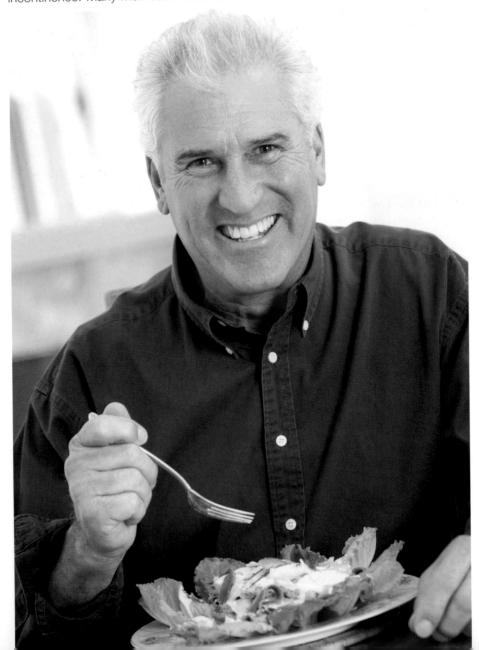

nerves and muscles with chronic diseases like diabetes. In the same way as women, many men with jumpy bladder will benefit from bladder retraining, medications and electrical stimulation.

Men also have their own special burden, the prostate gland, which sits just under the bladder. The prostate gland enlarges as men age, sometimes enough to slow the flow of urine.

The most common symptoms include an interrupted or dribbling urine stream, frequency, urgency or incontinence. Many of the same factors that influence ageing also make prostate enlargement more likely, including obesity, lack of physical activity, diabetes, smoking and a high-fat diet.

OPTIONS TO SUPPORT A HEALTHY PROSTATE

☑ Maintain a healthy weight. See chapter 9 for a range of options to assist you

☑ Increase physical activity. Regular and moderate physical activity is associated with lower rates of prostate enlargement, while inactivity and obesity makes it more common. See chapters 21 and 22 for guidance

☑ Eat foods that are naturally rich in antioxidants, especially those containing:
  > Lycopenes — red fruits such as tomatoes, watermelon, pink grapefruit, pink guava, papaya and rosehip
  > Isoflavones — fresh fruit, vegetables, soy, lentils, flaxseed and chickpeas

☑ Sulforaphane — broccoli, Brussel sprouts as well as other plants in the cabbage family

☑ Eat more onions and garlic — a healthy intake of these vegetables is associated with lower rates of prostate disease

☑ Eat less animal fat (especially fried, roasted, broiled, grilled or barbecued meat)

☑ Make an appointment to see your doctor about bladder problems. What good is a long life if it means long suffering too? A number of treatments are available to get the flow going again, including medications and surgical options

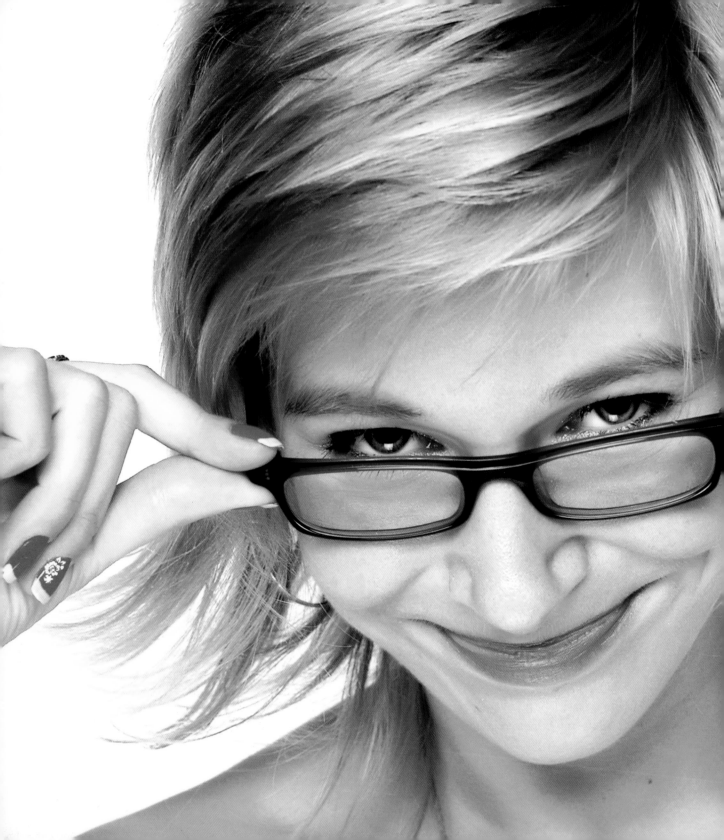

CHAPTER 36

EYES ON THE FUTURE
[EYES & AGEING]

Clear and comfortable vision is something most of us take for granted. Whether reading an email or keeping up with the children and grandchildren, we all need good eyesight to put our best foot forward - and not fall over! As we age, a number of changes may occur which can contribute to reduced eyesight or irreversible vision loss.

PRESBYOPIA

Apart from the typical long or short sightedness that results in having to wear glasses, the first time many of us are forced to acknowledge our ageing eyes is when we can no longer read the fine print. This is called Presbyopia or the 'short arm syndrome', since reading material must be held further and further away to focus. This helps for a while, but eventually the arms become 'too short' and reading correction in the form of reading glasses, bifocals or contact lenses is needed for close work.

DRY EYE

Another very common age-related change is ocular dryness, also known as 'dry eye'. We might notice this as stinging, burning, itching, scratchy, tired or bloodshot eyes. Often we just say it's too little sleep or too much stress. However, tear production tends to diminish as we get older, particularly in women after menopause, leaving eyes more vulnerable to drying out. Eyes can also dry out with certain medications, such as antihistamines, diuretics and pain killers, and in certain medical conditions, such as diabetes and rheumatoid arthritis.

Sometimes dry eyes can be caused by changes in the surface of the eye, called a pterygium. The exact cause is unknown, but it is more common in men and is associated with excessive exposure to UV rays, sand and wind (the typical Australian beach environment). The best prevention is wearing effective sunglasses that wrap around or have side shields.

Dry eye is easily treated with lubricating eye drops, many of which are available over-the-counter. An optometrist, ophthalmologist or chemist can help find the right solution for your needs.

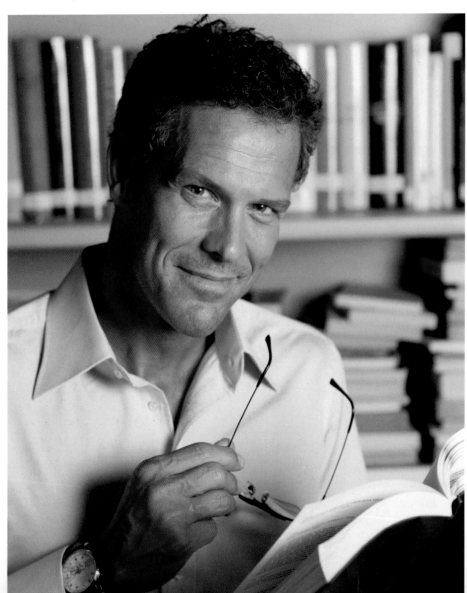

OPTIONS FOR TREATING THE SHORT ARM SYNDROME

Condition	Possible solution
Reading Glasses	Glasses used only for near work (must be taken off to see distance). Often wearing reading glasses (and never having a pair when you need them!) is som times just as frustrating as not being able to see things up close.
Monovision	One eye is corrected for near vision and the other eye is left to see things clearly in the distance. PRO: Very clear distance vision and very clear near vision. CON: Some people feel uncomfortable with the decreased depth perception and occasional fatigue that can occur when doing a specialised task for extended periods.
Multifocal contact lens	PRO: Quite natural vision where distance and near vision are reasonably clear in both eyes. CON: Neither distance nor near vision is perfectly clear. Generally not well suited to people requiring very high quality distance vision.
Laser vision correction	Now a very safe and predictable way to utilise monovision. However it is wise for prospective users of monovision to find a solution that is both comfortable and suits their needs before they undergo surgery. The main problem in using laser vision correction in this way is that our near vision prescription changes between the ages of 45 – 55.

CATARACTS

Cataracts are opacities in the lens of the eye that obstruct the passage of light. As we age, many of us will experience a degree of vision loss due to cataracts. Cataracts typically progress very slowly. Because they distort the lens, an early sign of a cataract forming may be near-sightedness. Yellowing of the lens can also reduce the perception of blue colours.

A number of different factors influence our chances of developing cataracts. The most common preventable cause of cataracts is diabetes (see chapter 6). Exposure to ultraviolet and infrared rays contained in sunlight also contributes to cataract development. Consequently, UV-B protecting sunglasses, wearing a brimmed hat and avoiding direct sunlight at the peak hours of solar radiation are important ways to reduce our risk of cataracts. There are now many ways to treat cataracts, such as lens replacement, but prevention is still a better alternative.

MACULAR DEGENERATION

Ageing in the retina is associated with accumulation of debris in focal deposits called drusen. An excess of drusen, just like an excess of garbage on the street, can disrupt traffic and make it unpleasant for those (cells) living nearby. An in-growth of new blood vessels in response to the drusen further accelerates the damage and visual loss. When these new vessels bleed or cause swelling of the retina, sudden permanent blindness can occur. However, visual impairment is more commonly insidious and often goes undetected until quite advanced. This form of damage, called Macular Degeneration, is a major cause of blindness as we get older.

There are several preventable risk factors for the development and progression of macular degeneration, including obesity, high blood pressure, diabetes and smoking. Modern research has shown that a low-fat diet rich in antioxidants and omega–3 fatty acids (through foods such as green leafy vegetables, whole grains, fish and nuts) appears to reduce the risk of age-related macular damage, while a diet high in animal fat makes vision loss from macular degeneration more likely. There is also some evidence that some antioxidant supplements can have beneficial effects on age-related eye disease (see chapter 8).

GLAUCOMA

Another disease that threatens our vision as we get older is glaucoma, in which painless damage occurs to the nerves that relay signals from the retina to the brain. This causes vision loss that starts in the periphery (tunnel vision) and works its way inward until eventually all vision is irreversibly lost. This damage most commonly occurs because of raised pressure inside the eyeball.

Important risk factors are age, diabetes and a family history of glaucoma. There are no special steps we can take to prevent it. However, regular eye checks performed by ophthalmologists and optometrists can detect it in its earliest stages, when it is easily treated. Because there are almost no symptoms until the final stages of the disease, waiting for visual loss to occur may be too late.

OPTIONS TO SUPPORT HEALTHY EYES

☑ Get an annual eye check-up – especially if you have a family history of eye disease. You should be tested for:
  > Vision (long and short sightedness)
  > Pressure inside the eye (main problem causing glaucoma)
  > Health of structures inside the eye such as optic nerve and the macular (macular degeneration and glaucoma)

☑ Diabetes is the main cause of preventable vision loss, so do whatever you can to prevent it (see chapter 6 for a range of options)

☑ Eat a low fat diet rich in fresh foods that are naturally high in antioxidants every day especially whole grain, whole fruit and vegetables. Eat a variety of richly coloured produce (see chapter 8 for a comprehensive range of options to boost your antioxidant intake)

☑ Eat more omega-3 fats from deep sea fish, seeds or supplements to reduce your risk of macular degeneration. Go to chapter 12 for a comprehensive range of options

☑ Wear good sunglasses and a hat — solar damage is a major cause of vision loss and can be prevented by taking very simple actions. Buy yourself a great hat that you will wear and an approve pair of sunnies that will wrap around or have side shields to reduce radiation exposure

☑ Wear eye protection — when shredding, grinding, mowing or hammering. Vision is precious, so don't risk losing it

☑ Stop smoking - even passive smoking will put your eyes at risk

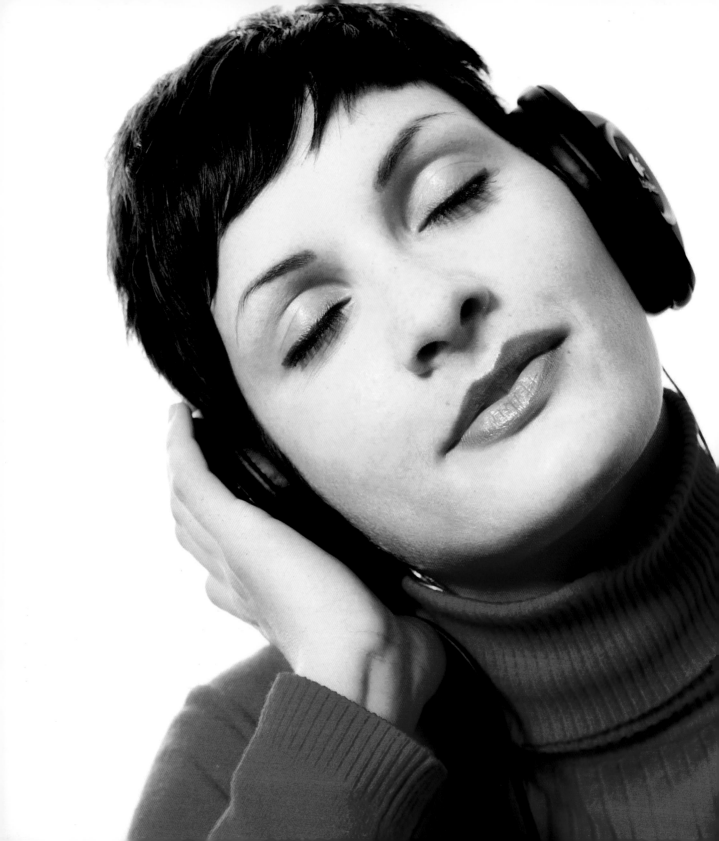

CHAPTER 37
ABOVE THE NOISE
[HEARING & AGEING]

Ageing sees slow deterioration in hearing (presbycusis). This loss can vary in severity from very mild changes to significant deafness. Hearing loss that is sufficient to impair communication will occur in at least half of all people aged over 60.

The most common complaint is not that we can't hear, but that we can't understand what is being said, particularly in loud environments, such as at the dinner table, in a crowd or in situations where there is competing background noise.

Presbycusis usually affects high-pitched sounds first. This means that some sounds are harder to hear than others and words that are quite different can sound the same, such as fine, shine and sign.

Rather than the world becoming quieter, hearing loss with age often makes things noisier, as different sounds blend into each other. Hearing loss can also manifest as ringing in the ears (called tinnitus). Other problems include a reduced ability to detect where a sound is coming from, which affects orientation.

When hearing deteriorates slowly, many people automatically find ways of minimising its impact, such as lip reading or using non-verbal cues, such as facial expressions, body language and gestures. Because of these coping mechanisms, and the fact that hearing loss happens gradually, other people may notice hearing loss before the person who has it.

As we age, there is selective damage to the most metabolically active areas of the inner ear. This is because the most demanding cells are also the most vulnerable to any factors that reduce supply, normally met by the circulation and metabolism. Consequently, disorders of the blood flow and metabolism, such as diabetes, obesity, heart disease and hypertension, all shorten the time it takes for age to have its effect. Equally, by preventing these other damaging factors, we can step back from the edge where time is no longer the enemy.

Exposure to an excessive amount of noise also causes damage to these same sensitive areas of the inner ear. Many believe that age-related hearing loss is largely the cumulative result of a lifetime of noise. The more exposure, the more damage, and the sooner we reach the threshold for dysfunction. For example, loud music exposure in our prime will make it more likely that we will have problems with our hearing during our retirement years.

Hearing tests are widely available. After the age of 65, or earlier if we have any risks for hearing loss, we should get a full hearing check at least every three years at our local hearing centre. For anyone who wonders if their hearing is not what it should be, a fifteen minute hearing screening is an easy way to find out more about your hearing and what can be done to help. Australian Hearing offers free hearing screenings at its centres nationally. Call 131 797 to be connected to your nearest centre.

RATHER THAN THE WORLD BECOMING QUIETER, HEARING LOSS WITH AGE OFTEN MAKES THINGS NOISIER, AS DIFFERENT SOUNDS BLEND INTO EACH OTHER

While protecting our hearing is the best way to preserve its function into old age, there are now many alternatives for its treatment, which can partially restore hearing and quality of life for sufferers. Most people can achieve enormous health and lifestyle benefits from a well-fitted hearing aid. These are now smaller, highly discreet, more sophisticated and can be personally designed to suit individual hearing losses. They can be matched to hair and skin colour, making them nearly invisible, and they are increasingly able to interconnect with other electronic devices, such as a phone or television using Bluetooth technology. If your hearing is poor, get fitted with a hearing device – they will open up your world.

OPTIONS TO KEEP YOUR HEARING

☑ Become aware of how well you are hearing
  > Listen to others if they tell you that you might be having trouble with your hearing. Don't put your head in the sand!
  > Stop making excuses for not being able to hear (such as that people are mumbling)
  > Pay attention if your family complains that the TV is too loud or you can't hear the phone ringing
  > Understand that hearing loss normally limits your ability to distinguish sounds in background noise – so you may find you avoid busy restaurants and bars

☑ Protect yourself from loud noise–the risk of hearing loss as we get older can be reduced by avoiding hazardous noise exposure or use of suitable hearing protection
  > Limit the amount of time you are exposed to very loud noise. Take time out periodically from loud concerts or other noisy environments
  > Wear properly fitted ear plugs or muffs if you are exposed to loud sounds at work or at play (e.g. loud concerts, guns, motor races, mowing the lawn, etc)
  > Give your ears frequent rest and take 'time out' in a quiet area.
  > Listen to your MP3 player at a volume that you can hear someone speak to you who is at arm's length. If you can't hear them, then the music is too loud, and potentially damaging your hearing

☑ If your ears 'ring' after you have been exposed to loud noise, or the world sounds a little quieter, then the noise level was probably hazardous to your hearing. You should limit the amount of time you spend exposed to loud noise If you have any concerns about your hearing, make an appointment to get your hearing checked

☑ Get your hearing checked, if you are over 65 or have an increased risk of hearing loss (diabetes, high blood pressure, family history of deafness, occupational noise exposure, etc)

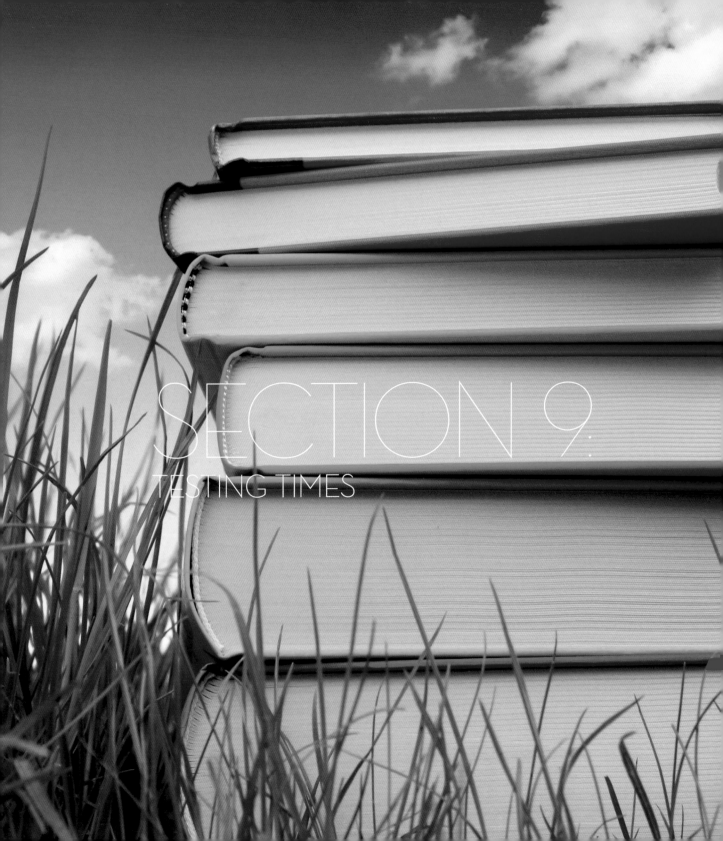

SECTION 9:
TESTING TIMES

CHAPTER 38: HOW OLD ARE YOU REALLY?
CHAPTER 39: WHAT TESTS SHOULD YOU DO?

SLOW begins with understanding and awareness. If you know where you are, you have a better idea of where you are heading (and can ask yourself whether you want to go there). This involves some soul searching and other forms of personal discovery. Some of this is just opening your eyes and looking at your relationships, your environment, your food and your activity as though your choices actually matter. But some things we can't see, at least not until it may be too late to make a difference. For these issues, we need to perform regular tests, measures or other evaluations of our health. You can spend thousands of dollars - or very little - in getting to know your ageing. This section looks at some of the practical ways to assess the ageing process and opportunities to use these results to slow ageing.

KATE'S EXPERIENCE
My doctor's job is to look for disease. My job is to be proactive and look for ways to find health. I want to keep tabs on my ageing and know if I am really on track - to stay in the driver's seat, learn what to test, when to test and why. There are many simple tests that everyone should do. New tests crop up all the time and it is important to investigate these, but don't get swayed by hype and end up spending money on tests that don't really tell you anything new. I keep copies of all my tests to follow my progress. Some tests are only available if you are 'at risk'; it's important to assess your individual risk and navigate your options with the right information at your fingertips.

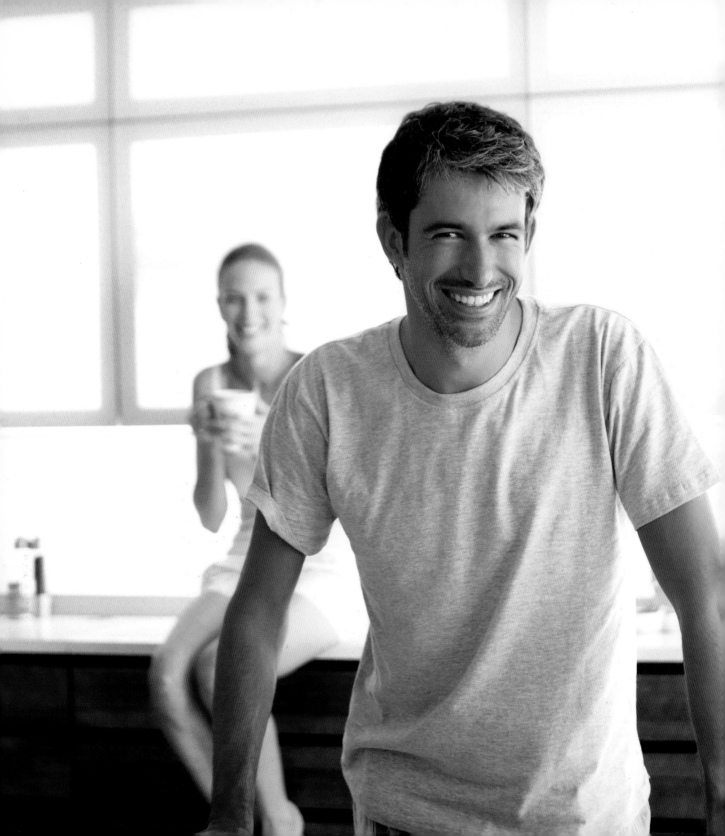

CHAPTER 38

HOW OLD ARE YOU REALLY?
[ASSESSING YOUR BIOLOGICAL AGE]

Why don't people believe us when we say we're only 30? How do they know we're not? And why can two people the same age look and feel totally different? Some people reach 80 with a similar health status to the average 50-year-old. Others experience extensive physical decline by the age of 60. The number of candles on our birthday cake is not a reliable indicator of our biological age. To determine our biological age, we need to look at a range of factors covering physical, mental and functional parameters and compare them with other people the same age. The more comprehensive the choice and assessment of parameters, and the more often they are measured, the better we are able to predict the cumulative effects of ageing, and ultimately control the outcomes. In this chapter we look at practical ways to assess how old we really are.

No consensus exists on a standard set of ageing biomarkers or their role in determining outcomes in individuals. Anti-ageing practitioners have traditionally considered the risk factors and early signs of disease as the most convenient way to measure biological age. However, while the presence of disease is important, the absence of disease does not guarantee quality of life or longevity. Biological age is also not the same thing as our health status. However, the healthier we are, the more likely we are to be 'biologically' younger than if we were unhealthy. There are many things we can do to be more healthy, and to have a positive impact on ageing. We can appear healthy, preserve our structures and functions, our looks and our strength, but we may be losing our reserves. Biological age looks at current functions, as well as how much we've got left in the tank. With this knowledge, we can anticipate, and potentially control, what happens next!

HOW OLD AM I REALLY?

Assessing some of the factors that drive our ageing can be very useful. For example, levels of oxidative stress, inflammation, stress or hormone levels can help us determine why we are ageing and provide specific targets for intervention. These and other tests are listed throughout this book and are summarised in chapter 39. However, while we can use these tests to help optimise our ageing, they are not a measure to tell us how old we are.

The decisions surrounding which tests to use are complex and specific to each individual. These choices are best made in concert with our health practitioner, and with a plan to act depending on the result. Knowing our age is a waste of money unless we use it to slow ageing. Don't be tempted to go it alone or buy tests over the internet. In choosing how to assess our biological age, most practitioners aim to cover the following questions:

WHICH MARKERS?

Not every test will cover all bases, but by choosing a variety of different tests, we can cover most of the crucial systems and functions of the body. Tests should be done on a regular basis. The huge numbers of tests now available are beyond the scope of this book, so instead we will focus on a few of the most informative markers.

CHOLESTEROL

Cholesterol levels are a good predictor of longevity. Keeping them at optimal levels is an important way to prevent heart disease. Testing our cholesterol fits nicely into the battery of tests required to document and predict our health, as well as providing a target to maintain it. Our levels of bad cholesterol (low density lipoproteins, or LDL) rise as we get older. The higher our LDL cholesterol levels, the higher our risk of heart attack and other diseases that shorten life expectancy. Levels of good cholesterol contained in high density lipoprotein (HDL) particles are used as a marker of the body's ability to remove bad cholesterol from blood vessels and transport it to safer storage sites. The higher our HDL cholesterol, the higher our capacity to reduce the effects of bad cholesterol, lowering our risk of heart disease.

GLUCOSE CONTROL

The ability to maintain glucose levels in an optimal range is another key requirement for health and longevity. This ability erodes as we get older, leading to impaired glucose tolerance and the onset of diabetes (see chapter 6). Long before we reach this stage,

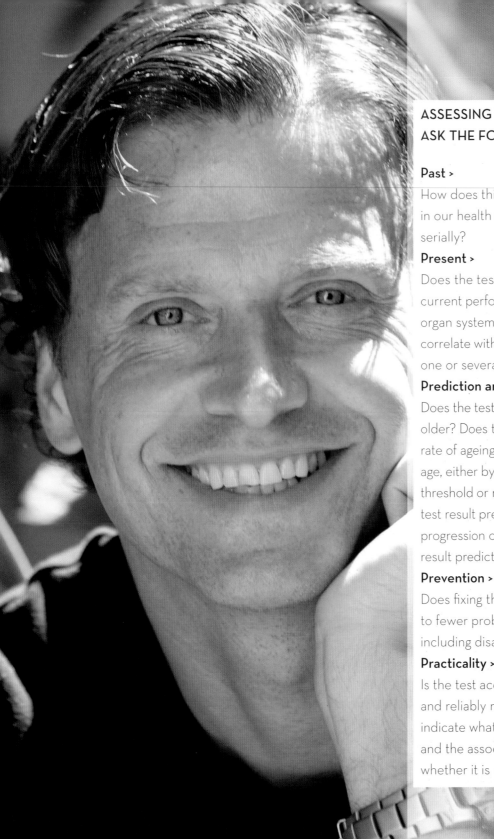

ASSESSING YOUR BIOLOGICAL AGE. ASK THE FOLLOWING QUESTIONS

Past >

How does this correlate with changes in our health status? Can it be tested serially?

Present >

Does the test result correlate with our current performance (in one or several organ systems)? Does the test result correlate with our functional reserve (in one or several organ systems)?

Prediction and prognosis >

Does the test result change as we get older? Does the test result predict our rate of ageing better than chronological age, either by showing reserve before threshold or rate of change? Does the test result predict the development and progression of disease? Does the test result predict lifespan and survival?

Prevention >

Does fixing the test result equate to fewer problems in advanced age, including disability, disease and death?

Practicality >

Is the test acceptable, minimally invasive and reliably measured? Does the result indicate what is healthy or unhealthy, and the associated risks (not just whether it is normal)?

it is possible to detect any loss of function with aglucose tolerance test (GTT). For this simple, non-invasive test, a large amount of sugar is taken orally or injected, and the effect of the sugar on the release of metabolic hormones is measured. Elevated levels of insulin denote a resistance to its effects. This is an early sign that the system is under strain, just like driving a car with the handbrake half on. Unless rectified, it will lead to loss of function. Another way to look at the body's capacity for sugar regulation is to measure the level of sugar modification on haemoglobin (called the HbA1c). The higher our HbA1c, the more sugar our body has been exposed to and the more susceptible we are to type 2 diabetes.

KIDNEY FUNCTION

The kidneys filter the blood, clearing it of toxins and maintaining the balance of our inner sea. Fortunately, we have two kidneys, providing a considerable buffer against losses due to ageing. People with impaired kidney function tend to accumulate toxins, such as AGEs, free radicals and damaged fats. This can accelerate ageing and many of the symptoms and diseases of old age. Even small changes in kidney function are associated with a risk of premature mortality. The capacity to filter the blood and clear it of toxins is estimated by measuring our Glomerular Filtration Rate (GFR). This is usually performed by a simple blood test. Another sign of early kidney damage is the presence of proteins, such as albumin in the urine, where they are not normally found. Increased levels of albumin in the urine, or a reduced GFR, are associated with early death, and those people with the highest levels of albumin excretion (albuminuria) and lowest GFR have the worst prognosis.

BODY COMPOSITION

Body composition is a key determinant of future health. Being overweight or obese shortens many lives (see chapter 9). Weight has traditionally been used as a marker of fatness and is an easy way to track the success of diet and exercise programs. The most widely used measure of body composition is the body mass index (BMI), which is our weight (in kilograms) divided by our height (in metres) squared. For example, if we weigh 68 kg and are 165 cm tall, then our BMI is 25 (68 divided by 1.65 squared). In white people, a BMI from 25 to 29 is considered overweight and a BMI of 30 or more is considered obese. In Asians, a BMI over 22.5 is considered overweight and over 27.5 is obese, reflecting ethnic differences in body shape. However, BMI does not take into account muscle mass, which can be very different in different people. For example, muscle loss as we get older can result in a lower BMI, and therefore complacency, yet body composition may still be highly abnormal.

An alternative is to simply measure our waist circumference with a tape measure at a point two finger breadths above the top of our hip bone. The deposition of fat around the waist, and particularly around the organs inside, is currently the best marker of compositional changes that result from too many calories and not enough exercise. Abdominal obesity is present if our waistline is:

Men > 102 cm (Asian men > 90 cm)
Women > 88 cm (Asian women > 80 cm)

Bioimpedance analysis is a novel way to look at body composition. This uses a small alternating current applied to the right hand and right foot to estimate a range of body components, including fat mass, lean body mass, water content and metabolic rate.

BLOOD PRESSURE

Systolic blood pressure is the highest pressure achieved by our beating heart. It is what we feel as our pulse. Systolic blood pressure is best measured by using a pressurised cuff to block off circulation in the arm. As the pressure in the cuff is lowered, the point at which the pulse is restored and blood first begins to flow is the systolic blood pressure. People with a lower systolic blood pressure often have a longer life expectancy. Interventions to lower blood pressure are effective in prolonging life. For every 1mmHg we reduce our systolic blood pressure, we reduce our risk of a heart attack by 2%. There is no ideal blood pressure. The lowest we can achieve will improve our health to the greatest extent, regardless of the raw value.

WEIGHT HAS T BEEN USED AS A MARKER OF FATNESS AND IS AN EASY WAY TO TRACK THE SUCCESS OF DIET AND EXERCISE PROGRAMS

Another way to look at the age of our blood vessels is to measure their stiffness. As we age, blood vessels generally become less elastic, commonly known as 'hardening of the arteries'. This is measured by using an ultrasound probe on our wrist or finger.

LUNG FUNCTION

Measures of respiratory function show a strong correlation with ageing. As we age, our lungs become stiffer, while the muscles required to expand them become weaker. This can be quantified by measuring how much air we can force out of our lungs in one second (Forced Expiratory Volume in 1 second, or FEV-1) or how much air we can breath in (Forced Vital Capacity, or FVC) using a spirometer. Both these parameters declineat the rate of about 1% per year and can be used as a marker of the ageing process. Of course, diseases of the lungs and muscle can also affect lung capacity, and these also impact on longevity.

STRENGTH AND FITNESS

Age-related declines in muscle mass and strength contribute significantly to age-related disability. By the time we reach our 80s, we have lost up to a third of our skeletal muscle mass. A simple strength test is the hand grip test. We hold a dynamometer in our dominant hand and give it a good squeeze. Grip strength is a good predictor of age, as well as disability, frailty and mortality. Adjustment for our height and fat mass further improves the ability of hand grip strength to determine our overall muscle mass.

As survival is generally longer in the fittest people, measuring our fitness level is one way to estimate our biological age. One measure of aerobic fitness is VO^2 max. Our body's maximum ability to use oxygen is determined while engaging in graded exercise. The walking test, beep test or step test are the most affordable, available and reliable tests. More expensive methods require making an appointment to see an exercise physiologist or other specialist. More simple markers of physical performance include walking distance, chair stands, walking speed and standing balance.

Flexibility is also a major determinant of physical performance, particularly as we get older. Many tests have been used to estimate flexibility. The sit-and-reach test measures the flexibility of our hamstrings and lower back. For this test, we sit on the floor with our legs straight out in front, then reach forward as far as possible. Other tests measure stiffness at multiple joints. Each has been shown to be useful in predicting functional capacity.

GRIP STRENGTH IS A GOOD PREDICTOR OF AGE, AS WELL AS DISABILITY, FRAILTY AND MORTALITY.

BONE INTEGRITY

Thinning of the bones is one of the best-known aspects of ageing. Reduced bone density indicates an increased risk of fracture and possibly osteoporosis. Bone density is usually measured by Dual Energy X-ray Absorptimetry (DEXA), which involves scanning of the spine, hip and sometimes wrist, as these sites fracture most often. By convention, bone density is compared to our maximum bone density when we are young. This is the T-score. A low T-score generally indicates a loss of bone density. The lower the T-score, the greater the risk of fracture. Bone density is

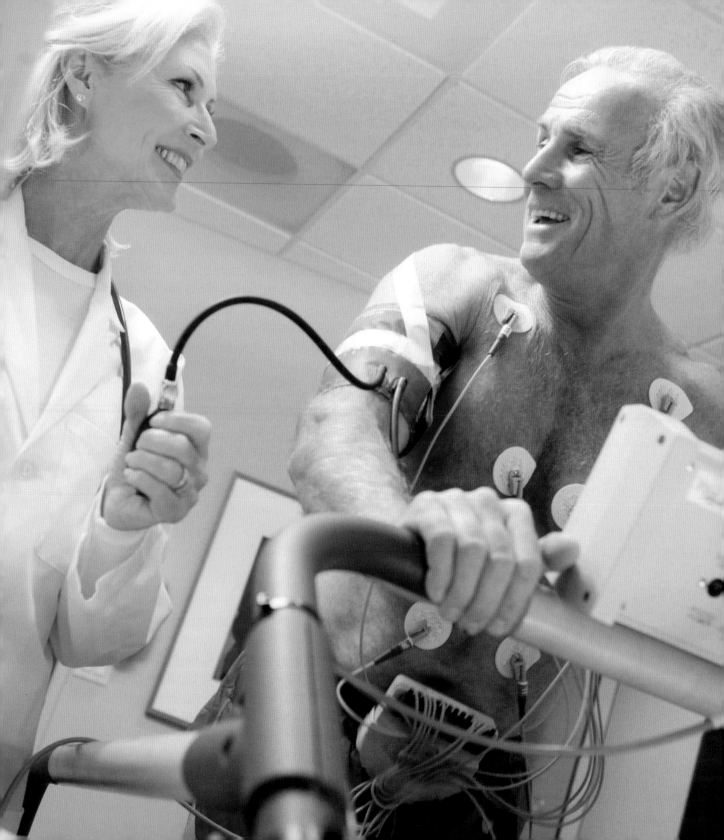

more commonly measured in women, as men have a greater peak bone density and it takes much more bone loss to lead to bone fragility and increased risk of fracture. However, men still experience bone loss and bone density can still be used to track the ageing process. In fact, in both men and women, there is a strong association between changes in bone density and age-related changes in other systems, including the lungs, heart and kidneys. Moreover, when compared to people of a similar age, those with a lower bone density (T-score) have a higher risk of cancer, heart disease and overall mortality.

A simple X-ray of the hand can also be used to identify age-related changes, including bone proliferations (spurs), reduced bone density, areas of scarring (sclerosis) and deformities of the joints. From these combined features, a score can be derived that approximates biological age and predicts longevity and mortality.

More recently, urinary N-telopeptide excretion (NTx) and Vitamin D levels have also been put forward as markers of future bone health.

BRAIN POWER

Batteries of cognitive tests that measure thinking power are widely used to examine the impact and rate of ageing. Ageing is associated with a decline in some cognitive tasks, such as short-term memory and spatial awareness. Memory loss, learning and other cognitive skills are highly variable between individuals. Nonetheless, there are many simple, standardised tests now available, many of them computerised, with alternate forms to allow accurate follow-up over time. Poor performance in these tests is associated with reduced quality of life and reduced survival, even after allowing for education and other factors.

GENETIC TESTS

When examining ageing, our family history must be taken into account. How long did our relatives live? Did they have any diseases that limited their life span, such as heart disease, cancer or diabetes? Of course, life today is very different to what it was even 50 years ago, so the things that made life short then may not be the same as today. Nonetheless, there is good evidence to suggest that some genes can be inherited, which influence predisposition to disease or the rate of ageing.

Only in the last few years has comprehensive genetic testing become possible and validated as a better marker of risk than family history. These genetic tests look for certain sequences in DNA that are associated with increased risk. These tests are usually performed on blood samples, but a scraping of the inside of our mouth is sufficient. Genetic test results are based on percentage predictions, telling us our risk of contracting a certain condition based on associations. Inheritance of certain gene sequences may increase or decrease our chances, although it does not ensure that a specific person will develop a specific problem. Most diseases result from a complex set of factors and genes are only one component. There is currently no genetic test for ageing.

TAKE THE TEST

Ageing affects all parts of the body, albeit at different rates in different areas for different people. Trying to get a handle on our age can be a protracted and expensive process. No single test can confirm we are on the right track. Tests must include markers of health, as well as disease, predictors of mortality and decline in function, parameters of current function, as well as functional reserve. To get an accurate indication of our age, the testing process must be comprehensive and reflect the processes of ageing across crucial tissues and organ systems. The necessity and frequency of the following tests is determined largely by our age, with some becoming more relevant as we get older. Most of the tests are recommended for those with average risk. For individuals at higher risk, such as those with a family history of problems or increased risk based on their lifestyle, additional or more intensive monitoring may be warranted in consultation with their health care provider.

TRYING TO GET A HANDLE ON OUR AGE CAN BE A PROTRACTED AND EXPENSIVE PROCESS. NO SINGLE TEST CAN CONFIRM WE ARE ON THE RIGHT TRACK.

CHOLESTEROL LEVELS

What to test?	LDL (bad) cholesterol, HDL (good) cholesterol
Who does it?	GP
How often?	Annually, or more often if we want to track our response to interventions
When?	Now

SUGAR CONTROL

What to test?	HbA1c, glucose tolerance test
Who does it?	GPs and medical specialists
How often?	Annually in those with impaired control or risks for it
When?	From 40

KIDNEY FUNCTION

What to test?	Glomerular filtration rate, albuminuria
Who does it?	GPs and medical specialists
How often?	Annually in those with impaired function or risks for it
When?	From 40

BODY COMPOSITION

What to test?	BMI, waist circumference, bioimpedance analysis (BIA)
Who does it?	We can measure our BMI and waist ourselves. Bioimpedence analysis is available through nutritionists, exercise physiologists and risk clinics, as well as many GPs
How often?	At least annually or more often if we want to track response to interventions
When?	Now

BLOOD VESSEL FUNCTIONS

What to test?	Systolic blood pressure, pulse wave velocity
Who does it?	GPs and medical specialists
How often?	Annually, or more often for those with vascular disease or risks for it
When?	From 40, or sooner for those with vascular disease or risks for it

LUNG FUNCTION

What to test?	FEV-1, FVC
Who does it?	GPs, medical specialists, exercise physiologists
How often?	Annually for those with vascular disease or risks for it
When?	From 50, or sooner for those with vascular disease or risks for it

STRENGTH, FITNESS AND FLEXIBILITY

What to test?	Hand grip test, VO· max, walking distance, chair stands, walking speed, standing balance, flexibility (eg. sit-and-reach test)
Who does it?	GPs and medical specialists
How often?	Annually
When?	From 40 or sooner if we want to track response to interventions

BONE INTEGRITY

What to test?	DEXA scans, NTx, bone x-rays
Who does it?	GPs and medical specialists
How often?	Every 5 years
When?	At or around the age of menopause in women. If indicated by an increased risk of fracture in men

BRAIN POWER

What to test?	Cognitive tests
Who does it?	Ourselves, in concert with our GP or medical
How often?	Annually
When?	From 40

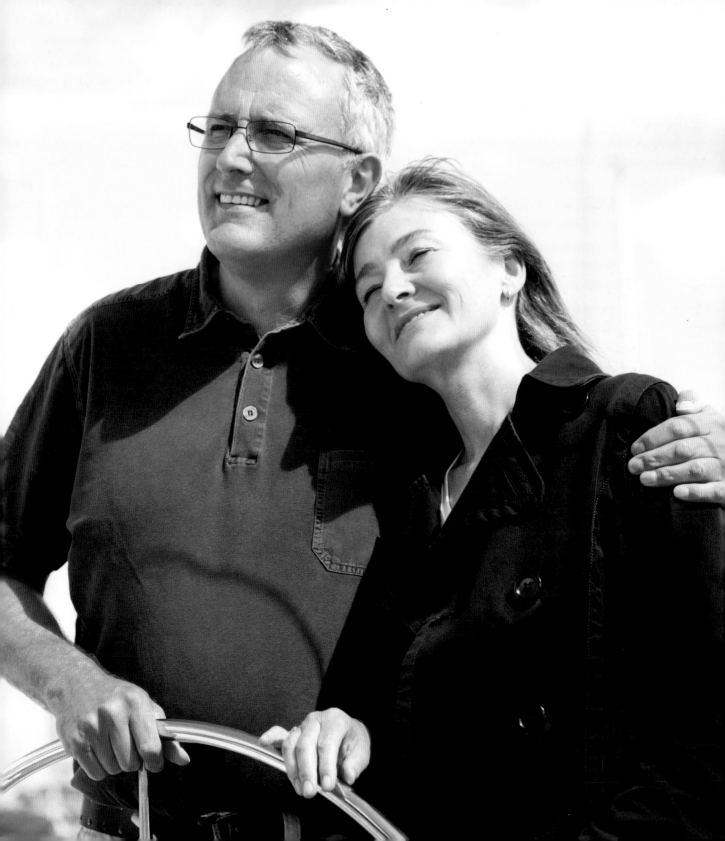

CHAPTER 39

WHAT TESTS SHOULD YOU DO?

SLOW begins with understanding and awareness. Knowing where we are is one way to get an idea of where we are heading (and asking ourselves whether we want to go there). Some of this is soul searching and other forms of personal discovery. Some of this is just opening our eyes and looking at our relationships, our environment, our food and our activity, as though these choices actually matter. But some things we can't see. At least, not until it may be too late to make a difference. For these issues we need to perform regular tests, measures or other evaluations of our health. Such tests can play a useful role in maintaining our health by:

> Identifying modifiable risks for disease or decline.
> Enabling us to detect problems early. Even before symptoms are recognised or increased risks are identified, screening tests help detect disease in its early and most treatable stages.
> Providing the opportunity for customised interventions based on our individual needs, rather than generic (one-size fits all) solutions.
> Identifying and reinforcing successful activities. The ability to quantify allows positive intervention with measureable results (the diet that reduces cholesterol and is shown to do so, or the gym program that improves BMI and reduces percentage of body fat).
> Improving resource allocation. Identifying non-essential or superfluous activities, seeing where the biggest gains can be made and where to allocate our limited time, energy and money.
> Providing an impetus and a focus for change. Even healthy individuals guard their health more closely when a test reveals the risk of a high cholesterol level, an abnormal Pap smear, a high level of oxidative stress or a glimpse of mortality. Test results will often be the best stimulus for people to take steps to reduce their risk of disease and disability. The most important part about testing is the act of looking, regardless of what we find.

It is important that any test and its result be connected to an opportunity for intervention or change. There is no benefit in screening to reveal a problem if it does not lead to action or allow us to implement targeted strategies to improve our health and wellbeing. In fact, it can be counterproductive if the weight of expectation becomes overwhelming when nothing can be done about it. Of course, no future can be predicted with certainty.

Trying to get a handle on our state of health, ageing and risks for certain diseases can be a protracted and expensive process. Some investigations are covered by Medicare or a health fund, but others are not. Consequently, we may find that some practitioners will select investigations based on their assumptions of our capacity to pay! The way around this is to stay connected to the process. Have a working knowledge of what tests you want to do on an ongoing basis and why. No test is so urgent that you don't have time to think it over and look at the options and rationale (if it was urgent, Medicare would cover it). Testing is a SLOW process too!

> AGEING, LIKE BEAUTY, IS IN THE EYE OF THE BEHOLDER, BUT IS THERE ANY WAY TO TELL US HOW TO GET AROUND THIS BIAS?

To be most effective in our testing, we need to keep track of all our investigations. We should aim to know more about ourselves than our doctor or health care provider, not the other way around, so we can more easily monitor and refine our progress and use it to ask more questions.

There are now an enormous number of tests available to measure every aspect of physical and mental function. To undertake them all is not only financially costly, but also unfocussed. Each will be more or less important in certain situations and in certain individuals. We must work our way through what is most important to us first, not those things that are most important to our healthcare provider. Get help to take the first steps. The best help comes from those who are willing to coach and guide us through our options, and who will listen and respond to our questions. Avoid falling to the latest fad that claims to have all the answers.

MILE MARKERS - MEASURES OF BIOLOGICAL AGE

Ageing is different for different people. It is far more than the passage of time or the number of candles on our cake. Some look and feel great at 40, others do not. Ageing, like beauty, is in the eye of the beholder, but is there any way to tell us how to get around this bias? As discussed in chapter 38, there are a number of tests (see table above) that can give us an idea of how we are tracking, physically and mentally. Each of these tests offer us useful information about disease risk and

System	Widely Available Tests
Cholesterol	LDL (bad) cholesterol, HDL (good) cholesterol
Sugar control	Glucose tolerance test, HbA1c
Kidney function	Glomerular filtration rate, albuminuria
Fat composition	BMI; waist circumference, bioimpedance
Blood vessels	Systolic blood pressure, pulse wave velocity
Lung function	FEV-1, FVC
Muscles	Hand grip strength
Fitness	VO· max, walking speed and distance, chair stands, flexibility tests
Bone	DEXA scan, T-score, Z-score, hand X-ray
Brain	Cognitive tests Quantitative EEG

age-related decline. However, to reflect overall ageing, we need to measure a range of factors from many systems, including physical, mental and functional parameters that vary with age. Ageing is the sum of a number of processes, so an estimation of our biological age, as well as any intervention strategy, must be determined by a range of processes. The answer to slow ageing is not found in a single pill or exercise regimen, and single measures of different factors often fail to accurately reflect changes in the whole.

In general, the more comprehensive our choice, the better our ability to predict the cumulative effects of ageing and its outcomes. The way to make the most of the available tests is not just to have them tested once, but have them repeated at intervals (every year or two, more often if they are abnormal). One test is a snapshot, two provides a trend.

BRAVING THE ELEMENTS

The changes of ageing are driven by a number of elements, including oxidative stress, glycation, inflammation and the calories we eat. Modifying these key areas is important to preserve structure and function, prevent disease and slow the ageing process. Many anti-ageing practitioners advocate measuring the strength of these elements, as one would gauge the wind or take the temperature or humidity to determine how long a structure will last. A number of different options are available: Like all tests, it is important not to over-interpret the results. For example, someone

Calories (Chapter 9)
Food diary
Waist circumference
Body fat assessment eg. bioimpedence
Fasting insulin levels

Advanced glycation (Chapter 10)
No standardised blood tests are currently available for clinical use
Skin fluorescence (AGE meters) are used in some clinics

Inflammation (Chapter 11)
Acute-phase proteins eg. C-reactive protein (CRP), fibrinogen
Cytokines eg. IL-6, TNF-alpha
Arachidonic acid to eicosapentaenoic acid (AA/EPA) ratio
White cell count and differentials

may have high levels of oxidative stress, but if they have high antioxidant defences, this may not be a problem. Equally, low levels of oxidative stress do not necessarily mean we would not benefit from antioxidants. The best of these tests allow us to track our success when we adopt some change or intervene in some way, such as increasing our physical activity. However, the absence of change does not mean our intervention has failed. It is vital not to get too caught up in numbers when health is priceless.

SCREENING FOR RISK AND DISEASE

Preventing the onset of age-related disease is the one effective way to improve the quality and quantity of our life into the future. While healthy ageing is far more than the absence of disease, any effective anti-ageing strategy must always also include participation in disease prevention programs and compliance with effective disease management. One of the most proven ways to prevent disease is to screen for its risk factors, as well as early signs of the disease itself.

System	Widely Available Tests
Skin	Check all areas of our skin, including areas not normally exposed to the sun. Look for changes in shape, colour or size of a pigmented lesion, or a new lesion (every three months)
Breast	Mammography, breast self-examination (annually for women over 40)
Cervical	Pap smears
Prostate	Digital rectal examination (annually for men over 50)
Colon	Flexible sigmoidoscopy (every 5 years for those over 50) or Air contrast barium enema (every 5-years for those over 50) or CT colonography (every 5 years for those over 50) or Faecal occult blood (annually for those over 50)

More frequent and/or earlier screening may be appropriate for people with an increased risk of specific cancers (eg. family history of cancers at an early age). Heart disease and stroke are accidents waiting to happen in our old age. One way to prevent this kind of accident is to identify and manage those (risk) factors that contribute to the narrowing and destabilising of blood vessels that can ultimately lead to heart attack and stroke. This should be done as early as possible before the damage is started, as some changes may be irreversible.

Risk Factor (Disease)	Widely Available Tests
Abnormal cholesterol levels (dyslipidemia)	LDL and HDL cholesterol Apolipoproteins and Lipoprotein(a)
Elevated blood pressure (hypertension)	Blood pressure sphygmomanometery Ambulatory BP monitoring
Abnormal sugar control (diabetes or impaired glucose tolerance, IGT)	Glucose tolerance test HbA1c
Too much fat (abdominal obesity)	Waist circumference Bioimpedance analysis
Too little exercise (sedentary)	Tests of physical fitness
Impaired kidney function (Chronic Kidney Disease, CKD)	Estimated GFR, albuminuria
Abnormal metabolism (hyperhomocystemia)	Homocysteine
Abnormal vascular function Applanation tonometry	Pulse wave velocity

It is recommended that these parameters be tested in everyone aged over 50, or earlier if there is a suggestion of greater risk, such as smokers, family history of heart disease, etc. Results in the normal range can then be repeated annually or biannually dependent upon the overall risk profile. Increased cardiovascular risk should be treated aggressively as this is the best way to prevent a heart attack or stroke.

TESTS FOR OPTIMISING NUTRITION

One important driver of disease and ageing is our diet, both what we consume and what we don't. While it is easy to see if we are taking too many calories (with a tape measure around our middle), detrimental changes in other nutritional parameters are less easy to spot. There is currently no simple test for an optimal diet, but there are many ways to find out where some problems may exist. This may be particularly relevant when considering the use of nutritional supplements (see chapter 17). The most basic way is to perform a detailed dietary history in conjunction with a dietitian or nutritionist, who can help us calculate our required daily intake of calories and essential vitamins, minerals and fatty acids.

A number of providers also offer tests that detect deficiencies of specific nutrients. The most widely used test is for iron levels, which often run low in women due to menstrual blood losses. Other important examples include measurement of serum B12, red cell folate and homocysteine. Vitamin D can also be measured, but this has more to do with sun exposure than diet. In fact, with current technologies, almost all the essential vitamins and minerals can be measured in blood samples. The theoretical value of this approach is to offer personalised dietary advice based on our current intake. However, most of this information can usually be obtained more cheaply from a simple dietary survey. Moreover, with the exception of a few specific cases, adopting a healthy and varied diet rich in whole and fresh foods is likely to be the answer in any case.

HORMONES AND AGEING

Given that ageing is all about achieving and maintaining balance, one of the most widely held theories of why we age suggests there could be a decline in the signals that keep things in check. Just like walking along a narrow log, it is the signals of our senses, their adaption and coordination that tell us how best to make the next move. Without coordination, the same passage can be dangerous or even life-threatening. In much the same way, adapting and coordinating our metabolism is important for health and wellbeing. In the human body, balance is the job of the hormones, including the sex hormones, growth hormone, cortisol and melatonin. As we age, there is an involution of these functions, resulting in decreased levels of hormones, or their inadequate regulation.

IN THE HUMAN BODY, BALANCE IS THE JOB OF THE HORMONES, INCLUDING THE SEX HORMONES, GROWTH HORMONE, CORTISOL AND MELATONIN.

The symptoms of low hormone levels are often very non-specific, including low physical, mental and sexual energy, low or fragile mood, reduced stress resilience and general aches and pains, all of which are often simply attributed to ageing. Because we can't readily tell on our own, a number of tests are available to measure the functions of key hormonal regulators of ageing, such as:

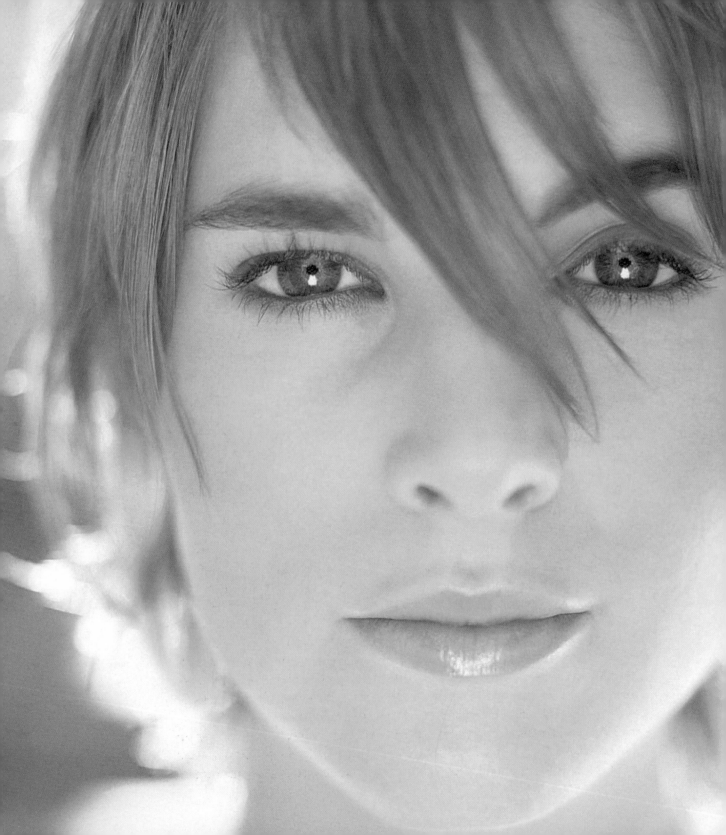

CORTISOL (CHAPTER 25)
Salivary cortisol tests (repeated a number of times through a day)
24-hour urinary free cortisol

FEMALE HORMONES (CHAPTER 28)
Menstrual history
Oestrogen
Progesterone
FSH

ANDROGENS (CHAPTER 29)
Screening questionnaires
Testosterone / Free Testosterone (performed on early morning blood tests)

DHEA (CHAPTER 30)
DHEAS levels (blood test)

GROWTH HORMONE (CHAPTER 31)
Insulin-like growth factor (IGF-1) (blood test)
IGF binding proteins (IGFBP-3) (blood test)
Arginine-stimulated growth hormone response (blood test)

MELATONIN (CHAPTER 28)
Sleep pattern questionnaires and surveys
Salivary melatonin levels

A number of providers also offer hormone tests performed on our saliva. This has the advantage of no needle usage (and is therefore less stressful and less painful). Unfortunately, such tests are not easy to standardise and the relationship between salivary and blood hormone levels, or symptoms of deficiency, may vary between and within individuals, adding to problems in their interpretation. However, repeated tests for one individual may deliver data on menstrual cycling, circadian rhythms or fluctuations in stress levels. Do not be tempted to buy a one-off kit over the internet and check the levels yourself. If you think you need to be tested, talk to a doctor or other qualified health care provider about the available options.

Finally, do not be overly concerned with numbers. The object is not to restore hormone levels to some arbitrary youthful value, but rather to ensure hormone levels are consistent with optimal function for you! You are the best judge of any intervention.

GENETIC TESTING

There is good evidence that some genes can be inherited that influence our risk of disease or rate of ageing. We are not on a level playing field and some people start with gene helpers and some with hindrances. When examining ageing, often the first question asked by our practitioner deals with our family history. How long did our relatives live? Did they have any diseases that limited their health span, such as heart disease, cancer or diabetes? Because the apple never falls far from the tree, this information can be used to screen earlier or more intensively for early signs of disease that can be nipped in the bud. An example of this is breast cancer, where a strong family history of breast cancer means that earlier and more frequent mammograms can be used to identity early lesions.

Only in the last few years has comprehensive genetic testing become possible and thus validated as a marker of future risk. For example, examining the genes that control cholesterol levels may be equivalent, or better than, testing cholesterol levels themsleves in predicting our risk of heart disease. These genetic tests look for certain sequences in DNA that are associated with increased risk. They are usually performed on blood samples, but a scraping of the inside of our mouth is also sufficient. Only for a handful of rare (single gene) inherited disorders or disease can it make precise predictions. Most genetic test results are based on percentage predictions, showing us whether we are at risk of acquiring one condition or another, based on previous associations. Inheritance of certain gene sequences increases or decreases the chance, although it does not ensure that a person with a 'bad' profile will develop a specific problem. Nor does it mean that those with a 'good' genetic profile can smoke and eat anything they like without effect. Most diseases result from a complex set of factors in which genes are only one small component.

Over the next decade, it will be possible for us to get our genes analysed in detail. If these findings only give us a time bomb to be worried about, they are not worth it. However, if finding a risk is the kick in the pants that we need to change our behaviour to improve our overall health, then by all means go ahead.

We must never test over the internet or on our own. If we find anything, we will immediately want to do something about it. Some practitioners are already using genetic testing as part of their drive to develop personalised interventions. However, it is advisable to have additional counselling before pursuing genetic testing. It may throw up more than what we are looking for and we need to be prepared to deal with it. Finally, always remember we are far more than the sum of our genes, so be wary of any practitioner who thinks our identity and our future is just in our genes.

Role of telomerase in ageing

It is believed by many people in the field that science and technology have reached a point where curing ageing can finally become a reality. According to Bill Andrews of Sierra Sciences, the main cause of ageing in humans is something called Telomere Shortening Disease. He believes it is the number one health risk in humans, causing not just ageing, but virtually every disease that is associated with advancing age.

The telomere is a region of DNA at the tips of our chromosomes. Every time our cells divide, our telomeres get shorter. They are about fifteen thousand bases in length when we're first conceived; they shorten to ten thousand bases by the time we're born; and they become progressively shorter throughout our lives as our cells divide. When they get down to about five thousand bases, our cells lose the ability to function, and that's when we typically die of old age.

Lengthening telomeres could prevent or reverse Telomere Shortening Disease. Scientists at Harvard, using this technology, have recently successfully reversed ageing in mice. They've turned old mice into young mice – not just young-looking mice, but young by every biomarker that was mentioned.

Two very recent studies have shown that telomere length is the single strongest predictor of how much longer a person will live. Measuring your telomeres will reveal your true biological age – a number much more useful and predictive than your chronological age.

For years, telomere length measurement has been an expensive and imprecise technology. But today, laboratories across the globe are making great strides in making this test more and more affordable and relevant as a diagnostic. The historical technique of measuring the average telomere length is being replaced by a more predictive method involving measuring the abundance of short telomeres in the body. These tests can predict the likelihood of developing various degenerative and age-related diseases, including heart disease, arthritis, COPD, and cancer.

Research has identified supplement regimens that will keep telomere shortening to a minimum; and there are a few supplements today that have been shown to induce our cells to produce telomerase, the enzyme that lengthens telomeres.

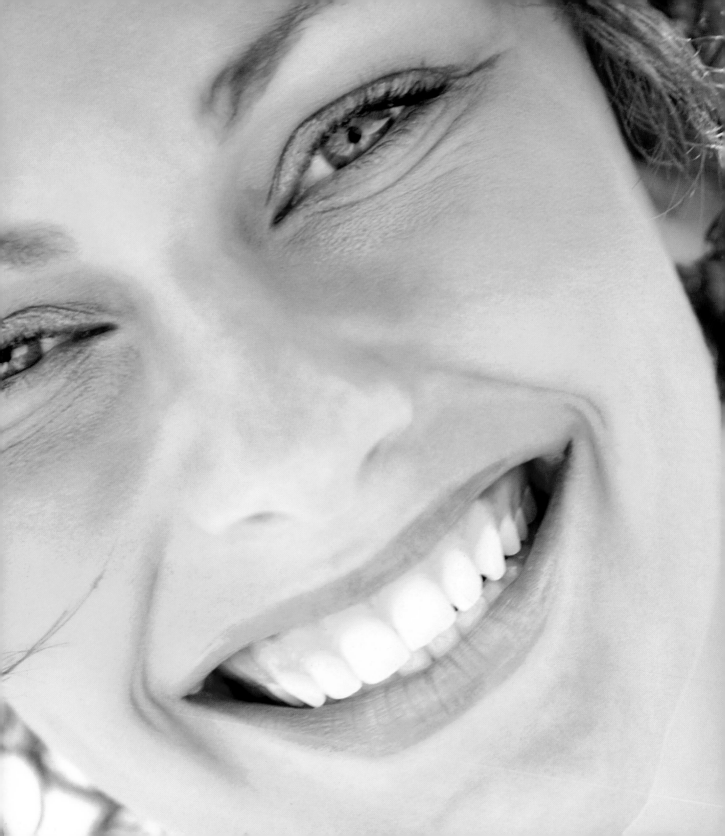

GETTING SPECIFIC

This book has looked at a number of specific areas impacted by the ageing process, as well as the choices we make along the way. Many of these are impacted by nutrition, oxidative stress and other elements of ageing, and some insight can be gained from testing in these areas as detailed above. But specific problems sometimes need specific solutions. We can perform additional tests as indicated by our personal situation and our evaluation of it. Some of these areas include:

ENVIRONMENTAL STRESS (CHAPTER 15)

> Intestinal dysbiosis
> Heavy metals toxicity testing

AGEING BRAIN (CHAPTER 23)

> Quantitative EEG

STRESS RESILIENCE (CHAPTER 25)

> Heart rate variability
> Questionnaires
> Salivary cortisol levels (repeated a number of times through a day)
> 24-hour urinary free cortisol

SLEEP (CHAPTER 26)

> Melatonin levels

BONES & JOINTS (CHAPTER 34)

> DEXA
> Urinary N-telopeptide excretion (NTx)

PELVIC FLOOR (CHAPTER 35)

> Assessment by a urogynaecologist or other pelvic floor specialist

VISION (CHAPTER 36)

Annual eye check for:
> Vision (long and short sightedness)
> Pressure inside the eye (main problem causing glaucoma)
> Health of structures inside the eye such as optic nerve and the mac lar (macular degeneration and glaucoma)

HEARING (CHAPTER 37)

> Full hearing check at local hearing centre (call 131 797 to be connected to your nearest Australian Hearing Centre)
> A screening test can be performed over the phone (Telscreen – phone 1800 826 500)

INDEX

moles 57
multivitamins 143, 148, 149, 152, 153, 154, 155
mycotoxins 130

N

nettle root 269
neurofeedback 109, 227, 229
niacin 149, 157
nutrigenomics 165
nuts 49, 62, 74, 75, 78, 83, 92, 99, 107, 111, 117, 118, 119, 120, 123, 132, 144, 147, 151, 152, 153, 162, 163, 174, 177, 178, 224, 228, 300, 313, 316, 328

O

obesity 86, 91, 112, 122, 126, 127, 140, 141, 162, 244, 283, 295, 307, 315, 322, 323, 328, 331, 341, 354
oestrogen 78, 128, 190, 275, 276, 277, 278, 281, 285, 286, 294, 311, 312, 316
olive 47, 53, 80, 83, 106, 111, 132, 164, 166, 167, 178, 179, 300
omega-3 49, 107, 110, 111, 166, 167, 168, 169, 224, 228, 279, 308, 317, 329
omega-6 110, 168, 169
organic 53, 130, 132, 138, 160, 166, 167, 168
orgasm 265, 266, 270, 282
osteoporosis 19, 21, 102, 111, 142, 151, 152, 164, 197, 275, 277, 288, 311, 312, 342
oxidative stress 48, 51, 55, 69, 71, 72, 73, 74, 75, 76, 78, 80, 96, 121, 129, 187, 197, 198, 224, 259, 285, 295, 301, 302, 338, 349, 351, 352, 361

P

pancreas 33, 50, 51, 52
parasympathetic 243, 244, 245, 251, 290
Parkinson's disease 138, 226, 293, 359
pelvic floor 275, 277, 297, 319, 320, 321, 322, 361
pesticide 130, 132, 160
photoageing 69, 71
physical activity 47, 52, 86, 91, 105, 141, 194, 195, 197, 199, 200, 205, 210, 211, 213, 228, 232, 249, 250, 257, 271, 279, 283, 291, 295, 311, 315, 317, 322, 323, 352
phytochemical 164, 165
plastic 31, 32, 60, 128, 135, 141
pollution 55, 128, 135, 308
polycyclic aromatic hydrocarbons 173
polyphenol 78, 80, 81, 166
probiotics 125, 126, 179, 184
progesterone 275
prolapse 320
prostate 62, 63, 67, 77, 80, 112, 164, 198, 282, 322, 323
protein 49, 65, 85, 88, 95, 96, 97, 103, 106, 107, 115, 116, 117, 118, 119, 127, 129, 132, 147, 160, 166, 167, 168, 169, 173, 179, 180, 232, 289, 352
psyllium 120, 121, 123
pyridoxine 146, 157

R

RDI 142, 143, 144, 145, 146, 147, 149, 151, 152, 153, 154, 157, 183, 184, 186, 190, 193
red wine 53, 77, 137, 138, 190
relaxation 107, 127, 187, 231, 233, 234, 235, 236, 239, 243, 245, 248, 249, 251, 257, 265, 271, 283
resistance training 48, 197, 199, 202, 209, 213, 215, 217, 218, 291
resveratrol 48, 77, 138, 190
retinoic acid 302, 305
retinol 137, 143, 190, 191, 193, 302
riboflavin 148, 149, 157
rutin 73, 75, 77, 145

S

saturated fat 48, 53, 93, 112, 140, 166, 316
selenium 73, 75, 153
sex 23, 61, 78, 80, 187, 250, 255, 256, 257, 260, 263, 264, 265, 266, 267, 268, 270, 271, 273, 274, 275, 276, 278, 280, 282, 285, 286, 311, 312, 316, 319, 321, 355
sexual dysfunction 265, 275, 281
skin 24, 38, 56, 57, 58, 59, 62, 67, 69, 71, 74, 76, 77, 85, 98, 106, 120, 127, 143, 144, 148, 149, 164, 168, 181, 187, 245, 259, 275, 280, 286, 287, 288, 293, 297, 299, 300, 301, 302, 303, 304, 305, 307, 308, 309, 313, 316, 332, 353
sleep 20, 26, 37, 39, 60, 107, 118, 135, 137, 150, 187, 198, 221, 224, 226, 227, 229, 234, 239, 241, 244, 248, 250, 251,

Bibliography is available at www.slowageingbook.com

KATE'S STORY

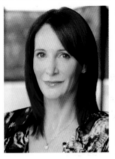

At 40, I was feeling old, fat and frumpy. I weighed 73kg, hardly exercised, ate poorly and drank too much. My marriage had broken down and an attempt to start a new business had failed. I was a single mum, stressed, unhappy and, hardly surprising, had a low sex drive. I was referred to a psychiatrist and diagnosed with postnatal depression. I felt I had no control in my life.

I started taking antidepressant drugs. In retrospect, I was lucky because I reacted badly to them and looked for alternative solutions.

Thus began my journey through the healthcare system and my own self-development, which became the impetus for this book.

I started by visiting a GP who specialised in nutrition and hormone replacement. After a comprehensive range of tests, I started on a hormone and supplement plan. My body seemed to 'wake up' and I found the energy to start walking three days a week and planning my life.

I decided that the first year was about removing my 'tuck-shop arms'. I thought about the future and my strategy for the next 30 years. How could I be where I wanted to be physically and mentally? How could I get healthy, stay healthy and slow down the ageing process? I wanted a long-term plan for staying well.

Within a relatively short period of time, I was feeling positive and alive. I was determined to make this feeling last forever. I didn't want to get old. I delved into the anti-ageing movement - reading books, attending conferences and researching online. I wanted guidance to help me look good, stay healthy and age slowly.

The problem was, and still is, there are no industry-validated and globally-recognised best practice protocols to guide practitioners in delivering anti-ageing medicine or advice. There is no reputable body that accredits, educates or examines doctors or other practitioners in anti-ageing medicine.

I found this very frustrating. I realised there was no evidence that any one thing you do will actually make you live longer or slow your ageing. You cannot 'anti-age'. There is no such thing. To try would be a losing battle.

However, there is evidence that you can increase the length of time that you are healthy, and help fend off disease and disability associated with age. I decided to create my own information source to guide me through the ageing process. I wanted to develop a set of principles (that I longed for, yet couldn't find) to help myself and others stay well. Ageing is a wonderful process that we should be positive and empowered about.

This book reflects my journey to good health (I lost 10kg and now have toned arms!) and I share the tools for planning your own slow ageing process.

Kate Marie

Kate is the driving force behind the 'Slow Ageing' collaboration. Drawing on her frustrations with established medical practice and the generic 'anti-ageing' industry, her work aims to provide transformational health information which gives all men and women the realistic means to control their own ageing and love getting old .

Professor Merlin Christopher Thomas MD, PhD

Christopher is a clinician scientist. His research focuses on the role of diabetes, glycation and oxidative stress in accelerating the changes of ageing, and finding a practical means for their control. Dr Thomas has published over 150 articles in many of the worlds leading medical journals. The Juvenile Diabetes Research Foundation, Diabetes Australia, the Australian NHMRC, Kidney Health Australia and the National Heart Foundation also support the work of Dr Thomas.